FALCONER'S CURRENT DRUG HANDBOOK 1980-1982

H. ROBERT PATTERSON, B.S., M.S., PHARM. D.
Professor of Microbiology and Biology
San Jose State University, San Jose, California

EDWARD A. GUSTAFSON, B.S., PHARM. D.
Pharmacist, Valley Medical Center, San Jose, California

ELEANOR SHERIDAN, R.N., B.S.N., M.S.N.
Assistant Professor, College of Nursing
Arizona State University, Tempe, Arizona

W. B. SAUNDERS COMPANY

W. B. Saunders Company: West Washington Square
Philadelphia, PA 19105

1 St. Anne's Road
Eastbourne, East Sussex BN 21 3UN, England

1 Goldthorne Avenue
Toronto, Ontario M8Z 5T9, Canada

RM300
.C8

Current drug handbook. 1958-
Philadelphia [etc.] W. B. Saunders Co.

v. 24 cm.

Annual, 1958-1961/62; biennial, 1962/64–
Compilers: 1958– M. W. Falconer, H. R. Patterson.
Alternate biennial revisions for 1962/64– also included in The drug, the nurse, the patient.

1. Pharmacology–Yearbooks. 2. Drugs–Yearbooks. I. Falconer, Mary W., comp. II. Patterson, H. Robert, comp.

RM300.C8 615.1 58–6390

Library of Congress

Falconer's Current Drug Handbook 1980–1982 ISBN 0-7216-3572-5

Last digit is the print number: 9 8 7 6 5 4 3 2

In memory of Mary W. Falconer, whose foresight, concern and determination resulted in the development and publication of the *Current Drug Handbook*.

PREFACE

This revision, as have past ones, presents specific information on approximately 1500 selected drugs in order to provide a handy source for quick reference. It supplies information supplemental to that in Part II of the textbook, *The Drug, The Nurse, The Patient.* As a general rule, active principles or individual drugs are considered rather than the myriad of mixtures available, and attempts have been made to include only drugs in general use regardless of their recognition by official publications.

Material has been organized with categories of usage similar to that of the *United States Pharmacopeia;* thus, drugs with the same use will be found grouped together in the handbook. In addition, the most recent U.S.P. monograph changes have been added to the index and cross-referenced to the appropriate place within the text.

The format has been planned in tabular form for ease in grasping all the pertinent facts at one glance. The material is to be read across the page.

The first column gives the names of the drug–generic, major trade names, and Canadian names when these differ from those used in the United States. The Canadian names are placed in parentheses with the letter "C" at the end. This column also gives the source of the drug, if this is not listed in the heading, the active principles (if any are therapeutically important), and the designation U.S.P. or N.F. if these apply. It should be remembered that there are some drugs with an almost unlimited number of names. Obviously, it has not been possible to include every one. In all cases the official names have been given preference. We have identified main or generic names by underscoring them.

In the second column are given the dosage, method, and times of administration, if the drug is usually given at definite times. The dosages are listed in the metric system. If the apothecaries' dose is desired the reader may consult the list of approximate equivalents in the back of the book.

The third column gives the major uses of the drug and sometimes the minor ones.

The fourth column states the action and fate (absorption, distribution, excretion) of the drug in the body insofar as this is known.

The fifth column covers the toxicity, side effects, contraindications, interactions and when applicable, the treatment of these. The sixth and last column is titled "Nursing Implications and Remarks" and includes important information that is not applicable under the other headings. This form has been used with only slight variations throughout, even though in some instances it has not been entirely satisfactory. The variations are self-explanatory. Since the tabular form has been used and brevity stressed, sentences are often incomplete. To conserve space and for clarity, interactions have sometimes been included in column 6 rather than, or in addition to, column 5. When they apply to an entire group, they have been placed across the page with general heading information.

The authors have drawn on a large number of sources for the information used, relying heavily upon such official publications as the *United States Pharmacopeia,* the *National Formulary,* and other sources such as *Drug Evaluations,* the *Modern Drug Encyclopedia,* the *American Hospital Formulary Service,* the *American Drug Index,* and, for the newest drugs, information provided by the pharmaceutical company preparing the medication.

In response to suggestions received from several sources we have included in this edition a tabulation of "Normal Laboratory Values of Clinical Importance," which appears immediately following the main body of the handbook.

Laws and regulations controlling the dispensing and administration of potentially addictive drugs and narcotics are undergoing intensive scrutiny as legislatures attempt to deal with drug abuse problems. On May 1, 1971, the federal "Comprehensive Drug Abuse Prevention and Control Act of 1970" went into effect in the United States. This act was known as the "Controlled Substance Act." As of October 1, 1973 the name of the control agency is "Drug Enforcement Agency" (DEA).

This act repeals the "Narcotic Acts" as well as the "Drug Abuse Control Amendments to the Federal Food, Drug and Cosmetic Act." The drugs that come under the jurisdiction of the act are divided into five schedules (I, II, III, IV, V). The greater the possibility of abuse and dependence the lower the classification number. Schedule I includes those drugs that have no accepted medical use in the United States and includes heroin, marijuana, etc. The remaining schedules have the former Class A, B, X narcotics, the amphetamines and amphetamine-like compounds, the barbiturates and hypnotic drugs.

The people working with these drugs should know in what schedule the various compounds are listed so that they can be handled as required by this act.

State laws are more stringent than federal laws in some cases. The student should become familiar with local regulations. Canadian students should refer to the books and pamphlets issued by the Department of National Health and Welfare such as *The Food and Drug Act and Regulations, Narcotic Control Act,* and *Controlled Drugs.* As with state laws, provincial laws may be more stringent than the dominion laws, in which case the student will need to know the local regulations. These laws are amended as circumstances indicate.

H. ROBERT PATTERSON
EDWARD A. GUSTAFSON
ELEANOR S. SHERIDAN

CONTENTS

Drugs included in this group are those used to destroy or to inhibit the development of microorganisms in the environment of the patient, or on the body surfaces. Some insecticides are also listed. Systemic anti-infectives are discussed later. These substances are all poisonous to a greater or lesser degree.

Name, Source, Synonyms, Preparations	Dosage and Administration	Uses	Action and Fate	Side Effects and Contraindications	Nursing Implications and Remarks
HALOGENS					
Only two of the halogen elements—chlorine and iodine—are commonly used as antiseptics and disinfectants.					
CHLORINE. *Gaseous element.*		For utensils, skin, mucous membranes, and sometimes food and water. Most common means of making water potable.	In insects, acts as contact and stomach poison. (In man, mainly central nervous system effects.)	Toxic in strong solutions, but poisoning rare in usual strengths. Irritating to skin; protect with oil or petrolatum.	The germicidal action of chlorine is decreased in the presence of organic matter or an alkaline pH.
Chlorinated lime (chloride of lime, bleaching powder).	5-20% solution. Environmental.	For excreta.	Other than chlorine gas, the chlorine-containing compounds act by the slow release of hypochlorous acid, which is bactericidal but also destructive to normal tissue.		
Halazone.	4-8 mg. to 1 liter. Environmental.	To render water potable.			After it is mixed with water, it should stand 1/2 hour before being drunk.
Sodium hypochlorite diluted solution, N.F. (hychlorite, modified Dakin's solution).	0.5% solution. Topical.	For wounds. Germicidal in action and dissolves clots.			Hygeol is twice the strength of Dakin's solution.
(Hygeol [C]). *Sodium hypochlorite solution,* N.F.	5% solution. Environmental			Too strong to use on the skin undiluted.	Some household bleaches are a 5% solution of sodium hypochlorite.
Succinchlorimide.	12 mg. to 1 liter. Environmental.	As above.	Same as Halazone.		
OXYCHLOROSENE. *Synthetic.* Derived from hypochlorous acid.					
Oxychlorosene (Clorpactin XCB).	0.5% solution. Topical, with contact time of at least 5 minutes.	Used to kill cancer cells in the operative field.	Thought to act by oxychlorination of the free cells.	None unless ingested.	
Oxychlorosene sodium (Clorpactin WCS-90).	0.4% solution. Topical. 0.1-0.2% solution in ophthalmology.	Used as an antiseptic, in urology and ophthalmology.	Contains 3-4% active chlorine.	Contraindicated when site of infection is not exposed to direct contact with solution.	

ANTISEPTICS AND DISINFECTANTS (Continued)

Name, Source, Synonyms, Preparations	Dosage and Administration	Uses	Action and Fate	Side Effects and Contraindications	Nursing Implications and Remarks
IODINE. *Kelp.*			These compounds are effective because of the presence of elemental iodine. Believed to act by their iodinating and oxidizing effects on microbial protoplasm.	Topical preparations are toxic if taken internally. Irritating in strong solutions or when skin is wet.	
Iodine solution, N.F.	2% solution. Topical.	Antiseptic for skin and wounds.			
Iodoform, N.F.	Powder. Topical.	Used for infected wounds and on gauze packings.			
Poloxamer-iodine (Prepodyne). Povidone-iodine N.F. (Betadine, Isodine) (Bridine, Provodine, PVP-I. [C]).	1% solution. Topical. 1% ointment, solution or gel. Topical, vaginal, surgical scrub, aerosols, foams and gauze.	Have longer antiseptic action than most iodine solutions; do not sting. Solutions used for scrubbing, mouth washes and douches. Ointment used for burns.			The complexes with povidone or poloxamer can be bandaged or taped following use.
Strong tincture of iodine.	7% alcoholic solution. Topical.	For skin; do not use in deep wounds.			
Thymol iodide.	Powder. Topical.	For skin and wounds; contains iodine and thymol from thyme.			
Tincture of iodine, U.S.P.	2% alcoholic solution. Topical.	For skin.			Tincture of iodine is irritating to wounds, probably because of 44-50% alcohol content.
Undecoylium chloride-iodine (Virac).	0.2-3.2% solution. Topical.	Similar to povidone-iodine.			
HEAVY METALS					
MERCURY. *Mineral.*		For skin, mucous membranes, and utensils.	Mercuric ion will precipitate plasma protein, but its antibacterial action probably results from its ability to inhibit sulfhydryl enzymes.	Local irritation from mercury products is not uncommon; severe dermatitis may occur. Stop drug and treat symptoms.	
Acetomeroctol (Merbak).	0.1% tincture. Topical.	For skin disorders.			
Ammoniated mercury ointment, U.S.P. (white precipitate).	5% ointment. Topical.	For skin disorders.			
	3% ointment. Topical.	For ophthalmic use.			
Merbromin. (Flurochrome K) (Mercurochrome). (Mercurescein [C]).	1-5% aqueous solution. Topical.	Used for skin or mucous membranes.			
	1-2% acetone-alcohol solution. Topical.	Used for skin only.			
Mercury bichloride (Mercuric chloride, corrosive sublimate).	1:20,000-1:1000 aqueous solution. Environmental.	Occasionally used as skin wash. Do not use on metals.			
Mercury cyanide.	1:4000 solution. Environmental.	As above; does not corrode metals.			
Mercury oxycyanide.	1:500 solution. Environmental.	As above; does not corrode metals.			

Nitromersol, N.F. (Metaphen).	1:1000 aqueous solution. Environmental. 1:2500-1:500 aqueous solution. Topical. 1:5000-1:200 tincture. Topical.	For skin and mucous membranes. For skin.			
Mercurial ointment, mild.	1% ointment. Topical.	Mainly for parasites.			
Thimerosal, N.F. (Merthiolate) (Thiomersal [C]).	1:1000 aqueous solution. Environmental. 1:1000 alcoholic tincture. Topical.	Also used for mucous membranes. For skin.			
Phenylmercuric acetate (Nylmerate).	0.2% topical (vaginally). 0.02% gel.				
Phenylmercuric nitrate, N.F. (Merphenyl nitrate, Phe-Mer-Nite).	1:1500 ointment or solution. Topical. 1:3000 ophthalmic ointment.	For skin. For eyes.			
Yellow oxide of mercury ointment, N.F.	1% ointment. Topical.	For eye infections.			
SILVER. *Mineral.*		For skin and mucous membranes, especially in infections due to the gonococcus.	Silver ion is a protein precipitant, but the concentrations that exhibit bacteriostatic action indicate that silver ions have an effect on some enzyme systems.	Strong solutions are caustic. Normal saline is antidote. If used repeatedly, watch for symptoms of argyria (silver poisoning): pain in throat and abdomen, vomiting, purging and graying of lips. Stop drug and treat symptoms.	
Toughened silver nitrate, U.S.P. (lunar, caustic, molded silver nitrate).	Pencils or applicators. Topical.	As styptic and caustic.			
Silver nitrate solution.	0.5-2% solution. Topical. 1:10,000-1:2000 solution. 1% solution. Eyes.	For skin and mucous membranes. Used in a 0.5% solution for treatment of burns. Instilled into conjunctival sac of newborn infants to prevent ophthalmia neonatorum.			Stains skin brown. When used for extensive burns, hypochloremia and hyponatremia may occur.
Silver picrate.	1-2% solution. Topical.	As above.		Watch also for picric acid poisoning (kidney or liver).	Picric acid stains skin yellow.

Name, Source, Synonyms, Preparations	Dosage and Administration	Uses	Action and Fate	Side Effects and Contraindications	Nursing Implications and Remarks
COLLOIDAL SILVER. *Mineral and protein.*		As above.	As above.	As above.	
Silver protein, mild, N.F. (Argyrol, Solargentum).	5-25% solution. Topical.	For skin and mucous membranes.			Mild silver protein contains more silver than strong silver protein, but is less astringent because of difference in ionization of solution. Trade names listed and others are similar to, but not always identical with, N.F. formula.
Silver protein, strong (Protargol).	0.25-1% solution. Topical. 1:2000-1:1000 solution. Topical.	For skin and mucous membranes.			
Silver iodide (Neo Silvol).	5% solution. Topical.	For skin and mucous membranes.			
OXIDIZING AGENTS *Synthetic.* Act by liberating nascent oxygen.			The nascent oxygen liberated from these compounds is capable of oxidizing susceptible components in cellular protoplasm, thereby affording bactericidal effect.		
Benzoyl peroxide, U.S.P. (Benoxyl, Persa-gel).	5-10% topical ointment, gel.	Treatment of acne.			
Hydrogen peroxide, U.S.P.	2.5-3.5% solution. Topical.	Antiseptic for skin and mucous membranes. Especially valuable for anaerobic organisms.		Toxic reactions are rare. Never instill in closed body cavities or abscesses from which the gas has no free egress.	Deteriorates on standing.
Potassium permanganate, U.S.P.	1:5000 solution. Topical.	For gastric lavage in certain cases of poisoning (alkaloid).		Toxic if taken internally, causing gastrointestinal disturbances. Evacuants, demulcent drinks, treat symptoms.	Dyes linens.
	1:2000-1:1000 solution. Topical.	For the skin; dyes skin brown.			
	1:10,000-1:5000 solution. Topical.	For mucous membranes.			
Sodium perborate, N.F.	2% saturated solution. 10-20% powder in dentifrices. Topical.	Antiseptic for mouth.		Toxic reactions are rare, but it can cause chronic glossitis from prolonged use.	Constituent of many dentifrices; should be used only on advice of doctor or dentist.
Zinc peroxide, medicinal, U.S.P.	5-25% ointment. 40% aqueous suspension, and as a dusting powder. Topical.	Antiseptic for skin.		Toxic reactions are rare.	Insoluble in water, but gradually decomposed by water to release oxygen.

PHENOL GROUP (carbolic acid) *Coal tar and crude petroleum.*		Disinfectant in strong solutions. Antiseptic in weak solutions.	Effect of phenols thought to result from their ability to denature protein. Some substituted phenols tend to be more effective depending on the position and the substituent. Phenol is bacteriostatic in concentrations of 1:800 to 1:500; in concentrations of 1:400 to 1:50 it is bactericidal. It is not effective against spores.	Caustic if too strong. Wash with alcohol.	
Cresol, N.F. (methylphenol).	1-5% solution. Environmental.	Largely replaced by saponified form.			
Saponated solution of cresol, N.F. (Creolin, Cresol compound, Cresylone, Hydrasol, Phenolor).	2-5% solution. Environmental. 0.25-5% solution. Topical.	For utensils, and for skin and mucous membranes. Disinfectant in strong solutions.			Cresol, vegetable oil, and soap. Cresol content 50%. Phenol coefficient 3.
Liquefied phenol, U.S.P.	85% solution. Topical.	As caustic.			
Phenol, U.S.P.	0.5-1% solution. Topical. 2-5% solution. Environmental.	As antiseptic and antipruritic. Soak for 1/2 hour or more.			
PREPARATIONS MADE SYNTHETICALLY FROM PHENOL					
Arylphenolic compounds (Amphyl, O-Syl, Staphene).	Varied. Topical, environmental. 0.5% strength is usual.	Used for utensils, environmentally, and in weak solutions for skin disinfection.		Some skin irritation in strong solutions.	
Metacresylacetate.	Varied. Topical. 0.5% strength is usual.	An antiseptic and analgesic used for ear, nose and throat.			
Betanaphthol.	5-10% ointment. Topical.	Antiseptic for the skin, especially in fungal infections.			
Hexachlorophene, U.S.P. (G-11) (Gamophen, pHisoHex, SurgiCen, Surofene) (Hexachlorophane, Dermohex, HexSurg, Ibaderm, Promani, Tersaseptic [C]).	0.5-3% soaps. Topical.	Mainly for skin antisepsis, and also for surgical scrubs.	Active primarily against gram-positive organisms, not gram-negative.	Warning–total body bathing of adults or children can result in absorption of toxic concentrations of hexachlorophene, especially in premature infants and those with dermatoses. Adverse reactions include dermatitis and photosensitivity.	Hexachlorophene should be discontinued at once if signs of cerebral irritability occur.
Pyrogallol.	5-10% ointment.	For skin disorders.		Toxic reactions rare in therapeutic strengths.	
Triacetylpyrogallol (Lenigallol).	6% powder or ointment. Topical.	Keratolytic, keratoplastic and antifungal.			

ANTISEPTICS AND DISINFECTANTS (Continued)

Name, Source, Synonyms, Preparations	Dosage and Administration	Uses	Action and Fate	Side Effects and Contraindications	Nursing Implications and Remarks
RESORCINOL GROUP					
Resorcinol, U.S.P. (Resorcin).	1-10% solution. Topical.	As above.			
Resorcinol monoacetate, N.F. (Euresol).	5-20% ointment and lotion. Topical.	As above.			
QUATERNARY AMMONIUM COMPOUNDS					
(Detergents). *Synthetic.* Soap-like substances.		Used for skin and mucous membranes and for utensils. Especially useful for pre- and postoperative skin disinfection and obstetrical procedures.	The exact mode of action of these agents is not presently known, but they do reduce surface tension and are thought to denature lipoprotein complexes.	Toxic reactions rare.	Inactivated by soap. Rinse thoroughly before using after green soap has been used.
Benzalkonium chloride, U.S.P. (Benasept, Germicin, Hyamine-3500, Phencen, Roccal, Zephiran Chloride) (Benzalchlor-50, Benzalide, Benzalkone, Drapolex, Ionex, Sabol [C]).	1:5000-1:500 aqueous. Environmental. 1:40,000-1:500 aqueous. Topical. 1:1000 tincture. Topical.	Utensils and skin must be completely rinsed after application.	Effective against gram-positive and gram-negative organisms, but some strains of gram negatives require a longer exposure time. These compounds are not tuberculocidal. Effect thought to be due to enzyme inactivation.	Serum and protein material decrease activity of benzalkonium chloride. The following substances are incompatible with benzalkonium: iodine, silver nitrate, fluorescein, nitrates, peroxide, $KMnO_4$, aluminum ion, kaolin, pine oil, zinc oxide, yellow oxide of mercury and soap.	
Benzethonium chloride, N.F. (Hyamine-1622, Phemerol Chloride, Phemithyn).	1:5000-1:1000 aqueous. Environmental or topical.	As above.			Used full or one-fourth strength as needed.
Cetylpyridinium chloride, N.F. (Ceepryn chloride) (Cepacol, Oracain [C]).	As above.	For skin; not reliable against spores.			
Hexetidine (Sterisol [C]).	0.1% gel. Topical.	Local antiseptic for bacteria, fungi, protozoa. Main use is in the treatment of vaginitis.		Toxic reactions are rare in topical application.	
Methylbenzethonium chloride, N.F. (Diaparene Chloride) (Amosept [C]).	1:25,000 solution. Environmental. 0.1% ointment, lotion or cream. Topical.	Especially for infants' diapers. For skin antisepsis.			

BISDIGUANIDE ANTISEPTICS *Synthetic.*					
Chlorhexidine gluconate. (Hibiclens) (Hibitane [C]).	4% solution.	Used for surgical scrub, skin wound cleanser and handwashing by health care personnel.	It is antimicrobial, effective against gram-negative and gram-positive bacteria. Somewhat less active against some strains of *Serratia* and *Pseudomonas* than other gram-negative bacteria. Not active against *Aspergillus.* The antimicrobial effect persists for over 6 hours on gloved hands. It is not appreciably absorbed from the skin.	Generally not irritating.	
TAR GROUP					
COAL AND OTHER TARS Coal tar ointment, U.S.P.	1% coal tar in zinc oxide paste. Topical.	For skin antisepsis. Keratoplastic and antipruritic.	This group has only slight antiseptic action; exact mode of action is not known, but tars are used empirically.	Toxic reactions rare.	May cause photosensitivity; protect treated areas from sunlight.
Coal tar solution, U.S.P. (Liquor carbonis detergens, Wright's solution).	20% diluted as required. Topical.				
Ichthammol ointment, N.F. (Ichthymall, Ichthyol).	10% ammonium ichthyosulfonate in petrolatum and wool fat. Topical.	Antiseptic, astringent and antipruritic.		Toxic reactions rare.	
Juniper tar ointment, N.F. (Cade oil).	15% cade oil in an oily base. Topical.	For skin.		Toxic reactions rare.	
Pine tar ointment, N.F.	5% pine tar in yellow wax and petrolatum. Topical.	For skin.		Toxic reactions rare.	
VARIOUS DYES *Crude petroleum* or *synthetic.*		For mucous membranes and skin antisepsis.	Bacteriostatic and bactericidal.	Harmful to body cells in strong solution but not in therapeutic strengths.	
Acriflavine.	1:8000-1:1000 solution. Topical.	For mucous membranes.			Watch for staining, as with any dye.

ANTISEPTICS AND DISINFECTANTS (Continued)

Name, Source, Synonyms, Preparations	Dosage and Administration	Uses	Action and Fate	Side Effects and Contraindications	Nursing Implications and Remarks
VARIOUS DYES *(Continued)*					
Methylrosaniline chloride (gentian, methyl or crystal violet).	1% solution. Topical. 0.4% vaginal inserts. 1.35% vaginal cream. 3-60 mg. Oral enteric-coated tablets are used, often for the relief of pinworms (see page 59).	For pyogenic and fungal skin infections, as an anthelmintic and for vaginal candidiasis.	Effective against gram-positive organisms but not against gram-negative organisms or acid-fast bacteria. Bactericidal effect thought to result from chemical combination of the dye with vital constituents in bacterial protoplasm.		
Scarlet red ointment.	4-8% ointment. Topical.	For skin—burns, ulcers and similar conditions.	Bacteriostatic; thought to aid healing and stimulate cell growth.	As above.	As above.
MISCELLANEOUS		*All of these preparations are synthetic unless otherwise noted.*			
Alcohol, U.S.P. (Ethanol).	70% solution. Topical.	For the skin and utensils.	Acts by coagulating protein; is bactericidal but not sporicidal.	Toxic reactions rare in topical application.	Wood alcohol (methyl alcohol) is not used except on utensils. Ethyl alcohol is from grain.
Alcohol, rubbing, N.F. (Alcolo, Lavacol, Nor-Co-Hol, Spiritex).	70% solution. Topical.	Used for skin disinfection and as a rubefacient.	As above.	As above. Toxic when taken internally.	Isopropyl alcohol is synthetic.
Acrisorcin (Akrinol).	2% cream. Topical. Apply twice daily for at least 6 weeks.	Used to treat mycotic infections caused by tinea versicolor.	Said to have the action of both 9-amino-acridine and hexylresorcinol.	Do not use around eyes. If irritation or sensitization develops, discontinue treatment.	Be sure to remove all soap from area and dry well before application of ointment.
Aluminum acetate solution, U.S.P. (Buro-Sol, Burrow's solution) (Acid mantle [C]). Chemical.	2.5-10% solution. Topical.	Used for treatment of various skin conditions.	An astringent and antiseptic.	None unless ingested.	Used alone and in various combinations either in solutions or ointments. Do not use around eyes.
Aluminum chloride hexhydrate, N.F.	2% solution.	Wet dressing therapy.	Has astringent soothing and cooling effect.		Dressing material and solution should be discarded daily and not reused.
Benzyl benzoate lotion. (Scabanca, Scabiol, Scabicide, Scabide [C]).	25-30% solution. Ointment. Topical.	For skin, especially for scabies and pediculi.	Exact mode of action is not known.	Toxic reactions rare in topical application.	
Boric acid (boracic acid), N.F. Mineral.	2.5% solution and ointment. Topical.	For skin and mucous membranes.	Very weak germicide but can be used because it is non-irritating. It can be	Toxic reactions rare in topical application. Toxic internally; use evacuants.	Do not use on denuded areas. Some authorities say this compound has no

			used on the cornea without ill effects.		place in modern medicine because of its doubtful therapeutic value and fatalities following accidental ingestion.
Chlordantoin (Sporostacin).	1% cream.	Vaginal candidal infections.	In vitro chlordantoin inhibits *Candida albicans* by an unknown mechanism.	Minor burning and sensitization have occurred.	
Chlorquinaldol (Sterosan [C]).	3% ointment or cream. Topical.	For topical treatment of superficial pyogenic and mycotic infections.	Mode of action is not well understood.	Toxicity low, but skin sensitivity has occurred.	Also available in combinations with hydrocortisone 1%.
Clotrimazole (Lotrimin, Gyne-Lotrimin, Mycelex).	1% cream. Apply b.i.d. 1% lotion. Apply b.i.d. Vaginal tablet. Every day for 7 consecutive days.	Topically for the following dermal infections: tinea pedis, tinea cruris and tinea corporis due to *Tricophyton rubrum, Tricophyton mentagrophytes, Epidermophyton floccosum* and *Microsporum canis.* Also for candidiasis due to *Candida albicans* and tinea versicolor due to *Malassezia furfur.*	Broad-spectrum antifungal agent that inhibits the growth of dermatophytes, yeasts and *Malassezia furfur.* Only small amounts appear to be absorbed following topical application.	Adverse reactions include erythema, stinging, blistering, peeling, edema, pruritus, urticaria and general irritation of the skin.	Has not been studied in 1st. trimester but has not been associated with ill effects in 2nd. and 3rd. trimesters of pregnancy.
Coparaffinate (Iso-Par).	17% ointment. Topical.	Used for mycotic infections of skin and genital or anal mucous membranes.	Same as above.	Toxicity low when used as directed.	Objectionable odor. Do not bandage part.
Crotamiton (Eurax).	10% cream. Topical.	Used to treat scabies and for symptomatic treatment of pruritus.	Scabicidic and antipruritic action. Both mechanisms unknown.	Toxicity low, but hypersensitivity has occurred. Avoid contact with eyes, mouth and urethral meatus.	Irritating if applied to denuded areas.
Diamthazole dihydrochloride.	5% ointment, alcoholic solution or powder. Topical.	For skin, especially for fungal infections.	For fungal infections. Also keratolytic.	Toxic reactions rare in topical application.	
Formaldehyde solution (Formalin, Formol) 37% solution of gas in water.	1-2%, mucous membranes. 2-10%, surgical instruments and gloves.	Disinfectant for excreta and utensils. (Also used in preparation of toxoids from toxins.)	In high concentration is capable of precipitating protein, and can also preserve tissue. Bactericidal effect thought to be through chemical reaction with protein present.	Irritant to mucous membranes and sometimes to skin. Avoid inhalation. Stop use of solutions; rinse area with water.	Effective disinfectant, but has a disagreeable odor.

Name, Source, Synonyms, Preparations	Dosage and Administration	Uses	Action and Fate	Side Effects and Contraindications	Nursing Implications and Remarks
MISCELLANEOUS (Continued)					
Gamma benzene hexachloride, U.S.P. (Gexane, Gamene, Kwell, Lindane) (Kwellade [C]).	1% cream, soap, or lotion. Topical. Leave cream or lotion on for 12 hours, but not for more than 24.	Used to treat scabies and pediculosis.	Exact mechanism of action is not known. Not readily absorbed through intact skin, but lipoid solvents enhance its absorption.	Toxicity relatively high but usually safe if used according to directions and not left in contact with the skin for too long. Small children more susceptible to toxicity.	Do not use in concentration greater than 1%. Avoid contact with mucous membranes and eyes.
Glutaral (glutaraldehyde, Cidex).	2% aqueous solution buffered with 0.3% $NaHCO_3$ to a pH of 7.5 to 8.5.	Disinfection and sterilization of endoscopic instruments and plastic and rubber apparatus used for inhalation and anesthesia.	Wide range of biocidal action; it is sporicidal and tuberculocidal. Can be used in the treatment of pre-existing lesions. hidrosis.	Main drawback to use is stability and cost. (Glutaral loses its stability after a period of 2 weeks.)	
Haloprogin (Halotex).	1.0% cream or solution. Topical. Apply b.i.d. for 2-3 weeks. Interdigital lesions may require 4 weeks.	Treatment of many fungal infections. Safe use in pregnancy not established.	Exact mechanism not known.	Local irritation, burning sensation, vesicle formation and increased maceration; pruritus and exacerbation of pre-existing lesions.	If no noticable improvement after 4 weeks of therapy, a rediagnosis is indicated. See insert for exact fungi covered. Keep out of eyes.
Miconazole nitrate (Micatin, Monistat 7).	2% cream. Intravaginal at bedtime for 14 days.	Treatment of candidiasis.	Alters cell permeability.	Burning, itching or irritation are the most frequent side effects. It is contraindicated in patients known to be sensitive to the drug.	See page 36 for I.V. product used systemically.
Nitrofurazone, N.F. (Furacin).	0.2-10% ointment. Topical. 0.2% cream. 0.2% powder. Topical.	For adjunct therapy of patients with second and third degree burns when bacterial resistance to other drugs is a problem. In skin grafting when bacterial contamination may cause graft rejection and/or donor site infection.	Tends to promote healing as well as destroy microorganisms. Nitrofuran derivative effective against certain fungi. Acts by inhibiting enzymes necessary for carbohydrate metabolism in bacteria.	Shown to cause mammary tumors in rats fed high doses; relevance of this to topical use in humans unknown. Sensitization reactions have occurred with topical use.	
Salicylanilide, N.F. (Salinidol).	4.5-5% ointment. Topical.	Antifungal preparation.	Action due to phenolic OH group. Also has some keratolytic effect.	Toxic reactions rare in topical application.	

Selenium sulfide, U.S.P. (Selsun).	2.5% lotion. Topical.	Treatment of tinea versicolor and seborrheic dermatitis of the scalp.	Mechanism unknown.	Avoid contact with eyes and mucous membranes. Detergent component may cause sensitization. Hair discoloration can occur; adequate rinsing can help prevent this.	Tinea-affected areas are covered with the lotion and lathered. It is thoroughly rinsed from body surfaces after 5 minutes and from facial areas after 10 minutes. Use daily for 4 days.
Sodium borate, U.S.P. (Borax).		For skin and mucous membranes.		Toxic reactions rare in topical application. Toxic internally; use evacuants.	Not so commonly used as boric acid.
Sodium caprylate.	10-20% solution.. Topical.	Used to treat mycotic infections of skin.	Exact mechanism is not known.	Toxicity low, but too frequent application may cause skin irritation.	
Sulfur precipitated, U.S.P.	10% ointment. Topical.	For skin, especially in fungal infections. Keratolytic.	Must be converted to some other form to be active. Fungicidal properties thought to be owing to conversion of water to pentothionic acid.	Toxic reactions rare in topical application. Occasionally causes local irritation. Stop drug.	
Tolnaftate (Tinactin, Afate).	1% solution, powder, gel, or cream. Topical. Apply b.i.d. for 2-6 weeks.	Treatment of mycotic infections. Infections of scalp, nails, soles and palms are usually chronic and do not respond well.	Exact mode of action not yet determined.	Keep out of eyes. Sensitization and irritation can occur.	Not effective against bacterial or candidal infections.
Triacetin, N.F. (Enzactin, Fungacetin) (glyceryl triacetate [C]).	33-1/3% aerosol, 25% cream or powder. Topical.	Used to treat mycotic infections of the skin.	Action due to slow liberation of acetic acid.	Toxicity low when used as directed.	Effectiveness of this preparation is questionable.
Copper undecylenate (Decupryl). Undecylenic acid, N.F. Zinc undecylenate, N.F. (Undesol).	Ointment. Topical. 2% ointment. Topical. 20% ointment, alcoholic solution, powder. Topical.	For the skin, especially for fungal infections.	Mechanism of action of these compounds is not known.	Toxic reactions rare in topical application.	Desenex is a combination of undecylenic acid and zinc undecylenate.

Name, Source, Synonyms, Preparations	Dosage and Administration	Uses	Action and Fate	Side Effects and Contraindications	Nursing Implications and Remarks

The first sulfonamide was azosulfonamide (Prontosil). It was a red dye discovered by a German chemist, Gerhard Domagk, about 1932, and could be given only orally. Neoprontosil was produced in 1935 and could be given either orally or parenterally. It was found that these drugs act by the liberation of sulfanilamide in the body. Sulfanilamide was first made in 1937. Since then many variations of the sulfonamides have been synthesized. The importance of this group has diminished as bacterial resistance to them has increased, and as more effective antibacterial agents have been developed.

INTERACTIONS: Sulfonamides potentiate oral anticoagulants, methotrexate, and oral hypoglycemics of sulfonylurea types. Increased sulfonamide blood levels may occur with urinary acidifiers, oral anticoagulants, phenylbutazone (Butazolidin), oxyphenbutazone (Tandearil), indomethacin (Indocin), sulfinpyrazone (Anturane) or salicylates. The potential for crystalluria may be increased when paraldehyde is administered concurrently. Decreased absorption of sulfonamides from the G.I. tract may occur if administered with antacids: administration with food appears to delay but not reduce absorption. Mineral oil interferes with antibacterial action of the nonabsorbable sulfonamides. Contraindications: history of hypersensitivity to sulfonamide and chemically related drugs; in patients with marked renal or hepatic impairment or with porphyria.

Name, Source, Synonyms, Preparations	Dosage and Administration	Uses	Action and Fate	Side Effects and Contraindications	Nursing Implications and Remarks
SULFONAMIDES *Synthetic.* Aminobenzene-sulfonamide rings with various radicals or compounds added.		Sulfas are used primarily in the treatment of lower urinary tract infections due to susceptible organisms, and in systemic infections caused by *Nocardia* sp. Other uses include locally on burns, in the eye and for vaginitis. Sulfas can also be used in treatment of chancroid, trachoma and lymphogranuloma venereum. Other specific sulfas are used for preoperative suppression of bowel flora, ulcerative colitis and dermatitis herpetiformis. They are used as adjuncts in the treatment of chloroquin-resistant strains of	The sulfonamides vary greatly in their rate of absorption. Most of these drugs are given orally, and some rapidly reach a high blood level, but others are so poorly absorbed as to render them useless for therapeutic purposes outside the gastrointestinal tract. The sulfonamides are changed (acetylated–conjugated) in the body, some much more than others. The degree of acetylation is important for in this form they are less effective and more difficult to eliminate. The acetylated sulfon-	Toxic symptoms include nausea, vomiting; oliguria, anuria, hematuria; cyanosis, anemia, leukopenia, granulocytopenia; dizziness, mental depression, drug fever, jaundice, skin rashes. Treatment symptomatic. If symptoms are serious, drug is stopped; if less serious, dosage is adjusted or type of sulfonamide is changed. Sulfonamides (especially the long-acting type) should not be given during the pregnancy or the nursing period because the sulfonamides pass the placental barrier and are	Sulfonamides will not eradicate group A streptococci and have not been demonstrated to prevent sequelae from such infections as rheumatic fever or glomerulonephritis. Fluid intake should be maintained at 1500 ml. a day.

		Plasmodium falciparum and in treatment of toxoplasmosis.	amides tend to form crystals in the urinary tract, and this produces some of the toxic symptoms. The easily absorbed sulfonamides are usually distributed through most or all of the body fluids. Of those absorbed, primary excretion is by the kidneys. The exact way in which the sulfonamide drugs act is not known, but their action is thought to be due to the ability to compete with PABA (para-aminobenzoic acid) for incorporation into PGA (folic acid or pteroyl-glutamic acid).	secreted with the milk and may cause kernicterus, hyperbilirubinemia and acute liver atrophy. The safe use of the sulfonamides during pregnancy has not been established. The teratogenetic potential of most sulfonamides has not been thoroughly investiga gated in either man or animals. Sulfonamides should not be given to infants less than 2 months of age, except in the treatment of toxoplasmosis as adjunct therapy with pyrimethamine.	
SULFONAMIDES, Short-Acting					
Sulfachlorpyridazine (Sonilyn) (sulfachloropyridazine, Cosulfa, [C]).	1.0 Gm. t.i.d. Oral	Urinary tract infections.			Continued therapy, at present, with sulfachlorpyridazine should not exceed 180 days.
Sulfacetamide, N.F. Isopto-Cetamide, [C]).	500 mg.-2 Gm. three to four times daily. Oral.	Urinary antiseptic; relatively nontoxic.			
Sulfacetamide sodium, U.S.P. (Bleph 10-30, Optiole S, Sulamyd sodium).	10% ointment. Ophthalmic. Four to five times daily. Topical. 10-30% solution. Ophthalmic. 1-2 drops three to four times daily. Topical.				
Sulfacytine (Renoquid).	500 mg. initially followed by 250 mg. q.i.d. for 10 days. Oral.	Acute, nonobstructive urinary tract infections caused by susceptible organisms.	As above.	Shares toxic potential of all sulfonamides	Not recommended for children under 14 years of age.
Sulfadiazine, U.S.P. (Diazoline, Solu-Diazine Sulfadets [C]).	500 mg.-2 Gm. five to six times daily. Oral	General anti-infective.			Total daily dose of sulfadiazine should not exceed 6 Gm.
Sulfadiazine sodium inj., U.S.P., Ph.I.	2.5-5 Gm. q. 6-8 h. I.V.				If precipitation of sodium solution occurs with diluent, discard preparation. Intravenous preparations must be diluted, preferably with sterile water, to a concentration of 50 mg. per ml. (5%) prior to administration.
Sulfamerazine, N.F. (Sumedine).	500 mg.-2 Gm. q. 4-8 h. 2-4 Gm. total daily dose. Oral.	General anti-infective, relatively nontoxic.			
Sulfamethizole, N.F. sulfamethylthiadiazole. (Microsul, Renasul, Sulfasol, Sulfastat, Sulfurine, Thiosulfil, Ultrasul)	250 mg.-2 Gm. Oral Adults, 500 mg. q.i.d. Oral.	Urinary antiseptic.			
Sulfathiazole (Sulfa-30, Sulfamul, Thiazol [C]).	500 mg.-1 Gm. q. 4 h. Oral 5% ointment. t.i.d. Topical. 5% jelly. Topical.	General anti-infective, relatively toxic, but very effective.			

Name, Source, Synonyms, Preparations	Dosage and Administration	Uses	Action and Fate	Side Effects and Contraindications	Nursing Implications and Remarks
SULFONAMIDES, Short-Acting *(Continued)*					
Sulfisoxazole, U.S.P. (Gantrisin) (sulfafurazole, Novosoxazole, Sulfizole [C]).	500 mg.-2 Gm. Usually 1 Gm. q. 4 h. Syrup, 5 ml. contains 500 mg. Oral.	General anti-infective. Relatively nontoxic. Dissolves in acid urine.			Preparations should be protected from light and moisture.
Sulfisoxazole acetyl, (Gantrisin acetyl, Lipogantrisin).	Children: 60-75 mg./kg. b.i.d. Adults: 4-6 Gm. $\bar{q}$ 12 h. Oral.				
Sulfisoxazole diolamine, N.F. (Gantrisin-diolamine).	5-10 ml. contains 2-4 Gm. q. 8-12 h. I.V. or I.M. 4% solution. 2-3 gtt. three or more times a day. Ophthalmic.				Caution should be observed when sulfisoxazole is given concurrently with methotrexate, since it decreases plasma protein binding of methotrexate and could result in methotrexate toxicity.
SULFONAMIDES, Intermediate					
Sulfamethoxazole, N.F. (Gantanol).	2 Gm. stat, then 1 Gm. two to three times a day. Oral	Used for urinary, respiratory, and soft tissue infections. Not recommended for newborn infants.	Widely distributed, crosses placenta.	Shares side effects of other sulfonamides.	Enhanced antibacterial activity in combination with trimethoprim (Bactrim, Septra). Maintain fluid intake at 1500 ml. daily.
Sulfaphenazole (Orisul, (sulphaphenazole [C]).	1-3 Gm. Oral	As above.		When administered concurrently with tolbutamide and sulfonylurea drugs, the hypoglycemic effect is potentiated.	
Sulfasalazine, N.F. (Azulfidine, Sulcolon) Salazopyrin [C]).	4-8 Gm. daily in divided doses. Oral. Maintenance therapy: 2 Gm. daily in divided doses. Oral.	Ulcerative colitis (chronic).	Poorly absorbed from G.I. tract. Drug and its metabolites excreted in urine and imparts an orange-yellow color to alkaline urine. Unabsorbed drug eliminated with feces.	Has caused agranulocytosis. In beginning therapy weekly white blood cell counts should be done. Watch for sudden sore throat or infections. Doctor must weigh risks against benefits in pregnancy and lactation.	Fluid intake should be maintained at 1500 ml. daily or more.

Silver sulfadiazine (Silvadene).	10 mg./Gm. cream. Topical. b.i.d. Keep wound cover 1/16 inch at all times.	Indicated for prevention and treatment of wound sepsis in patients with 2nd and 3rd degree burns.	Broad-spectrum antimicrobial activity. Acts on cell membrane and cell wall. Not a carbonic anhydrase inhibitor.	Burning, rashes, pruritus may occur. Some drug is absorbed so reaction similar to other sulfonamides may occur (see general statement). Safe use during pregnancy not established. Use in persons with glucose-6-phosphate dehydrogenase deficiency may be hazardous (hemolysis may occur). If renal or hepatic function is impaired, accumulation of drug may occur and may be necessary to discontinue it.	In considering use of topical proteolytic enzymes in conjunction with silver sulfadiazine, silver may inactivate the enzymes.
Sulfaguanidine.	50 mg./kg. of weight. q. 4 h. Oral	Poorly absorbed.			Has largely been replaced by sulfonamides that are more effective and less toxic.
Sulfanilamide (Streptocile [C]).	100 mg./kg. of weight daily in divided doses every 4 hours. Oral.	General anti-infective, relatively toxic; sodium bicarbonate given to combat acidosis.			
SULFONAMIDES, Long-Acting				Contraindicated in renal or hepatic impairment. Not recommended for generalized infections (including meningitis), pregnant women or nursing mothers. Do not use for children under 12 years or less than 100 pounds. Photosensitivity may occur.	Patients on long-term sulfonamides, such as sulfamethoxydiazine and sulfamethoxypyridazine (Midicel) should be watched for drug rashes; erythema multiforme exudativum (Stevens-Johnson syndrome) has been reported, with serious or fatal results.
Sulfameter (Sulfametin, Sulla) (sulfamethoxydiazine [C]).	1.5 Gm. first day, then 500 mg. Oral, preferably before breakfast.	Urinary tract infections (acute and chronic), caused by susceptible organisms.			
Sulfamethoxypyridazine, U.S.P. (Midicel) (Kynex, S.M.D. [C]).	As above. Suspension should be administered immediately p.c.				

Name, Source, Synonyms, Preparations	Dosage and Administration	Uses	Action and Fate	Side Effects and Contraindications	Nursing Implications and Remarks
SULFONAMIDES, Miscellaneous					
Phthalylsulfacetamide, N.F. (Thalamyd).	500 mg.-1 Gm. t.i.d. Oral.	Poorly absorbed. Used in gastrointestinal surgery or gastrointestinal diseases.			
Phthalylsulfathiazole (Sulfathalidine [C]). Succinylsulfathiazole.	500 mg.-1 Gm. four to six times daily. Oral. 1-3 Gm. six times daily. Oral.	As above. Not recommended for bacillary dysentery. Poorly absorbed. Used in gastrointestinal surgery or gastrointestinal diseases.		Extensive ulceration of colon may increase absorption.	After 3-4 days of therapy, intestinal coliform count is reduced and the patient has a soft tenacious, stringy stool of decreased bulk.
Sulfapyridine, U.S.P. (Dagenan [C]).	500 mg. -1 Gm. t.i.d. Oral.	Suppressant for dermatitis herpetiformis.		Toxic reactions frequent; include hematuria, methemoglobin formation and nausea.	Usual sulfonamide precautions.

ANTIBIOTICS

Penicillin was actually discovered by Sir Alexander Fleming at St. Mary's Hospital, London, in 1929. It did not come into general use until the period of World War II, about 1944-45. However, moldy bread has been used as a home remedy for infections for many years. Since the discovery of penicillin many other antibiotics have been discovered, and the search goes on. Antibiotics are all derived originally from molds or bacteria, which usually are soil organisms.

Penicillin is available in an endless number of preparations. Only representative ones are given here. Penicillin is prepared in salts of potassium and sodium. It is also made in a number of types (G, O, V), but types G and V are the ones most commonly used.

Penicillin and streptomycin are known as narrow-spectrum antibiotics; some of the others are called broad-spectrum antibiotics. The former are effective against a few organisms; the latter are effective against many organisms. Some antibiotics, though very effective in killing organisms in vitro, have only limited use in medicine because of their toxicity.

ESSENTIAL CONSIDERATIONS IN ANTIBIOTIC THERAPY

1. **Collection of cultures to identify the infecting organisms before antibiotic therapy is initiated. When known, organism susceptibility to antibiotics is checked to determine congruence with therapy.**
2. **Determination of the patient's previous responses to antibiotic therapy to determine history of hypersensitivity or allergy. If such a history is noted the drug is not administered and patient and staff are notified so that future administration is avoided.**
3. **Maintenance of adequate blood levels of the drug to prevent development of bacterial resistance. This means the drug must be given in the prescribed amounts at the directed times. When automatic stop orders are in effect, the physician is notified in sufficient time so that therapy can be continued without interfering with the drug blood level.**
4. **Support of the patient's defense mechanisms. Antibiotic therapy is directed at the causative organisms of the infectious disease and has no effect on the host's defense mechanisms.**
5. **Early detection of superinfection with non-susceptible bacteria or fungi that may occur.**

Warnings: Serious and occasionally fatal hypersensitivity (anaphylactoid) reactions have been reported in patients on penicillin therapy. Although anaphylaxis is more frequent following parenteral therapy, it has occurred in patients on oral penicillins. These reactions are more likely to occur in individuals with a history of sensitivity to multiple allergens. There have been reports of individuals with a history of penicillin hypersensitivity who have experienced severe reactions when treated with cephalosporins. Before therapy with any penicillin, careful inquiry should be made concerning previous hypersensitivity reactions to penicillins, cephalosporins or other allergens. If an allergic reaction occurs, appropriate therapy should be instituted and discontinuance of therapy considered. ***Serious anaphylactoid reactions require immediate emergency treatment with epinephrine. Oxygen, intravenous steroids and airway management, including intubation, should also be administered as indicated.***

Name, Source, Synonyms, Preparations	Dosage and Administration	Uses	Action and Fate	Side Effects and Contraindications	Nursing Implications and Remarks
PENICILLIN					
Mold. Penicillium chrysogenum. Also *Synthetic.*		Treatment of infections caused by alpha-hemolytic and beta-hemolytic streptococci, pneumococci, gonococci, meningococci, susceptible strains of staphylococci, *Treponema pallidium, Clostridium, Bacillus anthracis,* most strains of *Corynebacterium diphtheriae, Listeria,* some species of *Actinomyces,* fusobacteria, *Pasteurella multocida, Streptobacillus moniliformis, Actinomyces israelii* and some strains of *Bacteroides.*	Bacteriostatic and bactericidal. It acts by blocking the synthesis of the bacterial wall, and therefore is most effective on cells in rapid growth phase. Penicillin G 1/3 oral dose is absorbed from the intestinal tract, reaches peak level in 30–60 minutes. After injection reaches maximum level in 15-30 minutes. Widely distributed in body. 60-90% of I.M. dose excreted by the kidneys. Food may adsorb oral penicillin. It readily crosses the placenta and also appears in breast milk.	Actual toxic symptoms are rare, but allergic reactions do occur. These include direct reaction at the point of intramuscular injection, dermatitis of various types, delayed or immediate anaphylactic reactions. Local reaction may be due to the vehicle and not to the actual drug. Treatment as for any allergic reaction. Repetition of the drug may be unwise, if the reaction is severe. The most frequent adverse reaction of orally administered preparations are nausea, vomiting, epigastric distress, diarrhea and black hairy tongue.	Oral penicillin should be given 1 hour before or 2 hours after meals. Injections: After reconstitution, the solution may be stored under refrigeration for 1 week and is stable 24 hours at room temperature. Potassium Penicillin G, U.S.P. inj. contains 1.7 mEq. K and .33 mEq. Na per 1,000,000 units; Sodium penicillin G inj., U.S.P., contains 2 mEq. Na per 1,000,000 U. Parenteral administration may cause pain or sterile abscess at intramuscular sites and phelbitis or thrombophlebitis with intravenous administration.
PENICILLIN G					
Potassium penicillin G., U.S.P. crystalline buffered (Pentids, Pfizerpen) (benzyl-penicillin potassium, Abbocillin, Crystapen, Falapen, Hylenta, Ka-Pen, Megacillin [C]).	50,000–400,000-5,000,000 U. q. 2-3 h. day and night. Available in varied forms for oral, parenteral and inhalational use.				
Sodium penicillin G. (Crystapen [C]).	100,000-20,000,000 U. Oral, I.M., or I.V.			Hemolytic anemia, leukopenia, thrombocytopenia, neuropathy and nephropathy are rarely observed side effects and are usually associated with high I.V. dosage. In high doses (10,000,000 units) potassium penicillin should be given very slowly I.V. because of adverse effects of electrolytic imbalance due to potassium content.	Concomitant administration of probenecid 500 mg. q. 6 h. or phenylbutazone 600 mg. q.d. increases and prolongs penicillin serum levels.
Penicillins G and O, modified chemically and physically to increase duration of action by delay of absorption.					
Procaine penicillin G, U.S.P. (Crysticillin, Duracillin, Wycillin) (Ayercillin, Francacilline, Ibacillin [C]).	300,000-2,400,000 U. Given every 12-24–48 hours. Available in crystalline form and in oil; also with potassium penicillin for immediate and delayed action. I.M.				
Procaine penicillin G with aluminum monostearate, U.S.P.	300,000-1,200,000 U. I.M.			Interaction. Concomitant use of a bacteriostatic agent, such as a tetracycline,	
Benzathine penicillin G, U.S.P.	600,000-2,400,000				

(Bicillin) (benzethacil, Ben-P, Duapen, Megacillin [C]).	U. I.M. Given every 7-14 days; action prolonged due to slow absorption. 400,000-600,000 U. q. 4-6 h. Oral.			chloramphemicol or sulfa, is usually avoided since penicillin exerts its effect against organisms that are multiplying.	
PENICILLIN V					
Phenoxymethyl penicillin (Penicillin V, Pen-Vee, V-Cillin) (Ledercillin, Nadopen-V, Therapen V [C]).	200,000-500,000 U. q.i.d. Oral. 250 mg. considered equivalent to 400,000 U.		Better absorption than penicillin G after oral dose. More acid resistant. Gives Measurable blood level up to 4-6 hours after oral dose.	Same precautions as with penicillin.	
Potassium phenoxymethyl penicillin, U.S.P. (Compocillin-VK, Pen-Vee K, V-Cillin-K, Veetids).	200,000-800,000 U. q.i.d. Oral.				
Hydrabamine phenoxymethyl penicillin (Compocillin-V).	300,000 U. (180 mg.) q.i.d. Oral.				
SYNTHETIC PENICILLIN USED FOR RESISTANT STAPHYLOCOCCAL INFECTIONS					
Cloxacillin sodium, U.S.P. (Tegopen) (Orbenan [C]).	250-500 mg. q. 4-6 h. Oral.	Used for resistant staphylococcal infections.	Well absorbed by G.I. tract; food interferes with absorption. Primarily excreted in urine with some bile excretion.	Same precautions as with penicillin.	Give 1 h.a.c. or 2 h.p.c.
Methicillin sodium (Azapen, Celbenin, Staphcillin) (meticillin [C]).	1 Gm. q. 4-6 hr. I.M. or I.V.	As above.	Widely distributed but not to spinal fluid unless meningeal inflammation is present and then larger amounts are found here. Rapidly excreted by kidneys. Half-life for person with normal renal function, 6 hours. Crosses the placenta.	Same precautions as with penicillin.	Destroyed by stomach acid; must be given by injection. Methicillin should not be physically mixed with other agents. Methicillin, once diluted, should be administered within 8 hours but may be stored as concentrate 1 day at room temperature and 48 hours under refrigeration.

Name, Source, Synonyms, Preparations	Dosage and Administration	Uses	Action and Fate	Side Effects and Contraindications	Nursing Implications and Remarks
SYNTHETIC PENICILLIN USED FOR RESISTANT STAPHYLOCOCCAL INFECTIONS (Continued)					
Nafcillin sodium (Unipen).	500 mg.-2 Gm. q. 4 h. I.V. 500 mg. q. 6 h.I.M. 250-500 mg. q.4-6 h. Oral.	As above.	Peak blood level in 1 hour 60-70% plasma bound. 90% of I.V. dose exceted in bile.	As with penicillin.	Give oral dose 1 h.a.c. or 2 h.p.c.
Dicloxacillin sodium, U.S.P. (Dycill, Dynapen, Pathocil, Veracillin).	250 mg.-1 Gm. q. 6 h. Oral.	As above.	Crosses placenta.	Safety for use in pregnancy not established.	Best absorption on empty stomach at least 1 hour before or two hours after meals.
Sodium oxacillin, U.S.P. (Bactocil, Prostaphlin, Resistopen).	250 mg.-1 Gm. q. 4-6 h. Oral, I.M., I.V.	As above.	60% of oral dose absorbed. Peak blood level in 1 hour after oral dose. Excreted mainly by kidneys.	Pain at point of injection may occur. Neutropenia and an elevated SGOT have been reported.	Should be taken on empty stomach. Safety for use in pregnancy not established.
SYNTHETIC PENICILLIN WITH BROAD–SPECTRUM ACTIVITY					
Amoxicillin (Amoxil, Larotid, Polymox, Trimox).	250-500 mg. q. 8 h. Oral. Children, 20-40 mg./kg./day in divided doses q. 8 h.	Treatment of susceptible strains of gram-negative *H. influenzae, E. coli, P. mirabilis, N. gonorrhoeae,* gram-positive Streptococci (including *S. faecalis), D. pneumoniae,* nonpenicillinase-producing staphylococci.	Acts through inhibition of biosynthesis of cell wall mucopeptide. Stable in presence of gastric acid. Rapidly absorbed after oral administration. Diffuses in most body fluids and tissues except brain and spinal fluid. Half-life about 60 minutes. 60% excreted unchanged in urine. Excretion can be delayed by concurrent administration of probenecid.	Known sensitivity: urticaria, skin rash (cross-sensitivity with penicillin). Possibly nausea, vomiting, diarrhea; moderate rise in SGOT has occurred. Blood dyscrasias reported but rarely. Safe use in pregnancy has not been established.	Not resistant to destruction by penicillinase.
Ampicillin, U.S.P. (Omnipen, Penbritin, Polycillin, Polycillin-N, Principen) (Amcill, Ampen, Ampicin [C]).	250-500 mg. q.i.d. Oral. 250 mg.-2 Gm. q. 6 h. I.M. or I.V. Children: less than 20 kg.: 50-100 mg./kg./day in divided doses q. 6-8 h.	As above. Ineffective against penicillinase-producing organisms.	Appears in all body fluids except cerebrospinal. Excreted unchanged by the kidneys. High concentration found in bile. Crosses the placenta and appears in milk of nursing mothers.	Pain at point of injection may occur. Allergic reactions (see penicillin) and neutropenia have been reported. Safety for use during pregnancy not established.	See above.

Carbenicillin disodium (Geopen, Pyopen).	4-40 Gm. daily. I.M. or I.V.	Indicated in infections due to susceptible *Pseudomonas aeruginosa, Proteus species* (particularly indole-positive strains) and some strains of *E. coli.* Used in the treatment of severe systemic infections and septicemia, infections of the urinary and respiratory tracts and of the soft tissues.	Not absorbed orally. Following I.M. injections, peak blood levels are reached in two hours. As with other penicillins, probenecid will prolong the serum levels and also increase them somewhat. Widely distributed in body fluids including the cerebrospinal fluid. The drug is rapidly excreted in the urine.	Hypersensitivity (anaphylactic reactions have been seen). Such conditions as skin rashes, urticaria, pruritus, drug fever and nausea may occur. As with other penicillins, anemia, thrombocytopenia, leukopenia, neutropenia and/or eosinophilia can occur. SGOT and SGPT levels may become elevated. With high serum levels, convulsions or neuromuscular irritability may be seen. Vein irritation and phlebitis have been reported. Contraindicated in patients who have known penicillin allergy. Safety during pregnancy has not been established.	This is a synthetic penicillin with gram-negative spectrum. It is a benzylpenicillin derivative. Emergence of resistant organisms may lead to superinfections. When used with gentamicin I.V. the two must not be mixed together in the same infusion fluid. Used with caution in patients with sodium restriction.
Carbenicillin indanyl sodium (Geocillin).	382-764 mg. q.i.d. Oral.	Upper and lower urinary tract infections caused by susceptible strains of *E. coli, Proteus mirabilis* and *Pseudomonas.*	This salt is acid stable and well absorbed following oral administration. After absorption it is hydrolyzed to carbenicillin, which is primarily excreted in the urine.	See above.	
Ticarcillin disodium (Ticar).	3 Gm. every 3, 4 or 6 hours depending on weight and severity of infection. I.M. or I.V. Dose should be decreased in patients with renal insufficiency.	See carbenicillin disodium.	See carbenicillin disodium.	See carbenicillin disodium.	

Name, Source, Synonyms, Preparations	Dosage and Administration	Uses	Action and Fate	Side Effects and Contraindications	Nursing Implications and Remarks
SYNTHETIC PENICILLIN WITH BROAD-SPECTRUM ACTIVITY (Continued)					
Hetacillin and Hetacillin K (Veraspen and Veraspen K) (phenazacillin [C]).	225-450 mg. q. 6 h. in persons weighing over 90 pounds. Oral. Under 90 lbs. 10-20 mg./lb./day in 4 divided doses. Oral. Hetacillin K also given I.M. or I.V.	See amoxicillin.	The drug itself has no anti-bacterial activity, but it is converted by the body into ampicillin and as such is active against ampicillin-sensitive organisms during the stage of multiplication by inhibition of muco-proteins for cell wall synthesis. Well absorbed orally, but absorption is retarded by food so is best given on an empty stomach. Diffuses into most body tissues and fluids; crosses placenta and appears in human milk. Excreted in urine and bile.	See ampicillin. It is said to cause fewer gastrointestinal problems because it is con-verted by the body into the active substance. Periodic assessment of hepatic, hemopoietic and renal systems should be carried out when used on a long-term basis, especially in prematures, neonates and infants. Safe use in pregnancy not established.	The possibility of super-infections with mycotic or bacterial pathogens should be kept in mind. Contraindicated in patients with a history of penicillin or cephalosporin allergy.

CEPHALOSPORIN ANTIBIOTICS

The cephalosporins (derived from *Cephalosporium sp.*) are semi-synthetic antibiotic agents related chemically and pharmacologically to the penicillins. Chemically both contain a beta lactam ring. Pharmacologically they both interfere with the terminal step in bacterial cell wall synthesis. They are broad-spectrum antibiotics that are active in vitro against most staphylococci, both penicillin-sensitive and penicillinase-producing *Staphylococcus aureus,* most streptococci, including group A beta-hemolytic streptococci. *Streptococcus pneumoniae, Clostridium* species, *Escherichia coli, Proteus mirabilis, Neisseria gonorrhoeae* and some species of *Shigella* and *Salmonella.* They are considered the primary drugs in certain *Klebsiella* infections, yet many hospital-acquired *Klebsiella* infections are resistant to the cephalosporins.

Name, Source, Synonyms, Preparations	Dosage and Administration	Uses	Action and Fate	Side Effects and Contraindications	Nursing Implications and Remarks
Cefazolin sodium (Ancef, Kefzol).	500 mg.-1.0 Gm. q. 6-8 h. I.M. or I.V. Children, 10-20 mg./kg. up to 100 mg./kg. in severe infections.	Used in treatment of respir-atory, genitourinary, skin, soft tissue, bone and blood infections due to many susceptible organisms, both gram-negative and gram-positive. See above.	Not significantly absorbed from G.I. tract. Acts by blocking cell wall synthesis. 74-86% binds to serum proteins. 60% excreted unchanged by the kidneys in first 6 hours; up to 80% in 24 hours. Crosses	Anorexia, nausea, vomiting, oral candidiasis, pain and phlebitis at site of injection. Hypersensitivity reactions: fatal anaphylaxis, drug fever, rash, pruritus. Some blood dyscrasias reported. Positive direct and indirect	Safe use during pregnancy or in infants under one month of age not established. Patients with reduced urinary output should receive reduced dosage. A false-positive reaction to Clinitest tablets (Benedict's

			placenta and found in small amounts in milk of nursing mothers. Concentration in synovial fluid and bile about ½ that in serum. Concomitant administration with oral probenecid prolongs serum levels of cephalosporins.	Coombs' tests have occurred. Transient rise in SGOT, SGPT, BUN and alkaline phosphatase levels has occurred. Cross-sensitivity with penicillin may occur.	test) may be noted. Use any cephalosporin with caution in patients known to be allergic to penicillin. Allergic reaction to one cephalosporin C derivative contraindicates the use of all such derivatives.
<u>Cefadroxil monohydrate</u> (Duricef).	1 Gm. b.i.d. Oral.	Urinary tract infections caused by *Escherichia coli, Proteus mirabilis* and *Klebsiella* spp.	Rapidly absorbed from G.I. tract with serum concentrations present 12 hr. after administration. Over 90% excreted unchanged in the urine within 8 hr. Action as with cefazolin.	As with cephradine.	Administer with food to minimize G.I. effects. Watch carefully for adverse effects in renal patients.
<u>Cefamandole nafate</u> (Mandol).	Adults 0.5-1.0 Gm. q. 4-8 h. Parenteral. Children: 50-150 mg./kg. per day in divided doses.	Broad-spectrum activity as cephalosporins. Unlike earlier cephalosporins, is said to be more effective against anaerobic organisms.	As with cefazolin, relatively resistant to inactivation by penicillinase and cephalosporinase.	As with cefazolin.	Inject I.M. dose into large muscle to minimize pain.
<u>Cephalothin</u> (Keflin).	500 mg.-1Gm. q. 4-6 h. I.M. 2-6 Gm. daily. I.V. Can be given intraperitoneally in concentrations of 0.1 to 4% in saline.	See cefazolin.	Parenteral administration because of poor absorption from G.I. tract. Appears in all body fluids except cerebrospinal. 65-79% binds to serum protein. Excreted rapidly in the urine.	Pain at point of injection may occur. Allergic reactions including anaphylaxis have been reported. Also neutropenia and hemolytic anemia have been seen. Some patients (especially those with azotemia) have developed direct positive Coombs' test. Transient rise in SGOT and BUN and, in some patients, thrombophlebitis have occurred, especially in those receiving over 6 Gm. daily I.V.	Solutions may be stored 48 hours under refrigeration. If solution precipitates, it will redissolve on warming.

Name, Source, Synonyms, Preparations	Dosage and Administration	Uses	Action and Fate	Side Effects and Contraindications	Nursing Implications and Remarks
CEPHALOSPORIN ANTIBIOTICS (Continued)					
Cephaloridine, N.F. (Loridine) (Caporan [C]).	250 mg.-1.0 Gm. I.M., I.V. at equally spaced intervals. Range 1-4 Gm. daily. Children 30-50 mg./kg. in divided doses. 100 mg./kg. in severe infections. Do not exceed maximum adult dose.	Used in severe infections of bone, joints, blood stream, genitourinary tract. respiratory system and skin, if the organism is susceptible.	Parenteral administration because of poor absorption from G.I. tract. Peak blood levels of 7-15 mcg./ml. reached in ½-1 hour after I.M. injection of 250-500 mg. Measurable amounts persist for longer than 12 hours. These doses produce high urine concentrations (up to 1000 mcg./ml.).	Contraindicated in azotemia and hypersensitivity to cephalothin. Side effects: urticaria, skin rashes, itching, drug fever, rise in eosinophil count, leukopenia, elevation of transaminase and alkaline phosphatase, severe acute renal failure in some cases, especially with high dosage. Nausea and vomiting may occur. Safety during pregnancy, and for premature infants and infants under 1 month has not been established.	Because of renal toxicity, dosage should not exceed 4 Gm. daily. After mixing, store in refrigerator for not more than 96 hours.
Cephaloglycin dihydrate, N.F. (Kafocin).	250-500 mg. q.i.d. Oral.	Indicated only for urinary tract infections, both acute and chronic, due to susceptible strains of *E. coli, Klebsiella, Aerobacter, Proteus,* staphylococci and streptococci.	Is said to be acid stable and is absorbed orally. Food does not interfere with total absorption, but it can delay the time that peak urinary levels are reached. It is excreted almost entirely as the active metabolite desacetyl-cephaloglycin in the urine. Serum levels are not sufficient to be effective in any infections other than those of the urinary tract.	Gastrointestinal: nausea, vomiting, diarrhea. With allergy: rash, urticaria, etc. Others reported: malaise, fever, chills, headache, dizziness and vertigo. Eosinophilia has been reported. Contraindicated in known sensitivity to the cephalosporin drugs. Safe use during pregnancy or in children has not been established.	
Cephalexin monohydrate U.S.P. (Keflex).	1-4 Gm. daily in divided doses (usually 250-500 mg. q.i.d.). Oral. Children: 25-50 mg./kg. q.i.d.	Indicated for respiratory infections due to *S. pneumoniae* and hemolytic streptococci; in skin and soft tissue infections caused	It is acid stable and can be given without regard for meals. It is bactericidal because of its effect on cell wall synthesis.	Safe use during pregnancy or in infants under one year has not been established. Side effects: see cephaloglycin. Can cause positive	

		by staphylococci; and in urinary infections caused by *E. coli, Pr. mirabilis* and *Klebsiella sp.* Bone and blood infections due to susceptible organisms.	Well absorbed orally with peak serum level reached in an hour, and 90% is exreted unchanged in the urine in 8 hours.	Coombs' test and slight elevation of SGPT and SGOT.	
Cephapirin sodium (Cefadyl).	500 mg.-1 Gm. q. 4-6 h. I.M. or I.V.	Same as cefazolin. Closely related to cephalothin.	Same as cefazolin.	Same as cefazolin.	Reconstituted solution is stable for 12 hours at room temperature and for 10 days under refrigeration. Renal status of patient should be determined prior to and during therapy. Reduce dosage if renal function is impaired.
Cephradine (Velosef, Anspor).	250 mg.-1 Gm. q.i.d. Not to exceed 4 grams daily. Oral. Children 25-50 mg./kg./day. 250 mg.-1 Gm. q.i.d. I.M., I.V. Do not exceed 6 Gm. daily.	Used to treat respiratory, urinary, skin and soft tissue infections caused by a variety of gram-negative and gram-positive organisms.	Acid stable, well and rapidly absorbed after oral administration. Food in G.I. tract delays absorption but does not affect total amount absorbed. Over 90% excreted unchanged in urine within 6 hours after oral dose.	Mainly gastrointestinal disturbances and sensitivity reactions. Transient mild blood dyscrasias have occurred. Mild rise in SGOT, SGPT and total bilirubin reported. Transitory rise in BUN, which increases in patients over 50 years of age.	Safe use during pregnancy not established. Drug is excreted in milk of nursing mothers. A false-positive glucose urine test may occur (not in enzyme-based tests) and also a false-positive Coombs' test.
Cefoxitin sodium (Mefoxin)	1-2 Gm. q. 6-8 h. Parenteral.	See cefamandole. Appears more active against infections caused by *Bacteroides fragilis,* and *Providencia* spp.	As with cefazolin.	As with cefazolin.	With I.V. administration, use butterfly or scalp-vein needles to minimize risk of thrombophlebitis.

Name, Source, Synonyms, Preparations	Dosage and Administration	Uses	Action and Fate	Side Effects and Contraindications	Nursing Implications and Remarks
AMINOGLYCOSIDE ANTIBIOTICS					
	These drugs are organic bases with amino sugar groups. Hence, their group name, aminoglycoside antibiotics. They have similar activities, spectrums and side effects. They are not absorbed to any extent after oral administration. They are obtained from species of *Streptomyces* or are synthetic. The aminoglycosides are bactericidal antibiotics that exert their action by inhibition of protein synthesis. The site of this action is the 30S ribosomal subunit. By binding with this subunit they cause a misreading of the genetic code, which causes a wrong amino acid to be inserted into the peptide chain and results in formation of an inactive protein. **They all potentiate gallamine triethiodide and other muscle relaxant drugs used during anesthesia.**				
Amikacin sulfate (Amikin, Amikacin).	15 mg./kg./day in adults and older children with normal renal function, divided into 2 or 3 equal doses. Dose should not exceed 1.5 Gm./day even in heavier patients. Neonates: 10 mg./kg./day loading dose, then 7.5 mg./kg./day. In uncomplicated urinary tract infection 250 mg. b.i.d. may be used. Dose must be adjusted for patients with impaired renal function. I.M. or I.V.	Used in short-term treatment of serious infections due to susceptible strains of gram-negative bacteria, including *Pseudomonas* sp., *E. coli,* indole-positive and negative *Proteus, Providencia* sp., *Klebsiella, Enterobacter, Serratia* spp. and *Acinetobacter* (Mima-Herellea) species. Used in infections involving respiratory tract, bones and joints, CNS (including meningitis), skin and soft tissue, intra-abdominal infections, burns, postoperative infections and urinary tract infections. Also effective against staphylococcal infections and used in neonatal sepsis when other aminoglycosides cannot be used.	Readily absorbed after I.M. injection. Distributed almost entirely in extracellular fluid. Crosses the placenta. Not significantly metabolized. With normal renal function 91-92% of an I.M. dose is excreted unchanged in 8 hours and 98% within 24 hours. Not known whether it is excreted in human milk.	All aminoglycosides have the potential to cause oto-, nephro-, and neurotoxicity. Nephrotoxicity seen by albuminuria, presence of red and white cells, casts, azotemia and oliguria. Other side effects include skin rash, drug fever, headache, paresthesia, tremor, nausea, vomiting, eosinophilia, arthralgia, anemia and hypotension.	Avoid concurrent or sequential use of topically or systemically neurotoxic or nephrotoxic antibiotics, particularly all other aminoglycosides, cephaloridine, viomycin, polymyxin B, colistin and vancomycin. They should not be given concurrently with potent diuretics such as ethacrynic acid, furosemide or mannitol. They can enhance aminoglycoside toxicity by altering concentrations in serum and tissue.
Dihydrostreptomycin sulfate.	500 mg.-1 Gm. daily. I.M.	Most effective against gram-negative organisms and acid-fast bacteria.	Widely distributed but mostly in extracellular fluids. After I.M. dose 50-60% excreted unchanged in urine within first 24 hours, mostly in the first 12 hours.	Most serious side effect is neurotoxicity and ototoxicity with damage to eighth cranial nerve. Vertigo, dizziness, temporary loss of hearing, mental	Dihydrostreptomycin is a semi-synthetic preparation. It appears to be more toxic than streptomycin and is therefore used less. Streptomycin sulfate is

Streptomycin sulfate, U.S.P. (Strycin) (Strepolin [C]).	500 mg.-1-2 Gm. daily, but not usually continued on daily basis more than 3 to 4 weeks. Though available for subcutaneous and topical administration, by far the most common mode is I.M.	As above. Used concurrently with other antitubercular drugs.		depression; sometimes severe reactions such as fever, skin eruptions, and arthralgia. Treatment is symptomatic. Drug is usually reduced in amount or stopped. Crosses placenta and has been associated with hearing loss, multiple skeletal anomalies and eighth cranial nerve damage in the fetus. As above.	the most popular form of streptomycin. Should not be given with other ototoxic drugs or the diuretics, ethacrynic acid or furosemide. May give false positive results for urinary glucose tests utilizing cupric sulfate (Benedict's and Clinitest). Administer deep I.M. and alternate sites to minimize local irritation.
GENTAMICIN. *Bacterial. Micromonospora purpurea.* Gentamicin (Garamycin).	0.1% ointment or cream t.i.d. or q.i.d. Topical.	Used to treat various bacterial skin diseases. Primary: impetigo contagiosa, folliculitis, ecthyma, furunculosis, sycosis barbae, pyoderma gangrenosum. Secondary: infections in acne, pustular psoriasis, excoriations, wounds, burns.	Bactericidal. Slight absorption from G.I. tract, rapid absorption and wide distribution following injection. Appears in spinal fluid and crosses the placenta. Excreted unchanged in the urine	If sensitivity reactions, occur drug should be stopped. Gentamicin used parenterally is potentially ototoxic (both vestibular and auditory) and nephrotoxic. Monitoring of renal and eighth cranial nerve function during therapy is recommended. Other side effects include elevated SGOT and SGPT, increased bilirubin, anemia, granulocytopenia and thrombocytopenia. Fever, rash, urticaria, laryngeal edema, nausea and vomiting, lethargy, decreased appetite, headache, weight loss.	Not effective against fungi or viruses. Concurrent use of other neuro-and/or nephrotoxic drugs should be avoided. Dose must be adjusted in patients with impaired renal function. Safe use in pregnancy has not been established. See carbenicillin for interactions.
	Ophthalmic ointment 3 mg./Gm. or solution 3 mg./ml. b. or t.i.d.	Used for infections of the external eye caused by susceptible organisms.			
Gentamicin sulfate, U.S.P.	0.8-3.0 mg./kg. daily in 3 divided doses I.M. or I.V. Up to 5 mg./kg. in life-threatening infections.	Used parenterally in *Pseudomoas aeruginosa, Proteus sp., E. coli, Klebsiella, Enterobacter, Serratia sp.* and *Staphylococcus sp.* for infections of the central nervous system, urinary tract, upper respiratory tract, gastrointestinal tract, skin and soft tissues, including burns.			

Name, Source, Synonyms, Preparations	Dosage and Administration	Uses	Action and Fate	Side Effects and Contraindications	Nursing Implications and Remarks
AMINOGLYCOSIDE ANTIBIOTICS *(Continued)*					
Kanamycin sulfate U.S.P. (Kantrex).	15 mg./kg. in divided doses daily. I.M. Should never exceed 1.5 Gm. in one day. 1 Gm. q. 4-6 h. Oral. 15-30 mg./kg. daily in divided doses. Oral. Also prepared for intravenous or intracavitary use.	For tuberculosis and other infections. Active against a number of organisms. For preoperative disinfection of the intestines. For *Shigella* and *Salmonella* infections. For specific and usually severe infections.	Bactericidal. Action as for all aminoglycosides. Poorly absorbed from G.I. tract. 50-80% of parenteral dose excreted by kidneys in 24 hours, most in the first 6 hours. Diffuses into pleural and ascitic fluids but does not appear in amniotic fluid.	May cause nausea, vomiting, diarrhea. Adjust or stop dosage. Major toxic effect of parenteral kanamycin is its action on the auditory portion of the eighth cranial nerve. Safe use during pregnancy has not been established.	In patients with impaired renal function, the dose interval should be adjusted by the use of the following formula: serum creatinine (mg./100 ml.) x 9 = dose interval. As the creatinine clearance changes, dosage interval should be adjusted.
Neomycin sulfate, U.S.P. (Mycifradin, Neobiotic, Neocin [C]).	4.5-9 Gm. Divided doses 24-72 hours prior to surgery. Oral. 4-12 Gm. daily in divided doses. Oral. 10-15 mg./kg. in divided doses every 6 hours; not more than 1 Gm./day I.M. Treatment by I.M. should not be continued longer than 10 days.	For preoperative intestinal disinfection. For hepatic coma. For treatment of severe infections that do not respond to less toxic drugs. Effective against a number of organisms.	For mechanism see aminoglycosides. Oral dose poorly absorbed; 97% of such dose excreted in feces. After I.M. injection 30-50% excreted by kidneys.	Mild laxative action with oral use. With parenteral use there may be renal disorders, eighth cranial nerve involvement, or both. Adjust dosage or stop drug and treat symptoms. A potent neuromuscular blocking agent when given concomitantly with neuromuscular blocking agents or general anesthetics.	With I.M. use, frequent urinalyses and audiometry advised. May be given as retention enema in 1-2% solutions. May potentiate anticoagulant effect of warfarin, coumarin, and indandione derivatives.
Neomycin sulfate ointment and solution, U.S.P. (Myciquent).	1% solution or ointment once or twice daily. Topical.	For infections of skin and exposed mucous membranes.	Topical applications may be absorbed when applied to denuded areas.		
Paromomycin sulfate, U.S.P. (Humatin).	35-50 mg./kg. daily in divided doses for 5-7 days. Oral.	Amebicidic, antibacterial and some antihelminthic action. Used in treating enteric bacterial and amebic infections, and in preoperative suppression of intestinal flora.	Not appreciably absorbed from G.I. tract with recommended oral doses.	Diarrhea, abdominal cramps, pruritus ani. Treatment symptomatic.	Generally administered p.c.; overgrowth of some organisms may occur.

Tobramycin sulfate (Nebcin).	3-5 mg./kg./day administered in equal doses every 8 hours. Doses should not exceed 5 mg./kg./day unless serum levels are monitored. Neonates: 1 week of age or less up to 4 mg./kg./day in 2 equal doses every 12 hours. Dose must be reduced in patients with reduced renal function. I.M. or I.V.	See Amikacin.	Peak serum concentrations occur between 30 and 90 minutes following I.M. administration. Not appreciably absorbed from G.I. tract. Widely distributed in body tissues and fluids. Crosses the placenta. Excreted almost exclusively by the kidneys.	See amikacin. Safe use in pregnancy has not been established. Ototoxicity and nephrotoxicity are the most serious side effects.	The diluted solution (50-100 ml.) should be infused over a period of not less than 20 minutes to avoid serum levels over 12 mcg./ml. Manufacturer states that tobramycin injection should not be mixed with other drugs.

TETRACYCLINES

Tetracyclines, including chlortetracyclines, oxytetracycline and others, are all derived directly from a strain of *Streptomyces,* indirectly from chlortetracycline or are produced synthetically. They are mainly bacteriostatic. These drugs are effective against both gram-positive and gram-negative bacteria and many other types of microorganisms. They have a broad spectrum of activity. Tetracycline, oxytetracycline and methacycline may form a stable complex in any bone-forming tissue. No serious harmful effects have been reported thus far in humans. However, use of these drugs during tooth development–last trimester of pregnancy, neonatal period and early childhood–may cause discoloration of the teeth (yellow-grey-brown). The effect occurs most often during long-term use of the drug, but it has also been observed with the usual short-term therapy. It has also been associated with inhibited bone growth, micromelia and syndactyly in the fetus. Photosensitivity has occurred with all the tetracyclines and patients taking these drugs should be aware of this. **Any product containing aluminum, magnesium or calcium ions (antacids, milk and milk products) should not be taken the hour before or after an oral dose, since it can decrease absorption by as much as 25-50%.**

Chlortetracycline hydrochloride capsules, N.F. Chlortetracycline hydrochloride injection, N.F. Demeclocycline hydrochloride, N.F. (Declomycin) (demectocycline [C]).	50-500 mg. q. 6 h. Oral. 50-250 mg. q. 6 h., and only when unable to take medication orally. I.V. 30-150 mg. q. 6 h. Oral.	These drugs are used in the treatment of many diseases caused by microorganisms. Tetracyclines are among the drugs of first choice in infections caused by *Francisella tularensis, Pseudomonas pseudomallei, Vibrio cholerae, V. fetus, Hemophilus ducreyi, Donovania granulomatis, Mycoplasma*	The tetracyclines are bacteriostatic agents that exert their effect by blocking the attachment of aminoacyl transfer RNA to ribosomes and thus interfere with protein synthesis. As they do not affect cell wall synthesis they are effective against cell wall deficent organisms. Well absorbed and distributed	Side effects: slight gastrointestinal disorders, including diarrhea. Hypersensitivity reaction in the form of rash or fever. Transient and reversible vestibular side effects. If severe reaction accurs, drug is usually changed for another similar antibiotic. Side effects: they can cause an increase in BUN and	In renal dysfunction (especially during pregnancy) I.V. tetracycline therapy in daily doses exceeding 2 Gm. has been associated with deaths from renal failure. Therapy may result in superinfection.

Name, Source, Synonyms, Preparations	Dosage and Administration	Uses	Action and Fate	Side Effects and Contraindications	Nursing Implications and Remarks
TETRACYCLINES *(Continued)*					
		pneumoniae, all rickettsial infections, relapsing fever due to *Borrelia novyi* or *B. recurrentis* and all infections caused by *Chlamydia.* They are used as alternatives or combined with other drugs for the following: brucellosis, granuloma inguinale, plague due to *Yersinia pestis,* susceptible strains of *Shigella* and in any infection in which the infecting organism is susceptible and the agent of choice is not tolerated or is ineffective. Organisms usually susceptible include: *Streptococcus pneumoniae, Streptococcus pyogenes,* streptococci (most anaerobic, group A and group B), *Streptomyces anaerobius, Listeria monocytogenes, Bacillus anthracis, Erysipelothrix insidiosa, Fusobacterium fusiformis,* some strains of *E. coli, Hemophilus influenzae, H. ducreyi, Neisseria gonorrhoeae, Treponema pallidum, Malleomyces mallei,* some strains of *Acinetobacter, Clostridium tetani, C. welchii, Bordetella pertussis, Actinomyces israelii, Nocardia asteroides* and some *Bacteroides.*	to most body tissues and fluids after oral dose. Tetracyclines are concentrated in the liver and excreted in the bile and feces. They are also partially excreted in the urine.	depress plasma prothrombin activity. Tetracyclines cross the placental barrier, are found in fetal tissue and can have toxic effects on the developing fetus. They are also found in the milk of lactating mothers.	Since food interferes with absorption, administer oral dosages 1 h.a.c. or 2 h.p.c.

Doxycycline hyclate and monohydrate (Vibramycin).	25-100 mg. Oral. Usually 100 mg. q. 12 h. 1st day then 100 mg. q.d. or 50-100 mg. q. 12 h. Children less than 100 lb. 2 mg./lb. 1st day then 1 mg./lb.	As above.	Better absorption than some tetracyclines after oral dose. Absorption is not influenced by food or milk. Excreted slowly. Do not give with antacids. Much less is excreted by the kidneys than the other tetracyclines except minocycline. They may be used for extrarenal infections in patients with renal insufficiency with less chance of toxicity due to accumulation in the body, but the dose still may have to be reduced.	If renal impairment exists, usual dose may accumulate excessively and hepatic toxicity be induced.	Doxycycline hydrate comes in capsules; the monohydrate is a powder for oral suspension 25 mg./ml.
Doxycline hyclate (Vibramycin Hyrate).	100-200 mg./day I.V. children under 100 lbs. 2 mg./lb./1st day, then 1-2 mg./lb./day.				Avoid rapid administration. Consult brochure before giving this drug. Solutions should be protected from light and used within 12 hours at room temperature or 72 hours if kept under refrigeration.
Methacycline hydrochloride, N.F. (Rondomycin).	150 mg. q. 6 h. or 300 mg. q. 12 h. Oral. Children: 3-6 mg. per lb. in divided doses b.i.d. to q.i.d. Oral.			Side effects: same as others plus proctitis, vaginitis, dermatitis. If allergic reactions occur, stop drug at once. In renal impairment, dosage should be reduced.	In infants, intracranial pressure has occured. It clears with discontinuance of drug without known sequelae.
Minocycline hydrochloride (Minocin, Vectrin).	200 mg. 1st day, then 100 mg. q. 12 h. Oral; or I.V. 300 mg. single dose.		See doxycycline for use in renal patients.		Dairy products have not been shown to noticeably influence this particular tetracycline.
Oxytetracycline hydrochloride, U.S.P. (Terramycin) (Novoxytetra [C]).	50-250 mg. q. 6 h. Oral. 100-250 mg. q. 6 h. I.M. 250-500 mg. daily or q. 12 h. I.V.	As with chlortetracycline.		As with chlortetracycline.	Also available in preparations for topical use.
Rolitetracycline, N.F. (Syntetrin) (Reverin, Syntetrex [C]).	150-350 mg. q. 6 h. I.M. 350-700 mg. daily, I.V.				
Tetracycline hydrochloride, U.S.P. (Achromycin, Panmycin, Polycycline) (Cefracycline, Muracine, Neo-Tetrine, Sumycin, Tetrosol, Tetracyn [C]).	50-500 mg. q. 6 h. Oral. Also I.M., I.V., or as ophthalmic suspension 1%.	As above.		As above.	
Tetracycline phosphate complex, N.F. (Panmycin Phosphate, Sumycin, Tetrex).	150-500 mg. q. 6 h. Oral. Also I.M.				

Name, Source, Synonyms, Preparations	Dosage and Administration	Uses	Action and Fate	Side Effects and Contraindications	Nursing Implications and Remarks
CHLORAMPHENICOL GROUP					
CHLORAMPHENICOL. *Bacterial. Streptomyces venezuelae.* Also *synthetic.*	Adults, children and full-term infants over 2 weeks 50-100 mg./kg./day in divided doses q. 6-8 h.	Effective against many organisms, but especially the gram-negative organisms (colon-typhoid group). Useful in certain urinary infections and in many other conditions, but should be reserved for serious infections caused by susceptible organisms when less potentially hazardous therapeutic agents are ineffective or contraindicated.	Bacteriostatic and bactericidal. Believed to act by interfering with protein synthesis including enzyme formation. Rapidly absorbed. Widely distributed, but distribution not uniform. It is found in cerebrospinal fluid, aqueous and vitreous humor, snynovial fluid, pleural fluid, ascites and bile. Inactivated primarily by the liver and excreted by kidneys mainly as the glucuronide, only 5-10% in the biologically active form.	G.I. effects include nausea, vomiting, diarrhea, enterocolitis, unpleasant taste, dryness of mouth. Serious, even fatal blood dyscrasias with bone marrow depression may occur. Reduce or stop drug and treat as indicated. See manufacturer's bulletin for specific toxicology and contraindications. Found in milk of nursing mothers. Neurotoxicity may occur and is evidenced by headache, mental depression, confusion, optic neuritis, digital paresthesia, peripheral neuritis.	Frequent blood tests should be done during therapy. Can cause Gray syndrome or fetal death, since drug does cross placental barrier.
Chloramphenicol capsules, U.S.P. (Chloromycetin) (Chloroptic, Enicol, Mycinol, Novochlor, Novopoxide, Sopamycetin [C]).	50-250-500 mg. q. 6 h. Oral. 50-100 mg./kg. daily is usually adequate.				
Chloramphenicol palmitate, U.S.P. (Chloromycetin palmitate).	50-250 mg. Oral. As above.				
Chloramphenicol sodium succinate, U.S.P. (Chloromycetin succinate).	1 Gm. q. 8 h. I.V. As above.				
Chloramphenicol otic (Chloromycetin Otic).	5 mg./15 ml. in propylene glycol T. q.i.d.				
Chloramphenicol ophthalmic solution (Chloromycetin Ophthalmic solution).	0.5% solution.				
Chloramphenicol ophthalmic ointment (Chloromycetin Ophthalmic Ointment).	1.0%.				
POLYPEPTIDES					
BACITRACIN. *Bacterial. Bacillus subtilis.*		Effective against gram-positive organisms, the *Neisseria,* some spirochetes and *Entamoeba histolytica.* Used alone or in combination with other antibiotics.	Bacteriostatic and bactericidal. It has been reported to inhibit the incorporation of amino acids into bacterial protein with the accumulation of uridine nucleotide.	May cause nephrotoxicity. Adjust dosage, or discontinue and use another antibiotic. Anorexia, nausea, vomiting, diarrhea, rectal itching and burning and skin rashes may occur following I.M. administration.	Many of these antibiotics are used as powders and sprinkled directly on the wound or in solution as wet dressing.
Bacitracin ointment, U.S.P. (Baciquent).	500 u./Gm. p.r.n. Topical.				

				Pain sometimes accompanied by induration may occur at injection site. Allergic and hypersensitivity reactions have been reported.	
Bacitracin powder, U.S.P.	50,000 U.		Not absorbed from G.I. tract or intact skin. Widely distributed after injection with traces in spinal fluid. 10-40% excreted in the urine.		
Bacitracin solution, U.S.P. (Topitracin). Bacitracin ophthalmic ointment	10,000-20,000 U. t.i.d. I.M. 500 U./3.5 Gm.				Concurrent systemic use with other nephrotoxic drugs should be avoided. Bacitracin is known to inhibit neuromuscular transmission. Parenteral bacitracin may increase or prolong skeletal muscle relaxation produced by neuromuscular blocking agents.
COLISTIMETHATE SODIUM. *Bacterial. Aerobacillus colistinus.* Colistimethate sodium, U.S.P. (Colistin, Colymycin).	100-150 mg. I.M. or I.V. daily.	For the treatment of genitourinary or systemic infections caused by gram-negative organisms, particularly those caused by *Pseudomonas aeruginosa.* Not effective against *Proteus.*	Bactericidal; alters membrane permeability. Slightly absorbed from the G.I. tract, excreted primarily by kidneys following injection. Has serum half-life of 2-3 hours following I.M. or I.V. administration.	Both neuro and nephrotoxic, local irritation, nausea, paresthesia, leukopenia, fever, dermatitis, azotemia, pruritus and vertigo have been reported. *Used with caution in patients with impaired renal function.* This drug is transferred across the placental barrier. Safe use during pregnancy has not been established. Respiratory arrest has occurred following I.M. injection. Increased BUN has been seen, but returns to normal when drug is stopped.	See interactions with anesthetic muscle relaxants and aminoglycoside antibiotics under Streptomycin. See brochure for dosage calculation.
Colistin sulfate, N.F.	Dose on weight basis: 2 to 4 divided doses 2.5-5.0 mg./kg./day. Oral.				

Name, Source, Synonyms, Preparations	Dosage and Administration	Uses	Action and Fate	Side Effects and Contraindications	Nursing Implications and Remarks
POLYMYXIN B. *Bacterial. Bacillus polymyxa.* Polymyxin B sulfate, U.S.P. (Aerosporin).	1.5-2.5 mg./kg. in divided doses, b.i.d. but not over 200 mg. in any one day. Oral, I.M., or I.V. (500,000 U. is equivalent to 50 mg.)	Effective mainly against gram-negative organisms. Not given orally for systemic infections.	Bacteriostatic and bactericidal. Acts by rupture of cell membranes through cationic surface effect. Not absorbed orally. After parenteral administration, widely distributed in body fluids. Does not appear in C.S.F. or synovial fluid and does not cross placenta. Slowly excreted by kidneys after I.M. or I.V.	As above. May increase or prolong skeletal muscle relaxation produced by neuro-muscular blocking agents and/or anesthetics when given concurrently.	Available in preparations for topical use, but usually in combination products.
TYROTHRICIN. *Bacterial. Bacillus brevis.* Tyrothricin, N.F. (Hydrotricine [C]).	0.5-25 mg./ml. cream, ointment and spray for topical use.	Effective against gram-positive bacteria and some other organisms.	Bacteriostatic and bactericidal. Acts as cationic detergent which damages cell membranes.	Very toxic systemically. Used mainly topically.	Used alone or with other antibiotics.
MACROLIDES					
ERYTHROMYCIN. *Bacterial. Streptomyces erythreus.* Erythromycin, U.S.P. (Erythrocin, E-Mycin, Ilotycin) (Chem-Thromycin, Emcin, Ilosone [C]).	100-500 mg. q. 6 h. Oral. 100 mg. q. 8-12 h. I.M. 250 mg.-1 Gm. q. 6-8 h. I.V.	Active against most gram-positive organisms and a few gram-negative organisms, also against *Mycoplasma pneumoniae* (PPLO, Eaton agent) and certain *Actino-*	Inhibits protein synthesis without affecting nucleic acid synthesis. Bacteriostatic. Widely distributed. Excreted in bile and urine.	Usually slight. Treatment: symptomatic. The estolate ester (Ilosone) has been associated with an allergic type of cholestatic hepatitis (in adults). The effects	Available as the base and as several salts and in preparations for parenteral and topical use; also as chewables, especially for children. Safety during pregnancy has

	5 mg./Gm. ophthalmic ointment.	*myces* and *Treponema* species. Especially useful against penicillin-resistant staphylococci. The base is sometimes used with neomycin in preoperative reduction of bowel flora.		appear reversible on discontinuing the drug.	not been established.
OLEANDOMYCIN. *Bacterial. Streptomyces antibioticus.* Troleandomycin, N.F. (Tao).	250-500 mg. q.i.d. Oral.	Most effective against the gram-positive *Clostridium, Corynebacterium,* Pneumococcus, *Streptococcus* and some *Staphylococcus;* also effective against *Brucella, Hemophilus* and *Neisseria.*	Bacteriostatic. Exact mechanism is not known. Absorption incomplete. Widely distributed but not to brain and cerebrospinal fluid. Excreted in urine and bile.	May cause liver changes if administered for 2 weeks or longer. Hypersensitivity, nausea, vomiting, diarrhea, headache and anaphylatic reactions have occurred. Contraindicated in patients with liver disorders.	Should not be given for periods longer than 10 days.
ANTIFUNGAL POLYENES					
CANDICIDIN. *Bacterial. Streptomyces sp.* Candicidin, N. F. (Candeptin).	3 mg. tablet or ointment b.i.d. intravaginally for 14 days.	Treatment of vaginitis due to *Candida.*	Fungicidal.	Sensitivity may occur, but this is rare.	Store in a cool place. The tablet form is advised during pregnancy.
NYSTATIN. *Bacterial. Streptomyces noursei.* Nystatin, U.S.P. (Candex, Mycostatin, Nilstat).	100,000 U./Gm. cream or ointment. 500,000 U. once or twice a day. Oral. 100,000 U.Vaginal tablets. 100,000 U./Gm. Topical powder. 100,000 U./ml. suspension.	Antifungal; effective against intestinal moniliasis, vulvovaginal candidiasis, cutaneous or mucocutaneous infections caused by *Candida*.	Mechanism of action is believed to be by binding to sterols in the cell membrane with resultant change in membrane permeability. Poorly absorbed from intact skin or G.I. tract and excreted almost entirely in feces, unchanged.	Transient nausea and vomiting following oral use. Topical reactions rare, but sensitivities have occurred. Stop drug and treat symptoms.	In topical therapy, proper hygiene and skin care required to prevent spread or reinfection.
INJECTABLE ANTIFUNGALS FOR SYSTEMIC INFECTIONS					
AMPHOTERICIN B. *Bacterial. Streptomyces nodosus.* Amphotericin B, U.S.P. (Fungizone).	Begin with 0.25 mg./kg./day, increase to 1 mg./kg./day when possible. Available in 50 mg. vial. I.V.,	Used to treat deep-seated mycotic infections such as coccidioidomycosis, paracoccidioidomycosis, aspergillosis, chromoblastomy-	Fungistatic; acts by binding to sterol in the fungal cell membrane and interfering with membrane functions. Poorly absorbed from G.I.	Adverse reactions after I.V. use include chills, hyperhidrosis, fever, myalgia, arthralgia, general malaise, anorexia, abdominal cramps,	Should be given systemically only to hospitalized persons. The systemic side effects may be reduced if the rate of infusion is

Name, Source, Synonyms, Preparations	Dosage and Administration	Uses	Action and Fate	Side Effects and Contraindications	Nursing Implications and Remarks
AMPHOTERICIN B. (Continued)	3% ointment, lotion, powder. Topical.	cosis, systemic blastomycosis, histoplasmosis, cryptococcosis and candidosis.	tract, 90% bound by serum proteins. Excreted slowly by kidneys.	nausea, vomiting, diarrhea, headache, vertigo, phlebitis and thrombophlebitis. Those occurring only rarely include thrombocytopenia, leukopenia, agranulocytosis, hypotension, ventricular fibrillation, cardiac arrest (after rapid infusion), maculopapular rash, blurred vision, polyneuropathy, convulsions and anemia with prolonged therapy. Renal toxicity has also occurred with prolonged therapy and high doses. During therapy this is demonstrated by increased BUN, serum creatinine, decreased glomerular filtration and creatinine clearance.	reduced and the patient is given ancillary treatment such as heparin, antipyretic, antihistamines and antiemetics.
Miconazole (Monistat)	200-3600 mg./day depending on organism in divided doses t.i.d. I.V. Intrathecal dose of 20 mg. q. 3-7 days. Bladder irrigation with 200 mg. diluted solution for treatment of mycoses of urinary bladder.	Treatment of coccidioidomycosis, candidiasis, cryptococcosis, paracoccidioidomycosis and chronic mucocutaneous candidiasis.	Exact mode of action unknown. Metabolized in liver and about 14-22% excreted in urine. It fits a 3-compartment profile pharmacokinetically with biologic half-lives of 0.4, 2.1, and 24.1 hours. Same dose appears OK for patients with renal insufficiency, including those on renal dialysis.	Rapid injection of undiluted miconazole may produce transient tachycardia or arrhythmia. Side effects include phlebitis (29%), pruritis (21%), nausea (18%), fever and chills (10%), rash (9%) and emesis (7%). Transient decrease in hematocrit and serum sodium has been noted.	Drugs containing PEG 40 castor oil type vehicles are known to cause electrophoretic abnormalities of lipoprotein. It can interact with coumarin type anticoagulants to enhance their anticoagulant activity.
ORAL ANTIFUNGAL PREPARATION FOR SYSTEMIC FUNGAL INFECTIONS					
Flucytosine (Ancobon).	50-150 mg./kg./day at 6-hour intervals. Oral.	Used only in the treatment of serious infections caused	Acts by entering the fungal cell and inside the cell is	Nausea, vomiting, diarrhea, rash, anemia, leukopenia,	Nausea and vomiting may be reduced if capsules are

		by susceptible strains of *Candida* and/or *Cryptococcus.*	converted by an enzyme to 5-fluorouracil, which is the active metabolite. This enzyme is not present in human cells. It has in vitro and in vivo activity against *Candida* and *Cryptococcus.* It is not metabolized significantly when given orally and is excreted primarily by the kidneys. Only about 10% is converted to the active metabolite.	thrombocytopenis, elevation of hepatic enzymes, BUN and creatinine have been reported. Also seen: confusion, hallucinations, headache, sedation and vertigo.	given a few at a time over a 15 minute period. Must be used with extreme caution in patients with impaired renal function. Drug can affect hepatic and hematologic systems, and these must be monitored during therapy. Renal function should be determined before treatment is started. Safe use in pregnancy or nursing mothers has not been established.
ORAL ANTIFUNGAL PREPARATION FOR FUNGAL INFECTIONS OF SKIN, NAILS, HAIR					
GRISEOFULVIN. *Fungal. Penicillium griseofulvin* or *nigricans.* Griseofulvin, U.S.P. (Fulvicin U/F, Grifulvin, Grisactin) (Grisovin [C]).	125-500 mg. two to four times a day. Oral. Usually given four times a day in adult. It is also available in microcrystalline and ultra microcrystalline forms.	For treatment of mycotic infections by dermatophytes in hands, feet, nails, and scalp.	Fungistatic; acts primarily by arresting the metaphase of cell division. Absorbed from the duodenum and concentrated in the skin, hair, nails, liver, fat and skeletal muscles. Changed by the liver and excreted in feces, perspiration and urine.	Claimed to be mild and transient; heartburn, nausea, epigastric discomfort, diarrhea, headache. Discontinue if drug rash occurs. Patient's blood should be tested regularly for signs of leukopenia with prolonged therapy. Blood levels of griseofulvin may be lowered clinically to ineffective levels by concurrent or recent administration of phenobarbital, other barbiturates such as amobarbital, butabarbital, pentobarbital, secobarbital, and talbutal. If patient is on anticoagulants, the prothrombin times should be performed weekly until a stable level is found. This interaction does not occur in all patients.	Treatment usually prolonged (several months) owing to the mechanism of action involved. Safe use in pregnancy and in children under 2 years of age has not been established. Concurrent ingestion with alcohol reported to cause tachycardia and flushing; may potentiate effects of alcohol.

Name, Source, Synonyms, Preparations	Dosage and Administration	Uses	Action and Fate	Side Effects and Contraindications	Nursing Implications and Remarks
OTHER ANTIBIOTICS					
THE FOLLOWING ARE USED MAINLY IN TUBERCULOSIS OR AS RESERVE ANTIBIOTICS IN RESISTANT CASES					
Capreomycin sulfate (Capastat Sulfate). A polypeptide antibiotic obtained from *Streptomyces capreolus.*	1 Gm. daily, I.M. (not to exceed 20 mg./kg. per day) for 60 to 120 days followed by 1 Gm. 2 or 3 times a week for 18-24 months.	To be used with other anti-tuberculosis drugs in pulmonary infections caused by strains of *M. tuberculosis* sensitive to capreomycin when primary agents have been ineffective or cannot be used because of toxicity or resistant organisms.	Not absorbed in appreciable amounts from gastrointestinal tract. Must be given by injection. In patients with normal renal function 52% of a 1 Gm. dose can be recovered unchanged in the urine in 12 hours.	Nephrotoxicity is the most important side effect, shown by decreased creatine clearance, increased BUN and albuminuria. Other side effects include eosinophilia, ototoxicity, hepatotoxicity. Leucocytosis and leukopenia have been reported, as have urticaria and other skin rashes. Sterile abscess and excessive bleeding at point of injection have occurred. Use in patients with renal insufficiency or pre-existing auditory impairment must be undertaken with great caution. Safety for use during pregnancy or for infants and children has not been established.	Cross resistance occurs between capreomycin and viomycin and some has been reported with kanamycin and neomycin. After reconstitution, it may be stored for 48 hours at room temperature or for 14 days under refrigeration. Audiometric and renal function tests should be done before and during therapy.
Cycloserine, U.S.P. (Oxamycin, Seromycin). *Bacterial. Streptomyces orchidaceus* or *S. garyphalus.*	Initial dose: 15 mg./kg./day and increase by 250 mg./every 4 days until therapeutic serum levels are obtained.	Used mainly in severe pulmonary tuberculosis.	Competes with D-alanine as a cell wall precursor. Body distribution good. Excreted mainly in urine.	Neurotoxic, causes both neurologic and psychic disturbances in up to 10% of patients. Doses up to 100 mg. of pyridoxine t.i.d. may help prevent neurologic reactions, mental confusion, convulsions. Reduce dosage or stop. Contraindicated in epilepsy and severe renal insufficiency.	Safe use during pregnancy has not been established. Concurrent excessive use of alcoholic beverages should be avoided.

Rifampin (Rifadin, Rimactane).	600 mg. daily. Oral. For children: 10-20 mg./kg. daily. Oral. Not to exceed 600 mg. daily. Given once daily on an empty stomach.	For tuberculosis. Should not be given without at least one other antitubercular agent, such as isoniazid or ethambutol, or both.	Rifampin is believed to inhibit DNA-dependent RNA polymerase activity in susceptible cells (bacterial), but does not affect mammalian cells. Well absorbed from G.I. tract; widely distributed in body tissue and fluids. Crosses the placenta and found in maternal milk. Peak blood levels vary with individuals, but are usually reached in 2-4 hours after a 600 mg. dose. Half-life is about 3 hours. It is metabolized by the liver. Elimination is mainly through bile, but therapeutic concentrations are seen in the urine. Urine, feces, saliva, sputum, sweat and tears may be colored red-orange.	The drug may cause liver damage, especially in patients with impaired liver function. Should not be used with other hepatotoxic drugs for such patients. Liver function tests should be done frequently in such cases. Animal experimentation has shown the drug to be teratogenic; the effect in man is not known. Use in women of child-bearing age or during pregnancy should be carefully weighed—benefits against possible dangers. For other adverse reactions see brochure. Contraindication: The only known contraindication is sensitivity to the drug.	
	600 mg. daily for 4 consecutive days. Oral. For children: 10-20 mg./kg. daily for 4 consecutive days. Oral. Dosage for children under 5 years of age has not been established.	For meningococcal carriers.			The use of rifampin in meningococcal carriers should be limited to situations in which the risk of meningococcal meningitis is high. Patients on the coumarin-type anticoagulants may require increased amounts of anticoagulants.
VIOMYCIN SULFATE. *Bacterial. Streptomyces puniceus.* Viomycin sulfate, U.S.P. (Vinactane).	1-2 Gm. I.M. daily for 1-2 weeks, then 1-2 Gm. I.M. b.i.d. every third day or b.i.s.	Effective against acid-fast organisms. Used mainly in the treatment of tuberculosis.	Tuberculostatic. About 1/4 to 1/2 as effective as streptomycin in terms of clinical efficacy. It is a basic polypeptide. Good distribution. Excreted mainly by kidneys.	Nephrotoxicity associated with severe electrolyte imbalance, eighth cranial nerve damage (hearing and vestibular). Hypersensitivity reactions are rare but inadvertent I.V. injection may cause immediate shock-like state. Contraindicated in known renal disorders.	Audiometric tests should be conducted before and during treatment.

Name, Source, Synonyms, Preparations	Dosage and Administration	Uses	Action and Fate	Side Effects and Contraindications	Nursing Implications and Remarks
ANTIBIOTICS WITH VARIOUS USES					
FUMAGILLIN. *Fungal. Aspergillus fumigatus.* Fumagillin (Fugillin, Fumidil).	10-60 mg. daily in divided doses. Oral.	Used mainly in amebic dysentery. Also used in the treatment of certain neoplasms.	Has direct action on the amebae without effect on other intestinal flora.	Gastrointestinal disturbances, headache, rash. Effect upon blood not yet determined. Stop drug and treat symptoms.	Frequent blood tests should be done.
LINCOMYCIN. *Bacterial. Streptomyces lincolnensis var.* Lincomycin hydrochloride (Lincocin).	500 mg. three to four times a day. Oral. 600 mg. q. 12-24 h. I.M. 600 mg.-1 Gm. Given in 250 or more ml. of 5% glucose solution q. 8-12 h. I.V.	Used mainly in penicillin-resistant gram-positive infections, and in patients who are allergic to penicillin.	Bacteriostatic, interferes with protein synthesis of bacterial organism. Distributed in all body tissues except central nervous system. Good absorption and distribution. Body half-life about 6 hours. Excreted in bile, feces, milk and urine.	Loose stools or diarrhea, sometimes severe and persistent, with blood and mucus; nausea, vomiting, abdominal cramps, skin rash, rectal irritation, vaginitis, urticaria, pruritus and erythema multiforme; some resembling Stevens-Johnson syndrome have occurred. Neutropenia, leukopenia, agranulocytosis and thrombocytopenic purpura have been reported. Abnormal liver function tests, jaundice and hypotension following parenteral use, especially with rapid I.V. administration. Also, cardiopulmonary arrest has occurred after rapid I.V. infusion. Known *Candida* (monilial) infections should be treated concurrently with an antifungal agent such as nystatin.	Lincomycin must not be administered at the same time as kaolin-containing products since it may reduce absorption as much as 90%. Lincomycin should be given 1 hour before or 2 hours after eating. Not recommended for use in pregnant women or newborn infants.

<u>Clindamycin hydrochloride hydrate.</u> *Synthetic.* (Cleocin) (Dalacin [C]). Derivative of lincomycin.	150-600 mg. q. 6 h. (average 150 mg. q. 6 h.). Oral. 300-600 mg. I.M. or I.V. For children: 4-10 mg./lb./day in 4 divided doses. Oral.	*See* lincomycin. Bacteriostatic, interferes with protein synthesis. Well absorbed after oral administration. For beta-hemolytic streptococcal infections, treatment should be continued at least 10 days to diminish the likelihood of subsequent rheumatic fever or glomerulonephritis. Drug of choice in treatment of *Bacteroides fragilis.*	50% of oral dose is absorbed. Widely distributed in body fluids and tissues. Biological half-life is 2.4 hours. 10% of bioactive drug is excreted in the urine and about 3% in the feces. The remainder is excreted as bio-inactive metabolites. Crosses placenta.	*See* lincomycin. It is said to have more in vivo potency, better oral absorption and fewer gastrointestinal side effects than the parent drug. Safe use during pregnancy has not been established. Because of antagonism shown in vitro, clindamycin and erythromycin should not be administered simultaneously. I.M. injections may cause pain, induration and sterile abscess. I.V. injections may cause erythema, pain, swelling and thrombophlebitis. Physical incompatibility with aminophylline and with B complex vitamins. Causes increase in creatinine, phosphokinase and S.G.O.T. levels.	*Warning:* Can cause severe colitis, which may end fatally. Therefor, should be reserved for serious infections for which less toxic antimicrobial agents are inappropriate. Should not be used in patients with nonbacterial infections, such as most upper respiratory infections. Colitis is usually characterized by severe, persistent diarrhea and severe abdominal cramps and may be associated with passage of blood and mucus. Endoscopic examination may reveal pseudomembranous colitis. When significant diarrhea occurs, the drug should be discontinued or, if necessary, continued only with close observation of the patient. Large bowel endoscopy has been recommended. Antiperistaltic agents such as opiates and diphenoxylate with atropine (Lomotil) may prolong and/or worsen the condition. Diarrhea, colitis, and pseudomembranous colitis have been observed to begin up to several weeks following cessation of therapy with clindamycin. Deep I.M. injection recommended to minimize complications of administration. With I.V. injection, avoidance of prolonged use of indwelling catheter has been suggested.

Name, Source, Synonyms, Preparations	Dosage and Administration	Uses	Action and Fate	Side Effects and Contraindications	Nursing Implications and Remarks
RIFOMYCIN Rifomycin B. *Bacterial.* *Streptomyces mediterranei.*	1-2 Gm. I.M.	Effective mainly against gram-positive organisms and mycobacteria.	Exact mechanism of action not known.	Toxicity very low.	
SPECTINOMYCIN Spectinomycin dihydrochloride pentahydrate (Trobicin). Derived from *Streptomyces spectabilis.*	2 Gm. single dose I.M. for male patients. 4 Gm. for retreatment. 4 Gm. for female patients. (Usually divided between 2 gluteal injection sites).	Acute gonorrheal urethritis and proctitis in males. Acute gonorrheal cervicitis and proctitis in females when due to susceptible strains of *N. gonorrhea.*	Inhibits bacterial protein synthesis. Good absorption following I.M. injection giving peak concentration after 1 to 2 hours. Excreted in urine.	During single dose therapy, soreness at injection site, urticaria, dizziness, nausea, chills, oliguria, fever and insomnia may occur.	Can mask symptoms of developing syphilis. Serologic study should be done monthly for 3 months if syphilis is suspected. Safety in pregnancy not established.
VANCOMYCIN. *Bacterial. Streptomyces orientalis.* Vancomycin, U.S.P. (Vancocin).	500 mg. q.i.d. oral, I.V. Given with I.V. infusions.	Effective against infections caused by strains resistant to other antibiotics. Bactericidal for gram-positive cocci. Important drug for treatment of bacterial endocarditis and in other serious infections caused by staph, strep, or enterococci, especially in patients sensitive to the penicillins and cephalosporins.	Bactericidal, interferes with cell wall synthesis. Widely distributed in body tissue and fluids. Half-life in circulation 6 hours. Excreted mainly by kidneys. Only given orally for effect in G.I. tract.	It may cause eighth cranial nerve damage, renal disorders, or both. Contraindicated in reduced renal function. Other side effects include fever and macular rash. Safe use in pregnancy has not been established.	

ANTIVIRAL

PROPHYLAXIS FOR ASIAN INFLUENZA					
Amantadine hydrochloride, N.F. (Symmetrel).	200 mg. o.d. or b.i.d. capsule or syrup. Oral. Children: 1-9 yrs. 2-4 mg./lb. not to exceed 150 mg./day in divided doses t.i.d.; 9-12 yrs. 200 mg./day in divided doses t.i.d. 100 mg. up to b.i.d. Oral. 100-200 mg. q.d.	Used in the prophylaxis of Asian (A_2) influenza. For Parkinsonism and drug-induced extrapyramidal reactions.	Appears to act by preventing penetration of the virus into the host cell rather than as a viricide. 90% of oral dose excreted unchanged in urine, half within the first 20 hours. In Parkinson's disease action is believed related to the release of dopamine and other catecholamines from neuronal storage sites.	Contraindications: used with caution if at all in central nervous system disorders except parkinsonism, geriatric patients with arteriosclerosis or patients with epilepsy or history of other seizures. Side effects: ataxia, nervousness, insomnia, inability to concentrate and some psychic reactions have occurred. Dry mouth, gastrointestinal disturbances and skin rashes have been reported.	Not to be used in active cases of influenza of other respiratory disease or with central nervous system stimulants. Safety during pregnancy and lactation has not been established. Administer with caution to patients receiving other C.N.S. stimulant drugs. When administered with anticholinergic drugs, may increase the anticholinergic side effects.
HERPETIC KERATITIS					
IDOXURIDINE. *Synthetic.* Idoxuridine (Dendrid, Herplex, Stoxil).	0.1% solution or ointment. 1 gtt. q. 1 h. during day q. 2 h. during night in acute stage. Topical.	Used for herpes simplex of the lids, conjunctiva and cornea. Treatment should be continued for at least 2 weeks.	Mechanism of action is not known. Does not penetrate the cornea.	Irritation, pain, pruritus, edema of eye or lids, or photophobia may occur.	Use with caution in pregnancy or in women of childbearing age.
VIDARABINE. *Streptomyces antibioticus.* Vidarabine (Vira A).	3% Ophthalmic ointment. ½ inch of vidarabine into lower conjunctival sac 5 times daily at 3-hour intervals. If no improvement after 7 days or if	Used for treatment of acute keratoconjunctivitis and recurrent epithelial keratitis due to herpes simplex virus types 1 and 2.	A purine nucleoside. It possesses in vitro and in vivo antiviral activity against herpes simplex types 1 and 2, varicella-zoster and vaccinia viruses. Mechanism of action is by	Lacrimation, foreign body sensation, burning, irritation, superficial punctate keratitis, pain, photophobia and punctal occlusion and sensitivity have been reported.	Each mg. requires 2.22 ml. of I.V. solution to stay in solution; in some patients this volume could cause fluid overload. Vidarabine is teratogenic in rats and rabbits.

Name, Source, Synonyms, Preparations	Dosage and Administration	Uses	Action and Fate	Side Effects and Contraindications	Nursing Implications and Remarks
VIDARABINE. *Streptomyces antibioticus. (Continued)* Vidarabine (Vira A). (Continued)	complete re-epithelialization has not occurred by 21 days other forms of therapy should be considered. After re-epithelialization has occurred an additional 7 days of therapy at reduced dosage b.i.d. is recommended.		inhibition of viral DNA synthesis.		
	15 mg./kg./day I.V. for 10 days, given slowly.	Herpes simplex virus encephalitis.	Widely distributed after I.V. administration. Excreted by kidneys. Minimal absorption after oral dosage.	Principal reactions affect G.I. tract and are mild to moderate. C.N.S. disturbances such as tremor, hallucination, ataxia and psychoses reported. Blood effects include decreased Hgb., Hct., W.B.C. and platelet count.	As above. Not indicated in pregnancy or lactation.
ANTIBACTERIAL					
TUBERCULOSIS. See also antibiotics and antileprosy drugs.					
AMINOSALICYLIC ACID (PAS). *Synthetic.* Aminosalicylic acid, U.S.P. (p-aminosalicylic acid, Pamisyl, Parasal, PAS, PASNA, Teebacin Acid)	Daily doses total 12-16 Gm. as one dose or divided two to five times per 24 hours. Oral.	Used as adjunctive treatment with streptomycin or isoniazid in certain types of tuberculosis or alone when streptomycin is contraindicated.	Bacteriostatic only against *Mycobacterium tuberculosis.* Exact mode of action not known. Most effective in pulmonary tuberculosis. Delays emergence of resistant bacterial strains. Absorbed rapidly from the G.I. tract; widely distributed to most tissues and fluids. Diffusion into spinal fluid is less consistent and of lower concentration than other fluids.	Anorexia, nausea, vomiting, abdominal discomfort and diarrhea may occur. Treatment: symptomatic. Less frequent side effects are hypersensitivity, goiter and hypothyroidism. Electrolyte imbalance may occur with patients on restricted salt intake and those taking sodium aminosalicylic acid.	Available as several salts with isoniazid.

			Mainly eliminated in urine with small amounts in milk, bile and other secretions.		
Ethambutol hydrochloride (Myambutol).	Initial treatment: 15 mg./kg. as a single dose daily. Oral. Retreatment: 25 mg./kg. as a single dose. Oral. After 60 days reduce to 15 mg./kg.	One of prime drugs used in the treatment of tuberculosis.	Good oral absorption and distribution. Appears to inhibit the synthesis of one or more metabolites in growing bacterial cells, causing impairment of cell metabolism, arrest of multiplication and cell death. No cross-resistance with other available antimycobacterial agents has been demonstrated. Does not show any activity against fungi, viruses or other bacteria. 75-80% of oral dose absorbed. Has good distribution. Excreted in urine and feces.	May cause decrease in visual acuity, uni- or bilateral. Patient should promptly report any visual changes to the physician. Other adverse reactions include anaphylactoid reaction, headaches, malaise, anorexia, dizziness, fever, nausea, gastrointestinal disturbances, dermatitis, pruritus, numbness and tingling of extremities due to peripheral neuritis. Contraindicated in patients with optic neuritis. Cautions: Effect on fetus of this drug alone or in combinations is not known. Dosage should be reduced in patients with decreased renal function. With long-term therapy, renal, hepatic and hematopoietic tests should be routinely done.	Dose should not be used alone. Usually combined with isoniazid or isoniazid and streptomycin. If patient has cataracts or ocular abnormalities, a baseline should be established prior to treatment.
ETHIONAMIDE. *Synthetic.* Ethionamide (Trecator S.C.).	250 mg.-1 Gm. daily. Oral.	Used to treat pulmonary tuberculosis in patients with organisms resistant to isoniazid.	Mechanism is believed to be similar to that of isoniazid. Readily absorbed and distributed in body. Rapidly excreted by kidneys but less than 1% still in unchanged form.	Gastrointestinal disturbances may occur. Renal, hepatic and blood tests should be done during administration. Reduce dosage or stop drug if toxic reactions occur. Used with caution, if at all, in children under 12 years.	Used in conjunction with other antituberculosis drugs. This drug can potentiate psychotoxic effects of alcohol. Best taken with meals to minimize gastric irritation.

Name, Source, Synonyms, Preparations	Dosage and Administration	Uses	Action and Fate	Side Effects and Contraindications	Nursing Implications and Remarks
ISONIAZID. *Synthetic.* Isoniazid, U.S.P. (Laniazid, Niconyl, Nydrazid, Rimifon, Teebaconin, INH) (isonicotinic acid hydrazid, Isozide, [C]).	50-200 mg. t.i.d. or b.i.d. Oral.	One of the prime drugs used for treatment of TB. Also used to prevent development of active tuberculosis in recently converted tuberculin positive persons, or in individuals who have a high risk of developing active tuberculosis.	Bacteriostatic to *Mycobacterium tuberculosis.* Interferes with bacterial metabolism. Readily absorbed from oral and hypodermic doses. Widely distributed in body tissues and fluids including spinal fluid. Crosses the placenta, also appears in mother's milk. Metabolized by the liver, excreted primarily in the urine.	Peripheral neuritis is most common side effect. Other neurotoxic effects may occur and can be relieved by giving pyridoxine 50-100 mg./day. Convulsions, optic neuritis and sedation or incoordination may also occur. Constipation, difficulty in voiding, postural hypotension, dizziness, eosinophilia, agranulocytosis, hemolytic or aplastic anemia, skin eruptions, elevated SGOT and SGPT. Severe and sometimes fatal hepatitis associated with INH therapy may occur and may develop even after many months of therapy. This risk is age related and is increased with daily consumption of alcohol. Contraindicated when adrenergic drugs are being given, as well as in older patients and coexisting renal damage.	Patients who are genetically slow inactivators of isoniazid may experience diphenylhydantoin toxicity when taken concurrently. When given with PAS, isoniazid blood levels are increased due to competition for the same pathway of excretion. Pyridoxine is administered in conjunction with therapy in the malnourished, diabetic or adolescent patient.
PYRAZINAMIDE. *Synthetic.* Pyrazinamide (Tebrazid [C]).	20-35 mg./kg. of body weight. Three grams daily for 2 weeks before and after surgery. Oral.	Potent antituberculosis drug. Because of toxicity used for short-term therapy, such as presurgery and postsurgery.	Bacteriostatic. Organism develops resistance relatively fast. Thought to have action similar to that of isoniazid. Well absorbed after oral dose; primarily excreted by the kidneys.	May cause liver damage. Stop drug or reduce dosage and treat symptoms. Frequent tests for liver function should be made. Increases reabsorption of urates; routine blood uric acid evaluations recommended. Other effects include anorexia, nausea, vomiting, arthralgia, malaise and fever.	

LEPROSY. See also drugs used in the treatment of tuberculosis.					
SULFONE SERIES. *Synthetic.* Acetosulfone (Promacetin).	500 mg.-2 Gm. Oral.	Anti-infective. Especially effective in leprosy and tuberculosis.	Bacteriostatic. Slow acting. Slow excretion. Continued use will usually arrest disease and control symptoms.	Nausea and vomiting, mental confusion, headache, hepatitis, cyanosis, drug fever, allergic reactions and blood dyscrasias may occur.	Several of these compounds are being tried; their exact value has not been determined.
Dapsone, U.S.P. (Avlosulfon) (diaphenylsulfone, DDS [C]).	100-400 mg. twice weekly or 50-100 mg. q.d. Oral.	Anti-infective. Drug of choice in treatment of both lepromatous and tuberculoid types of leprosy in U.S.	Good oral absorption. Distributed to all body tissues. Excreted slowly in the urine.	Dapsone is excreted very slowly, thus cumulative poisoning may occur, but it is less toxic than most of the sulfone drugs. Nausea, vomiting, headache, dizziness, tachycardia, blood dyscrasias and allergic dermatitis may occur. Sometimes exfoliation with concurrent liver damage and lymphangitis. Patients with G6PD deficiency have a greater chance of hemolysis and significant hemolytic anemia. Erythema nodosum type of "leper reaction" is a common occurrence during sulfone therapy; characterized by malaise, fever, and painful inflamed induration of skin and mucosa. Therapy may be discontinued depending on severity of reaction.	Dapsone blood levels may be increased by as much as 50% by concurrent administration of probenecid so, if possible, these two drugs should not be given at the same time.
Glucosulfone sodium, U.S.P. (Promin).	1-5 Gm. daily 6 days a week with rest periods. I.V.	As above.			
Sulfoxone sodium, U.S.P. (Diasone).	165 mg.-1 Gm. One dose daily. Oral.	For leprosy and for maintenance in dermatitis herpetiformis.	About 50% absorbed from G.I. tract. See above.		Two week rest periods from therapy every 2 months are advisable.

Name, Source, Synonyms, Preparations	Dosage and Administration	Uses	Action and Fate	Side Effects and Contraindications	Nursing Implications and Remarks
LEPROSY (Continued)					
Thiazolsulfone (Promizole).	500 mg.-2 Gm. daily in divided doses. Oral. 330 mg. I.M. daily.	Also indicated for the treatment of dermatitis herpetiformis.			
ANTISPIROCHETAL AND ANTIPROTOZOAL DRUGS					
See also drugs used for amebiasis.					
ARSENIC. *Mineral.* Oxophenarsine hydrochloride, U.S.P.	40-60 mg. q. 4 to 7 days. I.V.	Anti-infective, especially useful in protozoal infections.	Arsenicals act as protoplasmic poison by their affinity for sulfhydryl groups. They are not used widely since the introduction of penicillin and other antibiotics that are effective and less toxic for treatment of treponemal infections. Distributed widely after I.V. injection, but not into central nervous system. Excreted mainly by the kidneys.	Immediate or nitritoid reactions: flushing of face, edema of lips, profuse diaphoresis, fall in blood pressure, feeling of anxiety. Stop drug, give adrenalin, treat symptoms. Intermediate or Herxheimer reaction: chills, fever, headache, malaise, nausea. Treatment: symptomatic. Delayed reaction: dermatitis (may be exfoliative), hepatitis, blood dyscrasias, hemorrhagic encephalitis. Treatment: symptomatic. For dermatitis, give sodium thiosulfate; for blood dyscrasias, give BAL (British antilewisite).	
ARSTHINOL (Mercaptoarsenol). *Synthetic. Trivalent arsenical.* Arsthinol (Balarsen).	10 mg./kg. daily. 50-100 mg. after breakfast for 5 days. Oral. Caution: Not over 500 mg. daily.	Effective in amebiasis and in yaws.	As above.	May cause abdominal cramps, diarrhea, skin eruptions. Reduce dosage or stop drug and treat symptoms.	Combination of arsenoxide and dimercaprol (BAL).

ANTIMONY POTASSIUM TARTRATE. *Mineral. Synthetic.* Antimony potassium tartrate, U.S.P. (tartar emetic).	40-140 ml. as a 0.5% solution. I.V. on alternate days. Usually given with sterile water or glucose. 8 ml. of 0.5% solution initially, increase dose given on alternate days by 4 ml. until maximum daily dose of 28 ml. has been reached.	Anti-infective. Especially effective in schistosomiasis, kala-azar and granuloma inguinale. Also used as expectorant and emetic.	The exact mechanism of action is not known, but is thought to be similar to that of the arsenicals. Excreted very slowly, primarily by the kidneys.	Coughing, muscular stiffness, and severe symptoms similar to arsenic poisoning. Treatment: symptomatic. Contraindicated: in presence of febrile infection, severe cardiac or renal disease and hepatic damage not caused by schistosomiasis.	Solutions must be freshly prepared in either water or D_5W.
BISMUTH. *Mineral.* Glycobiarsol, N.F. (Amoebicon, Milibis) (bismuth glycollylarsanilate [C]). 15% arsenic 42% bismuth	500 mg. t.i.d. for 7-10 days. Oral or topical. One vaginal suppository daily for 10 days.	Mainly used in amebiasis and in trichomonas vaginitis as vaginal suppositories.	Poor oral absorption limits its use in amebiasis to intestinal organisms.		
HYDROXYSTILBAMIDINE ISETHIONATE. *Synthetic.* Hydroxystilbamidine isethionate, U.S.P. (Stilbamidine).	2 mg./kg. daily for 8 days. I.V. Occasionally I.M.	Used to treat protozoal infections such as leishmaniasis and some fungal infections such as North American blastomycosis. Also used in the palliative treatment of multiple myeloma.	As antifungal and antiprotozoal. Exact mechanism is not known but is thought to be due to enzyme inhibition. It does not enter CNS and is too irritating if given intrathecally.	Fall in blood pressure, tachycardia, nausea, dyspnea, syncope, etc. Stop drug temporarily and proceed very slowly. Best prevented by giving the solution very slowly.	

Name, Source, Synonyms, Preparations	Dosage and Administration	Uses	Action and Fate	Side Effects and Contraindications	Nursing Implications and Remarks
LUCANTHONE. *Synthetic.*					
Lucanthone hydrochloride, U.S.P. (Miracil D).	200 mg. Usually given 15 mg./kg. daily in divided doses for 7 to 20 days. Oral.	Used for oral treatment of schistosomiasis. Most effective against *Schistosoma hematobium.*	Has been said to react with nucleoprotein and to inhibit mitosis. Readily absorbed orally. Most is degraded in body. About 10% appears in urine.	Side effects may include anorexia, nausea, vomiting, vertigo, or tremor. Convulsions may result from overdosage. Chronic toxicity may result in liver and kidney degeneration. Use with caution in cases of liver damage or impaired kidney function.	
MERCURY. *Mineral.*					
Mild mercurous chloride ointment (calomel ointment).	30% in oily base. Topical.	For venereal prophylaxis.			
STIBOPHEN. *Antimony compound. Synthetic.*					
Stibophen, U.S.P. (Fuadin).	7% solution 0.1-0.3 Gm. daily for about 2 weeks. I.V.	Used to treat schistosomiasis caused by *Schistosoma hematobium* and *S. mansoni,* not effective against *S. japonicum.*	Anti-infective. Action believed to be similar to that of arsenic.	Coughing, muscular stiffness, and severe symptoms similar to those of arsenic poisoning. Treatment: symptomatic. Contraindicated in severe renal or cardiac disease and hepatic disease not due to schistosomiasis.	Less toxic and easier to administer than tartar emetic.
ANTIAMEBIC DRUGS					
ARSENIC COMPOUNDS. *Synthetic, mineral.*					
Carbarsone, U.S.P.	250 mg. b. or t.i.d. for 7-10 days. Oral. Children: 7.5 mg./kg./day in 3 divided doses for up to 10 days.	Effective in amebiasis, especially that associated with the lumen of the intestine.	Amebicide with some trichomonacide activity. Contains approximately 29% arsenic. Well absorbed orally. Slowly	May cause gastrointestinal disorders, hepatitis, skin rashes, or visual disturbances, sore throat, polyuria, splenomegaly,	Should not be given to patients with liver or kidney disease or to patients with contracted visual or color fields.

	As retention enema 2 Gm. in 200 ml. of a 2% sodium bicarbonate solution h.s.		excreted in urine, so oral therapy should be interrupted.	hepatitis, jaundice, dermatosis, neuritis and edema. Exfoliate dermatitis, hepatic necrosis and hemorrhagic encephalitis have been reported.	Safe use during pregnancy not established.
BIALAMICOL HYDROCHLORIDE. *Synthetic.* Bialamicol hydrochloride (diallylamicol hydrochloride, Camoform hydrochloride).	250-500 mg. t.i.d. Oral.	Used to treat amebic infections.	A substituted cresol which has amebicidal activity. Rapid oral absorption, stored in high concentration in liver and lungs. Slowly excreted mainly in bile which gives prolonged fecal levels.	Relatively nontoxic but some nausea, vomiting, and abdominal distress reported at high doses; skin rashes also have been reported.	
GLAUCARUBIN. *Plant. Glycoside of Simarouba glauca.* Glaucarubin (Glarubin).	3 mg./kg. of body weight daily for 5-10 days. Maximum dose of 200 mg./day should not be exceeded. Oral.	Used in the treatment of intestinal amebiasis.	Has amebicidal action.	Anorexia, nausea, vomiting, abdominal pain, bloody stools, giddiness, difficulty in urination. Treatment: symptomatic.	
IPECAC. *Plant. Ipecacuanha, emetine, cephaeline.* Emetine-bismuth-iodide. Emetine hydrochloride, U.S.P. Ipecac.	200 mg. Oral. 30-60 mg. O.D. for 6-10 days. I.M. Bed rest essential during treatment. 300 mg. enteric capsules. Oral.	Especially effective in amebiasis. Also used as expectorant and emetic. Emetine is effective in amebic abscess.	Directly kills motile forms of *Entamoeba histolytica* but does not affect cysts. Absorbed readily but excreted slowly by the kidneys. May cause cumulative symptoms.	Rare in therapeutic dosage. Sweating and depression may occur. Watch for cumulative action. Nausea, vomiting, diarrhea, vertigo, tachycardia. Sudden cardiac failure may occur during or following therapy. Ipecac and its alkaloids are contraindicated in cardiac and metabolic diseases.	Emetine bismuth iodide is less reliable than the hydrochloride. Patient should be kept in bed and have vital signs monitored during therapy. Emetine hydrochloride must be protected from exposure to light. Multiple injection sites are recommended to prevent abscesses.

Name, Source, Synonyms, Preparations	Dosage and Administration	Uses	Action and Fate	Side Effects and Contraindications	Nursing Implications and Remarks
METRONIDAZOLE. Metronidazole, U.S.P. (Flagyl). *Synthetic.*	250 mg. t.i.d. for 7 days. Oral. 250 mg. t.i.d. for 7 days. Oral 750 mg. t.i.d. for 5 to 10 days. Oral. 500-750 mg. t.i.d. for 5 to 10 days. Oral. 35-50 mg./kg. of body weight per 24 hours divided t.i.d. for 10 days. Oral.	For trichomoniasis (male). For trichomoniasis (female). For intestinal amebiasis in adults. For amebiasis with liver abscess. For children.	Has direct trichomonicidal and amebicidal activity. Well absorbed orally, reaches peak serum concentration in about 1 hour. Excreted mainly in urine—unchanged or as various metabolites. Low concentrations are found in saliva and breast milk during therapy. For this reason, nursing mothers probably should not nurse during therapy. Recent studies in animals have shown that metronidazole is possibly carcinogenic, teratogenic and mutagenic.	Side effects are mainly gastrointestinal—anorexia, nausea, vomiting, diarrhea, epigastric distress. An unpleasant metallic taste is not uncommon. Monilial overgrowth may occur, giving a furry tongue, glossitis and stomatitis. A moderate leukopenia may occur, but usually returns to normal when drug is stopped. Contraindications: patients with history of blood dyscrasia or active organic disease of the central nervous system. It should not be given during pregnancy and the doctor should weigh the benefits against adverse effects before using it for trichomoniasis.	Patients taking metronidazole should be advised not to drink any alcoholic beverages, since they may experience a disulfiram-like reaction. Urine may be darkened in color, believed to be caused by the metabolites. When treatment for a patient is in conjunction with the treatment of his/her sexual partner, the medication should be taken by both partners over the same 10 day period.
OXYQUINOLINE-IODINE COMPOUNDS. *Synthetic.* Diiodohydroxyquin, U.S.P. (Yodoxin) (diiodohydroxyquin, direxiode [C]).	200 mg. Give 3 tablets t.i.d. for 20 days. Oral. Children: 40 mg./kg./day in 2 or 3 doses.	Amebicide. Especially effective in intestinal amebiasis and trichomoniasis.	Contains about 64% iodine. Exact mode of action not understood. Is not effective in amebic abscesses. Very little absorbed. Most passes unchanged in feces.	Gastrointestinal disorders. Treatment symptomatic. Rash, acne, slight enlargement of the thyroid gland. Optic neuropathy has occurred following use of diiodohydroxyquin.	Diiodohydroxyquin is less toxic and more effective than Chiniofon or Vioform. Will interfere with results of thyroid function test for several months following its use.

Iodochlorhydroxyquin, N.F. (Vioform) (iodochlorohydroxyquine, clinquinol, Domeform [C]).	250 mg. Give 3 tablets t.i.d. for 20 days. Oral. 3% topical.		Little if any absorption.		
Sodium iodohydroxyquinoline sulfonate (Chiniofon).	1.0 Gm. Give daily for 10 days. Oral. 2.5% solution 200 ml. Rectal.	Amebicide.	About 15% absorbed after oral dose. Most of absorbed drug eliminated in urine.		
ANTIMALARIAL DRUGS		*These are all synthetic drugs unless otherwise indicated.*			
Amodiaquine hydrochloride, N.F.	200-400 mg. o.d. Oral. 500 mg. daily for suppressive therapy.	To treat malaria. Also used to treat rheumatoid arthritis and lupus erythematosus, extra-intestinal amebiasis and giardiasis.	Similar to chloroquine. Most effective against estivo-autumnal malaria.	Nausea, vomiting, salivation. diarrhea and melanosis. Treatment: symptomatic.	Give with meals or antacids.
Chloroguanide hydrochloride	100 mg. q.d. Therapy is begun 2 weeks prior to entering malarial area and continued 8 weeks after return.	Prophylaxis for malaria.	Anti-infective. Especially effective in malaria caused by *Plasmodium falciparum.* Destroys parasites in the asexual-erythrocytic stage. Slowly absorbed after oral dose approximately 70-90%. Rapidly excreted in urine. 60% unchanged.	Nausea, vomiting, diarrhea. Megaloblastic anemia, anorexia and malaise.	Tends to cause resistant strains to develop.

Name, Source, Synonyms, Preparations	Dosage and Administration	Uses	Action and Fate	Side Effects and Contraindications	Nursing Implications and Remarks
ANTIMALARIAL DRUGS (Continued)					
Chloroquine phosphate, U.S.P. (Aralen, Nivaquine, Roquine).	Malaria: 600 mg. base followed by 300 mg. base in 6 hours, then 300 mg. base q. 6 h. for 2 days. Prophylaxis: 500 mg. orally once weekly beginning one week before departure and continuing for 6 weeks after return from malarious areas. Amebiasis: 1 Gm. daily for 2 days, then 500 mg. q.d. for 2-3 weeks.	Used to treat malaria and amebiasis.	Anti-inflammatory and anti-infective. Especially effective in malaria caused by *Plasmodium vivax* and *P. falciparum.* Destroys parasites in the asexual-erythrocytic stage. Complete absorption following oral dose. Widely distributed in body but concentrated by certain tissues such as liver, spleen, kidneys, lungs and leukocytes. Most degraded by body. Slowly excreted by the kidneys.	May cause pruritus, G.I. discomfort, nausea, diarrhea, rash, headache, CNS stimulation. Overdoses can cause acute circulatory failure, convulsions, respiratory and cardiac arrest. Contraindicated in patients with psoriasis and in patients with retinal or visual field changes, as irreversible retinal damage has been observed. Chloroquine crosses the placenta and can cause thrombocytopenia in the fetus.	Also available as the diphosphate. Does not discolor skin. Give with meals or antacids to minimize G.I. side effects. Large doses may antagonize effects of parasympathetic agents and produce quinidine-like effects on the heart. For suppressive therapy, the drug should be administered on the same day each week. Also used to suppress lupus erythematosus.
Chloroquine hydrochloride, U.S.P. (Aralen HCl).	160-200 mg. daily for 10-12 days. I.M. In no instance should the single parenteral dose exceed 5 mg./kg. in infants and children.	Used for patients unable to tolerate oral therapy.			
Hydroxychloroquine sulfate, U.S.P. (Plaquenil).	800 mg. initially, then 400 mg. in 6-8 hours; follow with 400 mg. on 2 successive days for total of 2.0 Gm. Oral.	Used to treat malaria and amebiasis. Has beneficial effect in lupus erythematosus and rheumatoid arthritis.	Effective against both intestinal and abscess forms of amebic dysentery. Absorption and excretion similar to chloroquine.	As above.	
	400-600 mg. daily initially, then reduced gradually to 200-400 mg. daily to weekly. Oral.	For maintenance in collagen diseases.			
Pamaquine naphthoate. (Plasmochin).	20 mg. daily. Oral.	To treat tertian malaria.	Anti-infective. Especially effective in malaria caused by *Plasmodium vivax.*	Anorexia, nausea, epigastric tenderness, diarrhea, cardiac arrhythmia, headache,	This drug has largely been replaced by pentaquine phosphate.

			Destroys exoerythrocytic forms and is effective against gametocytes.	pallor, subnormal temperature and blood changes. Treatment: symptomatic. Watch for cyanosis.	
Pentaquine phosphate. (Isopentaquine).	13.3 mg. t.i.d. for 14 days. Oral.	To treat tertian malaria.	Destroys exoerythrocytic forms and is effective against gametocytes.	Nausea, abdominal pain, anorexia, anemia, leukopenia, fever, cyanosis, jaundice. Treatment: symptomatic.	Usually given with quinine. More toxic when given with sulfonamides.
Primaquine phosphate, U.S.P.	15 mg. base. q.d. for 14 days. Oral. 17.5-26.5 mg. q.i.d. Oral.	Used to treat vivax malaria, especially relapses. For treatment of Southwest Pacific strains.	Considered more effective than most antimalarial drugs. Since it destroys the sexual exoerythrocytic forms, it therefore aids in clearing blood of parasites. Rapidly absorbed and most metabolized by the body.	Patients with glucose-6-phosphate dehydrogenase (G6PD) deficiency are more likely to suffer intravascular hemolysis manifested as acute hemolytic anemia. Patients whose ethnic origin suggests the possibility of this deficiency should be screened and the dose reduced accordingly. Other side effects include nausea, vomiting, headache, disturbance of visual accommodation and pruritus. Methemoglobinemia, leukopenia and agranulocytosis have been observed.	Has largely replaced pamaquine. Give with meals or antacids to minimize G.I. side effects. Quinacrine enhances the toxicity of primaquine, so the two should not be given together.
Pyrimethamine, U.S.P. (Daraprim).	50-75 mg. daily. Oral. 25-50 mg. weekly. Oral.	For toxoplasmosis. For malaria prevention. Used mainly to treat toxoplasmosis. Sulfadiazine is usually given at the same time. Also used as a malarial preventive and to treat chronic malaria.	Similar to Primaquine in preventing relapses. Causes patient's blood to become noninfective to mosquito. Absorption and excretion data variable, but compound has been found in body up to 30 days following a single 100 mg. dose.	Cumulative side effects: anorexia, diarrhea, bad taste, headache, weakness, gingivitis, rash, convulsions and blood dyscrasias. As this is a folic acid antagonist, frequent blood checks are advised.	This drug has produced anomalies in experimental laboratory animals. Its use during pregnancy must be weighed against possible risk to the fetus from the drug or from active toxoplasmosis in the mother.

Name, Source, Synonyms, Preparations	Dosage and Administration	Uses	Action and Fate	Side Effects and Contraindications	Nursing Implications and Remarks
ANTIMALARIAL DRUGS (Continued)					
Quinacrine hydrochloride, U.S.P. (Atabrine) (mepacrine hydrochloride [C]).	100 mg. q.d. Suppressive. Oral. For giardiasis: 100 mg. t.i.d. for 7 days. Oral. For tapeworm: 800 mg. for 2 doses, 30 minutes apart.	Used to treat and to prevent malaria, and to treat giardiasis and tapeworm infestations. Also used to suppress lupus erythematosus and to treat rheumatoid arthritis.	Anti-infective. Especially effective in malaria and giardiasis. Similar to quinine but considered to be more effective and less toxic. Rapidly absorbed, widely distributed in body and strongly tissue bound. Crosses the placenta. Slowly excreted from body, found in urine up to 2 months following therapy for malaria. Small amounts excreted in sweat, milk, saliva and bile.	Dizziness, headache, gastrointestinal disturbances. Has cumulative action. Treatment: symptomatic. Causes a temporary yellowish, harmless discoloration of skin; also discolors urine. Other side effects are infrequent and usually associated with chronic administration. These include urticaria, C.N.S. stimulation, blood dyscrasias, hepatitis and dermatitis. Rarely convulsions, toxic psychoses and retinopathy.	Has been largely replaced by chloroquine and amodiaquine. With alkaline urine, the excretion of the drug is slowed.
QUININE. *Active principle of Cinchona succirubra. Other active principles: quinidine, cinchonines, cinchonidine.* Quinine dihydrochloride, N.F. Quinine sulfate, U.S.P. (quinine acid sulfate). (Kinidine, Novoquinine [C]).	650 mg. q. 8 h. for 7 days. I.V. 1 Gm. o.d. Oral. Suppressive. 600 mg. o.d. Oral. 650 mg. q. 8 h. for 7 days. Oral.	Especially effective in malaria. Also used as a bitter tonic, antipyretic, analgesic, oxytocic and emmenagogue.	Anti-infective. Destroys the asexual forms of the malarial organism, but not the sexual. Most effective in tertian and least effective in estivoautumnal malaria. Rapidly absorbed. Metabolically degraded in body. Less than 5% excreted unchanged in urine. Excretion is twice as fast with acid as with alkaline urine.	Fullness in head, ringing in ears, slight impairment in hearing and heart and respiratory weakness. May cause skin eruption, visual disturbances, vertigo, gastric pain and vomiting. Quinine crosses the placenta and has been associated with deafness and thrombocytopenia of the newborn.	Quinidine is used as a heart depressant.
HELMINTHICS		*All these drugs are synthetic unless otherwise indicated.*			
Oleoresin of *Aspidium.* *Rhizomes of aspidium (Dryopteris filixmas).*	3-5 Gm. one dose. Oral. Follow with a saline cathartic. 2-3 h. later, then S.S. enema 2 h. after the cathartic.	Especially effective in tapeworm infestations.	Anthelmintic. Aids by paralyzing the muscles of the worm. Try to limit absorption by reduction of lipids in	Heart depression, colic, diarrhea, headache, dizziness, yellow vision, dyspnea, temporary blindness. Treat with evacuants, then	Avoid oils, fats and alcohol. Save all stools for examination. If not effective, do not repeat for at least 3 weeks.

			intestinal tract. Absorbed aspidium is excreted by the kidneys, but is irritating to them.	demulcents. Nonstimulating emetics, saline cathartics. Treat for shock. Contraindicated in debilitated patients, in disease of heart, liver, or kidney or during pregnancy.	
Bephenium hydroxynaphthoate (Alcopara) (benphenium embonate, Alcopar [C]).	2-5 Gm. one dose. Oral. 2.5-5.0 Gm. q.d. (Give 1 day for *Ancylostoma duodenale* and 3 days for *Necator americanus*.) Oral.	Used to treat hookworm and roundworm infestations.	Anthelmintic. Not absorbed in any appreciable amounts.	Toxic symptoms rare, but some nausea, vomiting, and soft stools have been reported.	No purge necessary following drug. Especially useful in severe infestations.
Carbon tetrachloride (Benzinoform).	2.5-3 ml. before breakfast with water or low fat milk followed in 2 hours with saline cathartic. Oral.	Effective in most infestations except tapeworm.	Anthelmintic.	Headache, insomnia, nausea, vomiting, colic, diarrhea, convulsive seizures may occur. May cause liver, kidney or heart damage. Treatment: symptomatic.	Avoid oils, fats and alcohol. May be repeated after 3 weeks.
Chenopodium oil. *Chenopodium ambrosioides vasanthelmiticum.*	1 ml. one dose. Oral.	Anthelmintic. Especially effective in hookworm, pinworm and roundworm infestations.	Thought to cause direct paralysis of the worm's muscles.	Irritation of the mucous membranes, circulatory depression, dizziness, nausea; sometimes vomiting, deafness, albuminuria and hematuria. Treatment: symptomatic. Contraindicated in nephritis, cardiac disorders, hepatic dysfunction, gastrointestinal ulcers and pregnancy.	

Name, Source, Synonyms, Preparations	Dosage and Administration	Uses	Action and Fate	Side Effects and Contraindications	Nursing Implications and Remarks
HELMINTHICS (Continued)					
Diethylcarbamazine citrate, U.S.P. (Banocide, Hetrazan).	2.0 mg./kg. of body weight t.i.d. for 7-14 days in wuchereriasis, 10 days in loiasis and 14-21 days in onchocerciasis.	Especially valuable in the treatment of filariasis. Kills microfilariae of *Wuchereria bancrofti* and *W. malayi* and kills or sterilizes adult females of these species. Also used for *Onchocerca volvulus* and *Loa loa,* but not as effective for adult parasites.	Exact mode of action not known. Readily absorbed from G.I. tract. Distributed to all body tissues except fat. Excreted in urine.	Headache, dizziness, fever, nausea. Destruction of microfiliariae in onchocerciasis may cause allergic reaction manifested by severe pedal edema, pruritus, dermatitis, fever, colic and lymphadenitis. An allergic encephalitic reaction has occurred.	Antihistamines and corticosteroids can be given concurrently to minimize the allergic reactions. Not administered to pregnant women since drug is thought to cause uterine contraction. Patients should be advised of hygienic measures for preventing reinfection.
Diphenan (p-amino-benzyl-phenyl carbamate chloride).	500 mg.-1 Gm. t.i.d. p.c. for 1 week. Oral.	Anthelmintic. Especially effective in pinworm infestations.	Hydrolyzed to p-benzyl phenol which is said to produce extreme contraction that kills the worms.	Toxic symptoms rare. Treatment: none usually required.	
Hexylresorcinol, N.F. (Caprokol, Crystoids).	1 Gm. One dose to fasting patient and follow in 2 hours with saline purge. Oral.	Anthelmintic. Effective in most infestations. Less potent but also less toxic than most drugs of this group.	Directly vermicidal to hookworms, ascarides and trichiuris. Approximately 1/3 absorbed after oral dose. Rapidly excreted in urine as ethereal sulfate, unabsorbed hexylresorcinol appears in feces unchanged.	Irritation of the mucous membrane. Treatment: none usually required. Capsules must be swallowed whole to avoid burning mouth. Contraindicated in patients with gastroenteritis or peptic ulcer.	Also an intestinal and urinary antiseptic. May be repeated in 3 days if needed. Can be used for debilitated patients and children unable to take far more potent drugs.
Mebendazole (Vermox).	100 mg. b.i.d. for 3 days. 100 mg. single dose. Oral. 200 mg. b.i.d. for 4 days. Oral.	For trichuriasis, hookworms, and ascariasis. For enterobiasis. For taenia.	Only slightly absorbed from gastrointestinal tract.	Diarrhea, abdominal pain. The drug is contraindicated during pregnancy because of teratogenicity shown in rats. It is not recommended for children under 2 years of age.	Considered drug of choice for whipworm.

Methylrosaniline chloride.	60 mg. t.i.d. p.c. for 1-2 weeks. Oral.	Anthelmintic. Especially effective in strongyloidosis.	Exact mechanism of action not established.	Nausea, vomiting, diarrhea, constipation, abdominal pain. Reduce or stop drug and treat symptoms. Contraindicated in heart, liver or kidney damage or during pregnancy.	Tablets should be swallowed without chewing. Preparations stain skin and clothing.
Methylrosaniline chloride solution (crystal violet, gentian violet, methyl violet).	1:1000 1% solution by duodenal intubation. Rectal.	For pinworms and threadworms.			
Piperazine citrate, U.S.P. (Antepar, Anthecole, Ascarex, Multifuge, Oxucide, Parazine, Ta-Verm, Vermago).	65 mg./kg. of body weight. Oral. q.d. for 7 days (maximum 2.5 Gm.)	Used in treatment of pinworm and roundworm infestations.	Readily absorbed from gastrointestinal tract, some of the drug is metabolized in the liver, partly excreted in urine. Piperazine also inhibits growth of ascarides and pinworms.	Rare in therapeutic dosage. May cause urticaria, vomiting, blurred vision, and weakness. Stop drug and treat symptoms. Contraindicated in patients with nephritis.	No starvation or purging required.
Piperazine tartrate (Piperate) (Various salts of piperazine: Ancazine, Entacyl, Piperzinal [C]).	50 mg./kg. of body weight. Usually given O.D. for 5-7 days. Repeat after 7 days if needed. Oral.				
Pyrantel pamoate (Antiminth) (Combantrin [C]).	11 mg./kg. of body weight. One dose. Oral. 1 Gm. total maximum dose. As above. But dose is given daily for 3 days.	Used in the treatment of ascariasis and enterobiasis. For treatment of hookworm.	The anthelmintic activity is probably due to the neuromuscular blocking property of the drug. It is partially absorbed with about 7% of the single dose found in the urine unchanged or as metabolites. More than 50% is recovered unchanged in the feces.	Side effects: nausea, vomiting, gastralgia, abdominal cramps, diarrhea and tenesmus. A transient elevation of SGOT may occur. Headache, dizziness, drowsiness, insomnia and rashes have been reported. Safe use in pregnancy has not been established.	This drug is non-staining. Pyrantel pamoate and piperazine have antagonistic modes of action and should not be administered concomitantly. Oral dosage may be mixed with milk or fruit juice.
Pyrvinium pamoate, U.S.P. (Povan) (viprynium, Pamovin, Pin Kill, Vanquin [C]).	50 mg./10 kg. single dose. Oral.	An anthelmintic of value in the treatment of pinworm infestation.	In low concentrations inhibits oxygen uptake by parasites; in higher concentrations inhibits anaerobic metabolism of parasite. No appreciable absorption.	Toxicity is low, but nausea and vomiting may occur. Safe use in pregnancy not established. Not used in inflammatory bowel disease.	May stain stool and vomitus a reddish-brown. Instruct patient to swallow, not chew, tablet.
Quassia infusion. *Plant. Quassia.*	Varied. Topical. Given as enema.	Anthelmintic.	Action is not well understood.	Nontoxic.	

Name, Source, Synonyms, Preparations	Dosage and Administration	Uses	Action and Fate	Side Effects and Contraindications	Nursing Implications and Remarks
HELMINTHICS (Continued)					
Tetrachloroethylene, U.S.P. (Perchloroethylene).	2-5 ml. administered in morning in fasting state. Oral.	Anthemintic. Especially effective in hookworm infestation.	Mechanism of action is not known.	Drowsiness, dizziness. Treatment: usually none required. Can cause hepatitis.	Avoid oils, fats and alcohol before therapy. May be repeated after 7-10 days.
Thiabendazole, U.S.P. (Mintezol).	25 mg./kg. b.i.d. Oral. Repeat in 7 days. 25 mg./kg. b.i.d. Oral on 2 successive days. As above and repeat after 2 days. Doses given preferably p.c. Recommended maximum dose 3 Gm.	Enterobiasis. Intestinal parasites. Larva migrans. Used for many conditions such as the above and uncinariasis, trichinosis and trichuriasis.	Broad spectrum anthelmintic. Exact mechanism of action is not known. Rapidly absorbed. Reaches maximum blood levels 1-3 hours after oral dose. Excreted rapidly by the kidneys.	Side effects include nausea, vomiting, dizziness, diarrhea, epigastric distress and many more. May impart odor to the urine; also crystalluria and hematuria and transient leukopenia have been reported. Stevens-Johnson syndrome has been observed following use of thiabendazole. Patient should be warned not to operate machinery or drive a car during therapy, since this drug causes drowsiness.	See commercial brochure for further information. Safety for use in pregnancy and lactation has not been established.
Thymol. *Plant. Thymol camphor.*	2 Gm. administered in morning in fasting state; follow in 2 hours by a saline cathartic. Oral.	Anthelmintic. Especially effective in hookworm infestation. Sometimes used for pinworm and whipworm infestations.	Action similar to that of hexylresorcinol.	Central nervous system depression; later, spinal cord may be affected. Treatment: evacuants; and symptomatic.	Avoid oils, fats and alcohol. May be repeated after 3 weeks.

BIOLOGICALS

Biologicals are attenuated or killed suspensions of microorganisms (vaccines), products of microorganisms (extracts, toxoids) or antibodies stimulated by microorganisms or their products (antitoxins, immune serum globulins). The term also applies to antigenic extracts of materials known to be allergenic (allergens), and solutions of antibodies to the venom of snakes and spiders (antivenoms). They are used for prevention or modification of diseases (vaccines, toxoids, antitoxins, immune serum globulins, allergens, antivenoms) and detection of susceptibility to or possible presence of disease agents (allergens, extracts).

BIOLOGICALS USED FOR THE PREVENTION OR MODIFICATION OF MICROBIAL DISEASES

Bacillus of Calmette and Guérin (BCG Vaccine). *Attenuated strain of Mycobacterium bovis.*	See manufacturer's brochure. Given I.D. or S.Q. Newborn: ½ adult dose, revaccinate after one year of age.	Prophylaxis of skin test–negative individuals with repeated exposure to persistently active cases of tuberculosis or in communities with excessive rate of new infections.	Active immunity. Recipients should be skin-tested 2-3 months after vaccination. If negative, they should be revaccinated.	Contraindicated in persons with impaired immune response and during pregnancy.	Vaccines are freeze-dried suspensions of organisms and should be used within 8 hours after reconstituting.
Botulism antitoxin polyvalent. *Plasma of immunized animals.*	10,000 units of each type at 4-hour intervals.	Treatment of suspected botulism.	Neutralizes the toxin. Passive immunity.	Anaphylaxis or serum sickness may result in sensitive patients.	Test for sensitivity according to manufacturer's instructions before administering.
Cholera vaccine, U.S.P. *Killed bacteria.*	0.5-1.0 ml. 1-4 weeks apart. S.Q.	Cholera prophylaxis for travelers to endemic areas.	Active immunity. Booster dose of 0.5 ml. every 6 months required.	Soreness, fever, malaise, headache may occur.	
Diphtheria antitoxin, U.S.P. *Plasma of immunized animals.*	1000-5000 U, I.M. 10,000-20,000 U, I.V.	For prophylaxis after exposure when immune status is uncertain or unknown. For treatment.	Passive immunity.	As with botulism antitoxin.	As with botulism antitoxin.
Diphtheria toxoid, U.S.P. *Chemically modified toxin.*	0.5-1.0 ml. S.Q. 3 doses at 4-week intervals.	Prophylaxis for susceptibles.	Active immunity.	Tenderness at injection site; fever, malaise may occur.	Precipitated and adsorbed preparations require only two doses.
Diphtheria and tetanus toxoids and pertussis vaccine, U.S.P. (Triogen, Tri-Solgen, Adsorbed, DTP). *Killed bacteria and toxoids of diphtheria and tetanus.*	Three doses at 4-6 week intervals and another one year after the third dose.	For primary immunization of infants.	Booster doses when beginning school, at exposure and every 10 years. Active immunity.		Volume of dose varies with the manufacturer.

BIOLOGICALS USED FOR THE PREVENTION OR MODIFICATION OF MICROBIAL DISEASES *(Continued)*

Name, Source, Synonyms, Preparations	Dosage and Administration	Uses	Action and Fate	Side Effects and Contraindications	Nursing Implications and Remarks
Tetanus and diphtheria toxoids (Td), U.S.P. Adult type. *Mixed toxoids.*	One dose I.M. every 10 years or on exposure.	Maintenance of active immunity and booster effect in potential exposure.	Active immunity.		Volume of dose varies.
Tetanus antitoxin (TAT), U.S.P. *Plasma of immunized animals.*	3000-5000 U, I.M. 20,000-50,000 U, I.M. or I.V.	For prophylaxis when immune status is uncertain or unknown. For treatment.	Passive immunity.	Serum sickness or anaphylaxis may result in sensitized patients.	As with botulism antitoxin. Use only if Tetanus immune globulin (human) is not available.
Tetanus and gas gangrene antitoxin, N.F. *Plasma of immunized animals.*	Dosage varies. Parenteral.	As above.	Passive immunity.	As above.	As above.
Tetanus immune globulin (human), U.S.P. (Homo-Tet, Hyper-Tet, IMMU-tetanus, Pro-Tet, TIG). *Plasma of immunized humans.*	250 U, I.M.	Prophylaxis when immune status is absent or uncertain.	Passive immunity lasting longer than with TAT. Crosses the placenta.		This is the passive immunity of choice; usually free of side effects of TAT.
Tetanus toxoid (T), U.S.P. *Chemically modified toxin.*	One dose I.M.	In case of predisposing wounds. Booster effect upon exposure.	Active immunity.		Used in wound prophylaxis only with history of prior immunization.
Gas gangrene anti-toxin, pentavalent, N.F. *Plasma of immunized animals.*	1-4 vials I.V. or 1 vial q. 4 h. I.M.	As adjunct to surgical management of dirty, traumatic wounds in prevention and treatment of gas gangrene.	Passive immunity. Adequate systemic antibiotic and sulfonamide therapy is also employed.	Hypersensitivity reactions may occur.	Test for serum sensitivity. I.M. injection may be given above infected area; treatment continues as long as there is evidence of gas bacillus infection.
Hepatitis B immune globulin (human) (H-B IG). *Plasma of immune humans.*	0.06 ml. per kg. of body weight as soon as possible after exposure (preferably within 7 days) and repeat in 28 days.	Post exposure prophylaxis following either parenteral exposure or direct mucous membrane contact.	Passive immunity.		Local pain and tenderness at injection site. Urticaria and angioedema may occur. Use with caution in patients with history or prior systemic allergic reactions to human immune globulin preps.

Immune serum globulin, U.S.P. (Gamastan, Gamulin, ISG). *Pooled human plasma.*	0.1 ml./lb. 0.02 ml./lb. 10 ml. followed in 1 month by a second 10 ml. 0.3-0.45 ml./lb.	Prophylaxis of measles. Modification of measles. Prophylaxis of serum hepatitis. Treatment of agammaglobulinemia.	Passive immunity lasting 6-12 weeks.	Rare serum sickness–type reaction may occur. There is a remote possibility of serum hepatitis developing after administration.	Local tenderness, pain and erythema at injection site have been reported. It is important to remember that viral diseases attenuated with immune globulin are still infectious and communicable; usual precautions must be observed.
Influenza virus vaccine, Bivalent. (Flu-Immune, Fluogen). *Inactivated virus from chick embryo.*	Two doses given 6 weeks apart. Subcutaneous.	Prophylaxis for persons at "high risk" from influenza, especially the chronically ill and aged.	Active immunity. Requires annual booster.	Contraindicated in patients known to be sensitive to eggs.	See manufacturer's instructions for dose volume and for children's doses.
Influenza vaccine, polyvalent. *Inactivated virus from chick embryo.*	1 ml. S.Q. 0.5 ml. to children under 12 yr.	As above.	Active immunity against component strains of influenza virus.	As above. High concentrations of inactivated virus may cause toxic symptoms, especially in children.	Local and systemic reactions are common but mild.
Measles virus vaccine, live, attenuated (Attenuvac, Lirugen, M-Vac, Rubeovax). *Attenuated virus from chick embryo or dog kidney cell culture.*	One dose not earlier than 13 mo. of age unless earlier exposure likely, then repeat at 13 mo.	For lasting protection.	Active immunity.	15% of vaccinees have rectal temperatures of 103° beginning 6 days post-vaccination and lasting up to 4 days. Contraindicated in conditions of altered immune states, pregnancy and hypersensitivity to eggs or dog dander.	Check manufacturer's instructions for dose volume. Also available in combination with mumps and rubella vaccines for multiple immunization (MMR).
Meningococcal polysaccharide vaccine, Group C (meningovax-C)	50 mcg. S.Q.	Provides immunity to group C *N. meningitides* in military and similar groups with documented increased rate of infection with group C meningococcus.	Active immunity.	Erythema at site of injection may occur for less than 48 hr. Infrequent systemic reaction. Hypersensitivity rarely.	Contraindicated in pregnant women.
Mumps immune globulin (human), (Hyparotin). *Plasma of immunized humans.*	2-10 ml. I.M. 1.5-4.5 ml. I.M.	For prophylaxis following exposure. For modification or treatment of mumps.	Provides passive immunity lasting for 6-12 weeks.	Rare serum sickness–type reaction occurs.	

BIOLOGICALS USED FOR THE PREVENTION OR MODIFICATION OF MICROBIAL DISEASES *(Continued)*

Name, Source, Synonyms, Preparations	Dosage and Administration	Uses	Action and Fate	Side Effects and Contraindications	Nursing Implications and Remarks
Mumps virus vaccine (Mumpsvax). *Live attenuated virus from chick embryo.*	One dose S.Q.	For lasting protection.	Active immunity.	Contraindicated during acute febrile illness, sensitivity to eggs, neomycin, depressed immune states or pregnancy.	May be administered at any age after 12 months. Also available in combination with measles and rubella vaccines (MMR).
Pertussis immune globulin (human), U.S.P. (Hypertussis). *Plasma of immunized humans.*	2.5 ml. I.M. for prophylaxis. 1.25 ml. daily for 3-4 days for treatment, I.M. or I.V.	Prophylaxis or treatment of pertussis when immune status is absent or uncertain.	Passive immunity.	Rare serum sickness-type reaction occurs.	
Pertussis vaccine. See Diphtheria and Tetanus toxoid and Pertussis vaccine (page 61).					
Plague vaccine, U.S.P. *Killed suspension of bacteria.*	Two doses of 0.5 ml. at 4 or more week intervals and 0.2 ml. 4-12 weeks after second dose.	Prevention for travelers and people working with the bacteria or living in enzootic areas.	Active immunity. Boosters needed every 6-12 months.	Mild pain, reddening and swelling at injection site. Fever, headache, malaise occur more often with repeated doses.	See manufacturer's instructions for children under 10 years of age.
Pneumococcal vaccine, polyvalent (Pneumovax)	0.5 ml. S.Q. or I.M.	Immunization against the 14 most prevalent pneumococcal types in individuals 2 years and older with increased risk of infection.	Active immunity.	Local erythema and soreness; low-grade fever for less than 24 hrs. Occurs occasionally.	
Poliomyelitis vaccine (Salk vaccine). *Inactivated virus.*	Two doses of 1 ml. 4 weeks apart, followed by one dose 6-7 months later and another 12 months after that. S.Q.	Prevention of poliomyelitis.	Active immunity.		Has largely been replaced by the oral type vaccine.
Poliovirus vaccine, live, oral, trivalent, U.S.P. (Diplovax, Orimune Sabin vaccine). *Attenuated virus.*	Two doses 6-8 weeks apart, followed by one dose 8-12 months after second dose. Oral.	Polio prevention against all three types of polio virus.	Lasting active immunity.	Contraindicated in conditions resulting in altered immune states. Should not be administered during the first trimester of pregnancy.	Usually started at 6-12 weeks of age but is effective in children and adults. Available also as monovalent vaccine for each type.

Rabies vaccine, U.S.P. (duck embryo vaccine, DEV). *Inactivated virus from duck embryo culture.*	Pre-exposure: two doses of 1 ml. I.M., 1 month apart and one dose 6-7 months later or three doses of 1 ml. at weekly intervals and one dose 3 months later. Post-exposure: 14-21 doses as determined by the physician.	Rabies prophylaxis. Pre-exposure immunization recommended only for high-risk personnel.	Active immunity.	Erythema, pruritus, pain and tenderness at injection site are common. Low-grade fever and, rarely, shock may occur late during treatment. Neuroparalytic reactions are rare with DEV.	DEV has largely replaced the Semple type which was of nervous tissue (rabbit brain) origin and caused a higher incidence of neuroparalytic reactions. Corticosteroids may interfere with development of immunity and should be avoided during vaccination.
Antirabies serum (equine origin), U.S.P. *Plasma of immunized horses.*	40 U./kg. S.Q.	Post-exposure rabies prophylaxis used in conjunction with rabies vaccine.	Passive immunity.	Serum sickness or anaphylactic reaction may occur.	Package instructions for sensitivity testing must be followed before administration.
Rabies immune globulin, human (HRIG, Hyperab).	20 I.U./kg., 50% to infiltrate the wound; remainder I.M. (not I.V.).	Used post exposure to rabies (known or suspected).	Passive immunity against rabies for patients hypersensitive to horse serum.	Slight soreness at site of injection and slight elevation of temperature. Rabies immune globulin is contraindicated in repeated doses once vaccine treatment has been initiated as it may interfere with full expression of active immunity expected from vaccine.	Antirabies serum and HRIG have been shown to suppress antibody response to rabies vaccine. When either is used, a series of 23 doses of vaccine is recommended and the antibody level should be monitored.
Rubella virus vaccine (Meruvax; Meruvax II). *Live, attenuated virus from duck embryo, or human diploid cell culture.*	0.5 ml. S.Q. between 1 year of age and puberty.	Rubella prophylaxis.	Lasting active immunity.	Rash, lymphadenopathy and joint pains occur in about 5% of vaccinees. Contraindicated in pregnancy, altered immune states, severe febrile illness or sensitivity to vaccine components.	Also available in combination with measles and mumps vaccines (MMR). The human diploid cell culture (strain RA 27/3) is more immunogenic than previously available rubella vaccines.
Smallpox vaccine, U.S.P. *Glycerinated or lyophilized vaccinia virus.*	One dose by multiple pressure, multiple puncture or jet injection.	Smallpox prophylaxis of hospital and medical personnel at high risk and travelers to endemic areas.	Active immunity. Requires revaccination at 3 year intervals for maintenance.	Rare encephalitis, vaccinia necrosum, eczema vaccinatum. Contraindicated in skin disorders, pregnancy and altered immune states.	No longer recommended as a routine pediatric immunization in the United States.

BIOLOGICALS (Continued)

BIOLOGICALS USED FOR THE PREVENTION OR MODIFICATION OF MICROBIAL DISEASES *(Continued)*

Name, Source, Synonyms, Preparations	Dosage and Administration	Uses	Action and Fate	Side Effects and Contraindications	Nursing Implications and Remarks
Tetanus. See Diphtheria and Tetanus toxoids and Pertussis vaccine (page 61).					
Typhoid vaccine, U.S.P. *Suspension of killed bacteria.*	0.25 ml. S.Q. for ages 6 mo. to 10 years, 0.5 ml. S.Q. for ages over 10 years; two doses at 4 week intervals. 0.5 ml. S.Q. or 0.1 ml. intradermally every 3 years as booster or on exposure.	Prophylaxis of typhoid fever. Given to persons traveling in endemic regions and in high-risk occupations.	Active immunity.	Local erythema, tenderness at site of injection, malaise, myalgia, headache and fever. Contraindicated in acute illness, debilitating disease, tuberculosis, agammaglobulinemia or patients receiving corticosteroids, antineoplastic or immusuppressive drugs.	Routine immunization is not recommended. Should be given to contacts of carriers, or on exposure or possible exposure.
Typhus vaccine, U.S.P. *Inactivated rickettsiae from chick embryo culture.*	Two doses 4 or more weeks apart.	Typhus prophylaxis for travelers to endemic areas and high-risk personnel.	Active immunity. Booster required every 6-12 months for maintenance.	Contraindicated in patients sensitive to eggs.	See manufacturer's instructions for dose volume.
Vaccinia immune globulin, (VIG). *Plasma from immunized humans.*	0.6 ml./kg. I.M.	Prevention or modification of smallpox or effects of vaccination.	Passive immunity. The antibody crosses the placenta and appears in human milk.	Rare serum sickness.	
Yellow fever vaccine, U.S.P. *Attenuated virus from chick embryo culture.*	0.5 ml. S.Q.	Yellow fever prophylaxis for high-risk personnel and travelers to endemic areas.	Long-term active immunity.	Contraindicated in pregnancy, altered immune states and sensitivity to eggs.	Available from the United States Public Health Service.

BIOLOGICALS USED FOR TESTING PRESENCE OF OR SUSCEPTIBILITY TO MICROBIAL DISEASE AGENTS

Name, Source, Synonyms, Preparations	Dosage and Administration	Uses	Action and Fate	Side Effects and Contraindications	Nursing Implications and Remarks
Benzylpenicilloyl-polylysine (PRE-PEN).	Scratch test and intradermal test. If intradermal test is needed a control must also be performed.	To test a patient's hypersensitivity to penicillin. (No test will completely assure that a reaction to penicillin therapy will not occur.) This is for persons who say they are allergic to penicillin but in whom there is no concrete evidence.	In allergic patients a scratch test will cause a pruritus and a wheal of from 5-15 mm. or more in diameter to form within 15 minutes. If negative, administer an intradermal test on the upper outer arm sufficiently below the deltoid muscle to allow placement of a tourniquet.	There is insufficient data to assess potential danger of sensitization to penicillin from repeated skin testing with this agent. With any agent of this type be prepared for sensitivity-type reactions. Contraindications: do not perform skin tests with penicillin or other penicillin-derived agents simultaneously with this agent.	This test should not be used in patients known to be extremely sensitive to penicillin.

Coccidioidin, U.S.P. *Extract of Coccidioides immitis.*	0.1 ml. of 1:100 or 1:10 dilution. Intradermal.	Diagnostic test for coccidioidomycosis (coccidioidal granuloma).		As above. Reaction read after 24 hr. and again in 48 hr.	
Diphtheria toxin, U.S.P. *Active toxin from bacterial culture.* (Schick test).	0.1 ml. intradermally.	The Schick test is for susceptibility to the toxin of diphtheria.		As above. In nonimmune persons, reaction occurs in 24–48 hrs. and is at its height in 48–72 hrs., remaining for 6–12 days. Reaction read after 4 days.	A negative test is an indication that the patient has sufficient circulating antibodies to neutralize the toxin and is thus immune.
Histoplasmin, U.S.P. *Extract of Histoplasma capsulatum.*	0.1 ml. of a 1:100 dilution. Intradermal.	Diagnostic test for histoplasmosis.		Reaction read after 24-48 hrs., but the maximum reaction may be delayed for 3 days.	
Frei Antigen, (Lygranum). *Extract from chick embryo culture of the specific strain of Chlamydiae.*	0.1 ml. intradermally.	Diagnostic test for lymphogranuloma venereum.			
Tuberculin, old, U.S.P. (Mantoux test, Mono-Vaco test, Tine test). *Products of bacterial growth.*	5 TU, intradermally.	Determining sensitivity to the causative agent.		Induration at site 48-72 hours after inoculation in positive test.	A positive tuberculin test indicates sensitivity to the bacterium. Sputum and/or chest examination may be required to rule out active disease. TU means "tuberculin units."
Tuberculin, PPD, U.S.P. *Purified protein derived from bacterial cells.*	1, 5, 250 TU, intradermally.	As above.		As above.	As above.

AGENTS USED FOR PREVENTION OR MODIFICATION OF NON-MICROBIAL CONDITIONS

Allergens (Anergex, Allpyral). *Extracts or suspensions of allergenic materials.*	Individually determined.	Single small doses used as test for sensitivity. A series of larger doses is used for desensitization.	Requires annual desensitization.	Severe allergic or anaphylactoid reactions may occur.	

Name, Source, Synonyms, Preparations	Dosage and Administration	Uses	Action and Fate	Side Effects and Contraindications	Nursing Implications and Remarks
Antivenom Crotalidae, polyvalent. *Plasma of immunized horses.*	15-75 ml. initially depending on size of snake and size and condition of patient. Parenteral.	Treatment for bite of rattlesnake, copperhead, moccasin, fer-de-lance and bushmaster.	Neutralizes the venom.	Serum sickness or anaphylaxis may occur in patients sensitive to horse serum.	Package instructions for sensitivity testing must be followed before administration.
Antivenom *(Latrodectus mactans). Plasma of immunized horses.*	2.5 ml. I.M.	Treatment for bite of the black widow spider.	As above.	As above.	As above.
Bothrops antitoxin. *Plasma of immunized horses.*	Dosage varies. Parenteral.	Treatment for bite of a South American snake.	As above.	As above.	As above.
Poison oak–ivy extracts. *Extracts of the plant material.*	Dosage varies. Oral or I.M.	Prevention and treatment of poison oak or ivy.	Requires annual doses for prophylaxis.	Allergic type reactions may occur.	
Rh_O (D) immune globulin (RhoGam) (human). *Plasma of immune humans.*	300 mcg. I.M. within 72 hours after delivery.	Prevents development of Rh antibodies by Rh negative mothers delivering Rh positive infants, thus preventing active immunization of the mother.	Neutralizes Rh antigen.	Infrequent slight soreness at injection site and/or slight fever. Contraindicated in patients who have developed antibodies from previous pregnancy or transfusion.	Should be administered within 72 hours after delivery or abortion. Is given to mother only, never to the father or infant. Effective only if the mother has not already built up antibodies.

DRUGS AFFECTING THE AUTONOMIC NERVOUS SYSTEM

SYMPATHOMIMETICS (SYMPATHETIC STIMULANTS, ADRENERGIC AGENTS)

Sympathetic stimulants act through what has been called adrenergic effector cells. In the late 1940s, it was shown that these effectors are made up of two distinct receptor types, which were given the names alpha (α) receptors and beta (β) receptors. Now it has been shown that there are two types of beta receptors: beta $(\beta)_1$ and beta $(\beta)_2$. The (α) receptors are located mainly in the heart and the (β) receptors in the blood vessels of the kidneys, skeletal muscles and lungs. The alpha responses are mainly vasoconstriction of the arterioles of the skin and splanchnic area, which results in an increase in blood pressure, relaxation of the gastrointestinal tract and dilation of the pupils. The $beta_1$ responses include cardiac acceleration and increased contractility. The $beta_2$ responses include bronchial relaxation, vasodilation of the arterioles supplying the skeletal muscles and uterine relaxation. These responses cannot be totally separated, but some agents can be classified primarily as alpha effectors (norepinephrine), $beta_1$ and $beta_2$ effectors (isoproterenol), primarily $beta_2$ effectors (metaproterenol) and those that affect both the alpha and the beta receptors (1 and 2) (epinephrine). The heart and lungs contain primarily beta receptors, whereas the arterioles have both alpha and beta receptors.

The sympathomimetic drugs act in a manner somewhat similar to that of the parasympathetic depressants. In certain specific instances they are more effective. In some respects, these drugs have actions similar to the antihistamines, and they are sometimes used for the same purposes. Some act systemically as central nervous system stimulants.

NATURAL SYMPATHETIC AMINES

EPINEPHRINE. *Animal glands. Synthetic.*		Used in number of conditions such as bronchial asthma, glaucoma, urticaria and other allergic conditions, shock, cardiac and respiratory failure, congestion of mucous membranes and to prolong action of local anesthetics.	Main action is vasoconstriction of peripheral blood vessels. There is usually a temporary rise in blood pressure. In large doses there is stimulation of the myocardium with increased cardiac output. Rapidly inactivated by enzymes catechol orthomethyl transferase and monoamine oxidase. Most excreted by kidneys after inactivation as metanephrine and 3 methoxy-4 hydroxy mandelic acid. Very short acting; extended by delaying absorption by making a suspension (Sus-Phrine). Following topical application to conjunctiva, a reduction in intraocular pressure may occur within 1 h., reach a low in 4-8 h. and persist for 12-24 h. Mydriasis occurs within a few minutes and lasts less than 1 h.	Tremors, nervous apprehension, palpitation, precordial distress. Severe symptoms may include acute cardiac dilation, pulmonary edema. Treatment: symptomatic. Epinephrine and some other sympathomimetics (levarterenol, metaraminol, methoxamine, ephedrine, mephentermine, and phenylephrine) can interact with cyclopropane and other halogenated hydrocarbon anesthetics to give cardiac arrhythmias. This interaction is dependent on the amount of sympathomimetic agent used and mode of administration. Epinephrine, when given with the tricyclic antidepressants, antihistamines or sodium 1-thyroxin, will give an enhanced adrenergic effect. When given to patients taking azapetine there is a reversal of the pressor effect of epinephrine. This hypertensive effect of epinephrine is antagonized by the phenothiazines and butyrophenones. Sympathomimetic drugs, when given to patients receiving monoamine oxidase inhibitors, may precipitate a hypertensive crisis.	Epinephrine hydrochloride cannot be given orally, as it is inactivated by the digestive juices. There is a warning on most sympathomimetic drugs that they should not be used for patients with heart disease, high blood pressure, diabetes or thyroid disease unless closely supervised by a physician.
Epinephrine bitartrate, U.S.P. (Epitrate, Lyophrin) (Adrenatrate, Medihaler-Epi [C]).	1% or 2% solution. Topical in eyes.				
Epinephrine hydrochloride, U.S.P. (Adrenalin, Epifrin, Intranefrin [C]).	0.06-1 ml. of a 1:1000 solution. Parenteral. 1:100 solution. Topical as spray. 0.2-1 ml. I.M. and topical as spray. 1:10,000 solution for intracardial use.				
Epinephrine, aqueous solution (Sus-Phrine).	0.1-0.3 ml. of a 1:200 solution S.Q. May repeat in 4 hours if required.				
Epinephrine, racemic mixture (Vaponefrin) (Dysne-Inhal [C]).	2.25% inhalation therapy.				

Name, Source, Synonyms, Preparations	Dosage and Administration	Uses	Action and Fate	Side Effects and Contraindications	Nursing Implications and Remarks
NATURAL SYMPATHETIC AMINES (Continued)					
LEVARTERENOL BITARTRATE. *Synthetic.* Levarterenol bitartrate, U.S.P. (noradrenaline, norepinephrine, Levophed)	1-10 micrograms p.r.n. I.V.	Used for acute hypotension that persists after adequate fluid volume replacement.	A potent vasoconstrictor that raises blood pressure markedly with increased cardiac output. Pulse rate is usually slowed. It is the salt of norepinephrine. Excretion data similar to epinephrine. The drug crosses the placenta.	Tremors, nervous apprehension, palpitation, precordial distress. Severe symptoms may include acute cardiac dilation, pulmonary edema. Treatment: symptomatic, antihypertensive drugs. Contraindicated with cyclopropane anesthesia or when myocardial ischemia is suspected. See epinephrine for interactions. Also the thiazide diuretics antagonize the hypertensive effect of this drug. Toxic to subcutaneous tissues. Avoid infiltration. Contraindicated in pregnancy.	I.V. dosage must be diluted, usually 4 ml. to 1 liter of solution. Vital signs are monitored q. 2-5 min. since rate of infusion is determined by patient's pulse and blood pressure. Avoid tissue infiltration since the drug causes tissue necrosis and sloughing if infiltrated. Rate of flow of medication should be monitored closely, preferably with an infusion pump.
ETHYLNOREPINEPHRINE HYDROCHLORIDE. *Synthetic.* Ethylnorepinephrine hydrochloride (Bronkephrine).	2 mg. q. 3-4 minutes. S.Q. or I.M.	Used for severe asthma.	Bronchodilator similar to epinephrine but without significant pressor effects.	Generally well tolerated. May produce changes in blood pressure or pulse, palpitation, headache, dizziness or nausea.	
Isoetharine (Dilabon–A component of Bronkosol).	By inhalation usually q. 4 h. is sufficient. Used full strength or diluted with three parts saline or other suitable solution.	Treatment of bronchial asthma and bronchospasm associated with emphysema, bronchitis and chronic broncho-pulmonary disorders.	Acts as a bronchodilator.	Same as for others of this group. Should not be used with epinephrine but can be used alternately.	

SYNTHETIC SYMPATHETIC AGENTS	*Sympathetic agents used as pressor agents. These are all synthetic preparations.*				
Also see under Natural Sympathetic Amines.					
Angiotensin amide, N.F. (Hypertensin).	2.5 mg. in at least 250 ml. infusion. I.V.	Used for treatment of shock and collapse when blood pressure must be restored quickly.	Produces rise in blood pressure owing to constriction of peripheral blood vessels with increased peripheral resistance. Agent degraded by peptidases present in serum and plasma. Has mainly alpha response.	Too rapid or too great a rise in blood pressure. Use antihypertensive medication. Not given in myocardial infarction.	Check blood pressure every 1 to 5 minutes until stabilized.
Dobutamine hydrochloride (Dobutrex)	2.5 to 10 mcg./kg./min. and rarely up to 40 mcg./kg./min. to obtain desired effect. Parenteral.	Short-term treatment of cardiac decompensation due to depressed contractility. For shock only when it is caused by inadequate cardiac contractility.	A direct-acting inotropic agent whose primary activity results from stimulation of beta receptors of the heart while producing mild chronotropic, hypertensive, arrhythmogenic and vasodilative effect. Onset of action between 1-2 min., with up to 10 min. for peak effect. Plasma half-life is 2 min. Eliminated in urine after metabolism.	Increased heart rate, systolic blood pressure and ventricular ectopic activity. These effects are dose related. Nausea, headache, anginal pain, nonspecific chest pain, palpitations and shortness of breath have been reported in 1-3% of patients. Contraindicated in idiopathic hypertrophic subaortic stenosis. Safety and effectiveness not established in patients with myocardial infarction, in pregnancy or in children.	ECG and blood pressure should be continuously monitored during therapy as well as pulmonary wedge pressure and cardiac output when possible. Hypovolemia should be corrected before therapy is begun. Dobutamine may be ineffective if a beta-blocking drug has been recently given.

Name, Source, Synonyms, Preparations	Dosage and Administration	Uses	Action and Fate	Side Effects and Contraindications	Nursing Implications and Remarks
SYNTHETIC SYMPATHETIC AGENTS (Continued)					
Dopamine hydrochloride (Intropin).	2-5 mcg./kg./min. in diluted solution, I.V. to begin. May be gradually increased to 20-50 mcg./kg./min. If doses greater than 50 mcg./kg./min. are used and urine flow decreases in absence of hypotension, dosage probably should be decreased.	Used to correct hemodynamic imbalance in shock syndrome due to myocardial infarction, trauma, endotoxic septicemia, open heart surgery, renal failure, cardiac decompensation as in congestive failure.	Exerts an inotropic effect on the myocardium resulting in increased cardiac output. Increased systolic and pulse pressure with little or no effect on diastolic pressure. Blood flow to peripheral vascular beds may decrease while mesenteric flow increases. Reported to dilate renal vasculature, which increases glomerular filtration rate, renal blood flow and sodium excretion. Increased urinary excretion usually not associated with decrease in osmolality of urine.	Ectopic beats, nausea, vomiting, tachycardia, anginal pain, palpitation, dyspnea, headache, hypotension, vasoconstriction. Rarely: aberrant conduction, bradycardia, piloerection, widened QRS complex, azotemia, elevated blood pressure. Contraindications: patients with pheochromocytoma. Safety and efficacy for use in children has not been established. Use during pregnancy: doctor must weigh benefits against possible adverse effects on fetus.	Solutions must be diluted and nonalkaline as dopamine is inactivated in alkaline solution. Patients who have recently received or concurrently are receiving monoamine oxidase inhibitors should be started at about 1/10 usual dose as dopamine is metabolized by monamine oxidase. Prior to treatment with dopamine, hypovolemia should be fully corrected, if possible.
Mephentermine sulfate, U.S.P. (Wyamine [C]).	15-35 mg. p.r.n. I.V. or I.M.	Used mainly to raise blood pressure in shock and hemorrhage.	Acts predominantly by release of endogenous norepinephrine. Causes rise in blood pressure due to peripheral resistance. For fate see ephedrine.	Can cause euphoria, drowsiness, weeping, incoherence and convulsions. When patients have been receiving reserpine or guanethidine there is a diminished response to this drug.	May increase uterine contraction; thus should not be administered to pregnant women.
Metaraminol bitartrate, U.S.P. (Aramine).	2-10 mg. p.r.n. S.Q. or I.M. 15-100 mg. Usually given in dextrose. p.r.n. I.V.	Used mainly in postsurgical or other pathologically induced hypotension. It is not very effective in idiopathic hypotension, but has been used in paroxysmal atrial tachycardia.	It has a powerful and prolonged vasopressor action. As with most of these drugs action is mainly due to constriction of peripheral blood vessels. Excretion similar to ephedrine.	Severe hypertension. Give antihypertensive drugs. When patient is on reserpine or guanethidine, metaraminol can give a diminished response from what is expected.	Safe use in pregnancy has not been established. Prolonged use may deplete norepinephrine stores and tachyphylaxis may develop.

Methoxamine hydrochloride, U.S.P. (Vasoxyl).	5-20 mg. p.r.n. I.M., I.V.	Used to raise blood pressure in shock and collapse.	Strong vasopressor action due to constriction of peripheral blood vessels with increased blood pressure. Excretion similar to ephedrine. Can be used during surgery with cyclopropane as it does not increase irritability of the cyclopropane sensitized heart.	Rare, but watch for too high blood pressure. Stop drug and give antihypertensive drugs. May cause restlessness, anxiety, nervousness, weakness, dizziness, precordial pain, tremor, respiratory distress or pallor.	Has only α (alpha) stimulation effects. I.V. infusion flow rate must be monitored closely. Vital signs monitored closely during therapy and after its discontinuance.
Sympathetic stimulants with local vascular and bronchial effect, and used mainly for local or systemic vasoconstriction or bronchial dilation. These are all synthetic preparations except as noted.					
Cyclopentamine hydrochloride, N.F. (Clopane).	0.5% solution. Topical.	Used for nasal congestion as vasoconstrictor and vasopressor.	Stimulation of the sympathetic nervous system. Vasoconstriction, especially of superficial blood vessels; dilation of bronchial tubes; hemostatic when applied locally.	Headache, dizziness, palpitation, anxiety. Severe symptoms include cardiac depression, tremors, diaphoresis, fainting. Treatment: symptomatic. Should be used with caution in patients with cardiac disorder.	
EPHEDRINE. *Active principle of Ephedra vulgaris and E. equisetina (ma huang). Synthetic.*					
Ephedrine hydrochloride, N.F. (Ephedra, Neo-Fedrin [C]). Ephedrine sulfate, U.S.P. Etafedrine hydrochloride (Nethamine, Nethaprin) (Acepifylline [C]).	15-25-50 mg. q. 3-4 h. Oral. p.r.n. as nasal jelly. Topical. 25-50 mg. q. 3-4 h. p.r.n. Oral, I.M. or I.V. 3% solution. Topical. 12-24 mg. q. 3-4 h. p.r.n. Oral.	Used in hypotension, asthma and other allergies, narcotic poisoning, narcolepsy; as a mydriatic, and with neostigmine in myasthenia gravis.	In small dosage stimulates the heart, increasing rate and force of beat. Raises blood pressure by constriction of muscles and blood vessels. Ephedrine and most other noncatecholamines are effective orally and are longer acting than the catecholamines. They resist inactivation by enzymes—monoamine oxidase and catechol orthomethyl transferase. They are widely distributed in body and 50-75% is excreted unchanged by the kidneys.	Headache, dizziness, palpitation, anxiety. Severe symptoms include cardiac depression, tremors, diaphoresis, fainting. Treatment: symptomatic. Patients on long-term reserpine therapy may not respond adequately to normal pressor doses of ephedrine. See epinephrine for interaction with anesthetic agents and the monoamine oxidase inhibitors. Ephedrine interferes with the hypotensive effect of guanethidine.	Ephedrine, unlike epinephrine, can be given orally since it is not destroyed by the digestive juices. Available in preparations for topical and parenteral use. When used topically as a nasal decongestant, rebound congestion and tachyphylaxis may occur in a few days. Blood pressure of patients receiving parenteral therapy should be monitored closely.

Name, Source, Synonyms, Preparations	Dosage and Administration	Uses	Action and Fate	Side Effects and Contraindications	Nursing Implications and Remarks
SYNTHETIC SYMPATHETIC AGENTS (Continued)					
Hydroxyamphetamine hydrobromide, U.S.P. (Paredrine hydrobromide).	0.25-1% solution, p.r.n. Topical. 20-400 mg. daily in divided doses. Oral.	Used to relieve congestion of mucous membranes, as a mydriatic, and as a vasoconstrictor. Orally for postural hypotension, carotid sinus syndrome and heart block.	Action same as that of cyclopentamine. See Ephedrine for excretion data.	Toxic symptoms are rare in therapeutic dosage. Treatment: none usually needed.	
Pseudoephedrine hydrochloride, N.F. (D-Feda, Gyrocaps, Isophedrine, Novafed, Sudafed).	30-60 mg. q. 3-4 h. p.r.n. Oral. 6-120 mg. extended release capsules q. 12 h.	Used to relieve congestion of the mucous membranes and for bronchodilator properties.	Stereoisomer of ephedrine but is virtually without pressor effects in normotensive patients. Metabolized in liver and metabolites excreted in urine.	Mild C.N.S. stimulation. Use only on doctors' orders for patients with hypertension, heart disease, diabetes mellitus, thyroid disease.	Often given in combination with phenobarbital and antihistamines. Safety for use in pregnancy and lactation has not been established. Elderly patients may be especially susceptible to the side effects.
Isoproterenol hydrochloride, U.S.P. (Aludrin, Isuprel, Norisodrine-H) (isoprenaline, isopropylnoradrenaline, isopropylarterenol, Iso-Intranefrin, Isovon [C]). Isoproterenol sulfate, N.F. (Isonorin, Norisodrine-S).	10-15 mg. Oral; sublingual. q.i.d. but not more than 60 mg. in one day. 1:200-1:100 solution. p.r.n. Topical or by inhalation. 0.2-1 mg. I.M. or I.V. 10% solution. p.r.n. Topical by nebulizer. 5 mg. suppository. Rectal.	Used in a number of conditions, such as bronchial asthma, shock, bradyarrhythmias, allergic conditions, cardiac and respiratory failure, congestion of mucous membranes and to prolong action of local anesthetics.	A strong bronchodilator. Has direct action on the myocardium. Increases cardiac output by increasing strength of contraction and, to a lesser degree, the rate of contraction. It facilitates expectoration of pulmonary secretions. Topically, a decongestant. This is a catecholamine. Absorption and excretion similar to epinephrine.	Tremors, nervous apprehension, palpitation, precordial distress. Severe symptoms may include acute cardiac dilation, pulmonary edema. Treatment: symptomatic. The effect of isoproterenol can be blocked by propranolol, so patients on propranolol will not receive the desired effects from the drug. Tolerance may develop with too frequent or prolonged use.	Should not be administered simultaneously with epinephrine. With sublingual tablets, patient should hold saliva in mouth as long as possible. Absorption is variable and undesirable cardiac effects may result. May be used along with theophylline derivatives for additive effects. Frequent use of sublingual tablets causes damage to the teeth because of the acidity of the drug.

Metaproterenol sulfate (Alupent, Metaprel).	20 mg. t.i.d. or q.i.d. Oral. 0.65 mg. per inhalation. Not to exceed 12 inhalations per day. Children under 60 lb. 10 mg. t. or q.i.d.	Used mainly as a bronchodilator in asthma. Also for reversible bronchospasm associated with bronchitis and emphysema.	Similar to isoproterenol. Well absorbed from G.I. tract with only 40% reaching circulation because of metabolism by liver. Excreted primarily as glucuronic acid conjugates.	Similar to isoproterenol. Contraindicated in patients with cardiac arrhythmias associated with tachycardia. Used with caution in patients with hypertension, coronary artery disease, congestive heart failure, hyperthyroidism or diabetes mellitus.	Safe use during pregnancy or for children under 12 years of age not established. Care should be taken with respect to concurrent administration of additional sympathomimetic agents.
Methoxyphenamine hydrochloride, N.F. (Orthoxine).	50-100 mg. q. 4 h. p.r.n. Oral.	Used as a bronchodilator and antiallergic agent. Has minimal vasopressor effect.	See Uses. Absorption and excretion similar to ephedrine.	Rare in therapeutic dosage. Treatment: none usually required.	Also added to cough syrups.
Methylaminoheptane hydrochloride (Oenethyl).	50-100 mg. p.r.n. I.M. or I.V.	Used mainly to treat hypotension.	Vasoconstriction, with resulting rise in blood pressure.	Rare, but watch for too high blood pressure. Stop drug and give antihypertensive drugs.	
Naphazoline hydrochloride, N.F. (Clera, Privine) (Albalon, Vasocon [C]).	0.05-0.1% solution. p.r.n. Topical as drops or nebulae. 0.05% jelly. p.r.n. 0.012% solution eye drops. Topical.	Used locally to reduce nasal congestion. For relief of red, irritated eyes.	Decongestant due to local vasoconstriction. Effects occur within 10 min. and may last 2-6 h.	Occasionally causes too much blanching of the mucous membrane. Stop drug.	Do not put in aluminum container. Caution against too frequent use. Rebound congestion may occur. Avoid contamination of dropper or dispenser.
Oxymetazoline hydrochloride, N.F. (Afrin hydrochloride) (Nafrine [C]).	1:2000 solution. Topical, either 2-4 gtt. or as nasal spray.	Main use is in allergic rhinitis.	Decongestant. Effects occur within 5-10 min. and persist 5-6 h. with gradual decline over the next 6 h.	Side effects rare, but temporary nasal irritation may occur.	Rebound congestion with prolonged use. Not recommended for use by children less than 6 years old. Avoid contamination of dispenser.

Name, Source, Synonyms, Preparations	Dosage and Administration	Uses	Action and Fate	Side Effects and Contraindications	Nursing Implications and Remarks
SYNTHETIC SYMPATHETIC AGENTS (Continued)					
Phenylephrine hydrochloride, U.S.P. (Almefrin, Isophrin, Neo-Synephrine) (Deca-Nephrine, IsotoFrin, Prefrin [C]).	10 mg. q. 3-4 h. p.r.n. Oral. 1-10 mg. p.r.n. Parenteral. 0.125-0.5% solution. q. 3-4 h. p.r.n. Topical. 2-10% solution drops in eye q.i.d. As a mydriatic p.r.n. q. 1 h.	Used as a decongestant in vasomotor rhinitis, sinusitis and hay fever. Used to prolong action of spinal anesthetics, to maintain blood pressure and to treat orthostatic hypotension and paroxysmal atrial tachycardia. Also used in eye with other agents when mydriasis is desired without cycloplegia or when local vasoconstriction is desired.	Like all these preparations it is a decongestant locally but a stimulant and vasoconstrictor systemically. See ephedrine for excretion data. Acts primarily on alpha receptors.	Rare, but watch for too high blood pressure. Stop drug and give antihypertensive drugs. For eye, use with caution in patients with glaucoma. Also use with caution in diabetes or known hypertension.	Safe use in pregnancy has not been established.
Phenylpropanolamine hydrochloride, N.F. (Propadrine).	0.5-1% solution. p.r.n. Topical. 25-50 mg. q. 3-6 h. p.r.n. Oral.	Used as a mucous membrane decongestant and to treat allergic conditions.	Topical decongestant as a result of vasoconstriction. Systemic vasoconstrictor.	Rare in therapeutic dosage. Does not have the untoward effect of ephedrine.	
Phenylpropylmethylamine (Vonedrine).	0.5% solution. Topical by inhaler. p.r.n.	Used mainly as a local decongestant.	Topical decongestant as a result of vasoconstriction.	Rare in therapeutic dosage. Treatment: none usually required.	
Propylhexedrine, N.F. (Benzedrex).	Dosage varies. Topical by inhaler.	Used as a local decongestant.	Topical decongestant as a result of vasoconstriction.	Rare in therapeutic dosage. Rebound congestion may occur with prolonged use. Should not be used longer than 3-5 days.	Container should be warmed in the hands before administration to increase volatility of the drug.
Protokylol hydrochloride (Ventaire).	2-4 mg. t.i.d. to q.i.d. Oral.	Used as a bronchial dilator in reversible bronchospasm associated with acute and chronic asthma.	Local decongestant. Systemic action: vasoconstriction and bronchial dilation. Well absorbed from G.I. tract,	May cause palpitation, tachycardia, tremors, tension, insomnia, dizziness, nausea and vomiting.	Can be used for long-term treatment of asthma. Often effective when other drugs fail.

			with onset of action 30-90 min. and duration of 3-4 h. Appears to be metabolized by liver and excreted in urine as these metabolites.	Safe use in pregnancy not established.	Caution: as with other sympathomimetic amines of this class.
Terbutaline sulfate (Bricanyl sulfate, Brethine).	0.25 mg. S.Q. into lateral deltoid area. If significant improvement does not occur, repeat in 15-20 minutes. 0.5 mg. total should not be exceeded in a 4 hour period. 2.5-5 mg. q. 6 h. (t.i.d.). Oral. Total daily oral dose should not exceed 15 mg.	Used as a bronchodilator in asthma and for reversible bronchospasm occurring with bronchitis and emphysema.	A beta-adrenergic receptor agonist. Main effect on $beta_2$ adrenergic receptors (based on animal experimentation). Maximum effect in 30 to 60 minutes, can last for 90 minutes to 4 hours. Partially metabolized in the liver; about 60% excreted in the urine, 30% in the feces via bile.	Similar to epinephrine: increased heart rate, nervousness, palpitation, dizziness; sometimes headache, nausea, vomiting, anxiety. Contraindications: patients known to be sensitive to sympathomimetic amines. Safe use during pregnancy and for children not established. Used with caution in patients with diabetes mellitus, hypertension or hyperthyroidism.	Concomitant use with other sympathomimetics not recommended because their combined effect may be deleterious to the cardiovascular system.
Tetrahydrozoline hydrochloride, N.F. (Tyzine, Visine).	0.05-1% solution. Topical in nose or eyes.	Used as a topical decongestant.	Vasoconstriction with resulting decongestion.	Same as for others of this group. Rebound congestion may occur.	Not recommended in presence of glaucoma or other eye disorders.
Tuaminoheptane sulfate, N.F. (Tuamine sulfate) (Rhinosol [C]).	1.0% solution. Topical and inhalational.	Used mainly as a local decongestant.	Vasoconstriction with resulting decongestion.	Rare in therapeutic dosage. Treatment: none usually required.	Safe use during pregnancy has not been established.
Xylometazoline hydrochloride (Otrivin; Sine-off; Sinex, long acting).	0.1% solution q.3-4 h. Topical in nose.	Used mainly as a local decongestant.	Vasoconstriction with resulting decongestion. Effects occur within 5-10 min. and persist 5-6 h.	Rare in therapeutic dosage.	Rebound congestion with prolonged use.

SYNTHETIC SYMPATHETIC AGENTS (Continued)

Sympathetic amines that produce peripheral vasodilation by relaxation of the smooth muscles of the arterioles. Increase rate and force of heart and may relax uterus.

Name, Source, Synonyms, Preparations	Dosage and Administration	Uses	Action and Fate	Side Effects and Contraindications	Nursing Implications and Remarks
Isoxsuprine hydrochloride (Vasodilan).	10-20 mg. three to four times daily, oral, or two to three times daily I.M. I.M. doses greater than 10 mg. are not recommended.	For symptoms due to peripheral and cerebral arterial insufficiency or cerebral vascular disease associated with arteriosclerosis and hypertension. Also for uterine hypermotility, primary dysmenorrhea, threatened abortion and premature labor.	Vasodilator and uterine relaxant. Acts directly on smooth muscles of blood vessels and uterus. Rapidly absorbed from the G.I. tract. Partially conjugated and excreted in urine.	May cause palpitation, vomiting, dizziness, weakness, tachycardia and hypotension. Adjust dosage or change to another drug. Treat symptoms.	With I.M. administration the patient should be cautioned about postural hypotension.
Nylidrin hydrochloride, N.F. (Arlidin) (buphenine hydrochloride, Pervadil [C]).	6-12 mg. three to six times daily. Oral.	Peripheral vasodilator used to lower blood pressure.	A sympathomimetic drug whose main clinical action is peripheral vasodilation. Rapidly absorbed and has prolonged action. Excreted in the urine.	Toxicity apparently low. Chief side effect is palpitation which disappears with continued use.	Safe use in pregnancy not established.

SYMPATHOLYTICS (SYMPATHETIC DEPRESSANTS, ADRENOLYTIC AGENTS)

These drugs are antagonistic to epinephrine and similar drugs. They cause vasodilation and increase tone of alimentary tract muscles and of other smooth muscle tissue. They vary in their effects, and some will be discussed in areas of important therapeutic activity. These are synthetic preparations except as noted.

Name, Source, Synonyms, Preparations	Dosage and Administration	Uses	Action and Fate	Side Effects and Contraindications	Nursing Implications and Remarks
Azapetine phosphate (Ilidar) (azepine [C]).	25 mg. t.i.d. individually adjusted. Oral.	Used in peripheral vascular disease in which vasospasm is predominant.	Adrenergic blocking agent similar to tolazoline hydrochloride. It can reverse the pressor effect of epinephrine and reduce the vasoconstrictor effect of norepinephrine.	Rare in therapeutic dosage but may cause drug fever, nausea, vomiting, postural hypotension and syncope. Dosage adjustment is usually sufficient treatment. Contraindicated when fall in blood pressure is dangerous and in coronary disorders.	Safe use in pregnancy has not been established.

Phenoxybenzamine hydrochloride (Dibenzyline).	10-20 mg. q.d. up to q.i.d. Dosage individually adjusted. Oral.	Used to treat peripheral vasospastic vascular diseases. Control or prevention of paroxysmal hypertension and sweating in patients with pheochromocytoma.	Alpha-adrenergic blocking agent. Following oral administration, approximately 30% absorbed. Gradual onset of action. With continual therapy, effects cumulative for 7 days. May accumulate in fat; excreted in urine and bile.	Nasal congestion, miosis, tachycardia, postural hypotension. Reduce dosage or stop drug. Contraindicated when sudden fall in blood pressure might be dangerous.	As above. G.I. irritation may be reduced by giving with milk or in divided doses.
Phentolamine hydrochloride, N.F. (Regitine hydrochloride) (Rogitine [C]).	50 mg. four to six times a day. Dosage individually adjusted. Oral.	For diagnosis and for prevention or control of hypertensive episodes in patients with pheochromocytoma. Prevention and treatment of dermal necrosis and sloughing following I.V. administration or extravasation of norepinephrine.	Alpha-adrenergic blocking agent. Causes peripheral vasodilation and decreases peripheral resistance. Stimulates beta-adrenergic receptors and produces a positive inotropic and chronotropic effect on the heart and increases cardiac output.	Side effects are rare. Tachycardia has been reported. Myocardial infarction, cerebrovascular spasm and cerebrovascular occlusion have been seen, usually in association with marked hypotensive episodes with shock-like states which follow parenteral administration.	As above. Weakness, dizziness, flushing, orthostatic hypotension, nasal congestion, G.I. effects are common with long-term administration.
Phentolamine mesylate, U.S.P. (Regitine mesylate).	3 mg. I.M. 1 mg. I.V.	Mainly used to test for pheochromocytoma and for blood pressure control during surgery.	As above.	As above.	The mesylate is also used in small amounts with norepinephrine to reduce damage from extravasation when this cannot be avoided.
Tolazoline hydrochloride (Priscoline, Tazol, Tolavad, Tolpol).	25-75 mg. q.i.d. Oral or parenteral.	Used in spastic peripheral vascular disorders including acrocyanosis, acroparesthesia, arteriosclerosis obliterans, Buerger's disease, causalgia, diabetic arteriosclerosis, gangrene, endarteritis, frostbite (sequelae), thrombophlebitis, Raynaud's disease and scleroderma.	Adrenergic blocking agent causing dilation of peripheral arterioles, presumably from competitive interference at the pressor receptor.	Rare in therapeutic dosage. When toxic symptoms do occur they are similar to the mild toxic symptoms of the nitrites. Stop drug and treat symptoms. Contraindicated in collapse or shock. Given cautiously, if at all, in cases of coronary disease or peptic ulcers.	

Name, Source, Synonyms, Preparations	Dosage and Administration	Uses	Action and Fate	Side Effects and Contraindications	Nursing Implications and Remarks
ERGOT. *Claviceps purpurea.* *Semisynthetic and synthetic.*					
Dihydroergotamine mesylate (DHE45).	1 ml. at onset of headache then q. 1 h. up to 3 ml. I.M. Or 2 ml. in buffered solution. I.V.	Used to treat migraine syndrome and various types of vascular headache. Also for postherpetic pain.	Various active principles produce different results. Ergotamine and ergotoxine stimulate smooth muscle tissue, and tend to raise blood pressure. Ergotoxine has greater ecbolic action than ergotamine. Both are adrenergic blocking agents. Ergonovine has greater ecbolic action and does not tend to raise blood pressure. It does not act as an adrenergic blocking agent but rather appears to stimulate the effector cells connected with adrenergic nerves; it does not paralyze them. Metabolic fate unknown.	Acute: nausea, vomiting, thirst, tingling of extremities, uterine bleeding and abortion if patient is pregnant. Late: face and limbs swell, abnormal skin sensation occurs and there is pallor. Terminal: temperature falls, convulsions, coma and death occur due to cardiac and respiratory failure. Treatment: lavage, enemas, purgation, central nervous system stimulants. Toxic symptoms: chronic–dry gangrene may occur, and cataracts may form. Spasmodic–vertigo, tinnitus, headache, muscle tremors and abnormal skin sensations occur. Treatment: symptomatic, but prognosis is poor.	
Dihydroergotoxine mesylate (Hydergine)	1 mg. sublingual t.i.d.	Used in geriatric patients to treat cerebrovascular insufficiency.			Therapeutic response is gradual, and beneficial effects with elderly may not be observed until after 3-4 weeks of therapy.
Ergonovine maleate, U.S.P. (Ergotrate, ergosterine, ergometrine)	1-2 mg. two to three times daily. Oral. 2 mg. once for uterine bleeding. I.M. or I.V. Severe hemorrhage may require more than one dose.	Mainly used as an ecbolic.			
Ergotamine tartrate, U.S.P. (Femergin, Gynergen, Ergostat, Ergomar).	0.25-0.5 mg. and repeat in 40 minutes if not relieved. I.M. or I.V. Not more than 2 mg. weekly. 2-6 mg. (two to six 1 mg. tablets) used per attack. Oral. 2 mg. sublingual. No more than 10 mg. weekly.	Used to treat vascular headaches.		Ergotamine and dihydroergotamine are contraindicated in peripheral vascular diseases, angina pectoris and hepatic or renal dysfunction.	Also available as inhaler: Medihaler–ergotamine. Often used in combination with caffeine (Cafergot); it is postulated that caffeine acts synergistically with ergotamine, lowering the dose of ergotamine necessary for effectiveness.

SEMISYNTHETIC PREPARATIONS					
Methylergonovine maleate, U.S.P. (Methergine).	0.2 mg. three or four times daily for postpartum bleeding. Oral. 0.2 mg. after third stage of labor. I.M. or I.V.	Used mainly for postpartum hemorrhage and to hasten uterine involution.	As above. Stimulates contraction of uterine and vascular smooth muscle.	Methylergonovine should not be administered I.V. routinely because of the possibility of inducing sudden hypertensive and cerebrovascular accidents. In emergency, it can be given slowly over a 60-second duration with careful monitoring of blood pressure. Most common side effects include nausea and vomiting.	Not used for induction or augmentation of labor.
Methysergide maleate (Sansert).	2-4 mg. t.i.d. with meals. Oral. For each 6 month period of taking drug, there should be a 3 or 4 week rest period.	Used prophylactically in vascular headaches in patients whose headaches are frequent and/or severe and uncontrollable and who are under close medical supervision.	A potent antiserotonin agent. Inhibits vasoconstrictor and pressor effects of 5-Ht but mechanism of action unknown.	Mild nausea, heartburn and occasional vomiting have been reported. Contraindicated or used with caution in pregnancy, coronary artery disease, severe hypertension, peripheral vascular disease, arteriosclerosis, collagen diseases, fibrotic diseases, valvular heart disease or impaired renal or hepatic function. Warning: retroperitoneal fibrosis, pleuropulmonary fibrosis and fibrotic thickening of cardiac valves may occur in patients on long-term therapy.	Before discontinuing the drug, dosage is decreased over 2-3 wks. to prevent "headache rebound."

Name, Source, Synonyms, Preparations	Dosage and Administration	Uses	Action and Fate	Side Effects and Contraindications	Nursing Implications and Remarks
SYNTHETIC PREPARATIONS					
Clonidine hydrochloride (Catapres).	0.1-0.8 mg. Daily. Oral. Maximum dosage (rarely used) 2.4 mg./day.	Used to reduce high blood pressure. Prior and concomitant use of a diuretic is recommended to give better therapeutic response.	Appears to stimulate alpha-adrenergic receptors in C.N.S., causing inhibition but not blockade of sympathetic vasomotor centers. Brings about reduction of blood pressure, bradycardia, and fall in cardiac output. Pressure declines within 30 to 60 minutes, maximum effect in 2 to 4 hours, lasts approximately 6 to 8 hours. Plasma ½ life 12 to 16 hours. Clonidine is well absorbed and widely distributed and its metabolites are excreted mainly in the urine. Tolerance may develop in some.	Dry mouth, drowsiness, sedation. Constipation, dizziness, headache, fatigue have been reported. Safe use during pregnancy has not been established. Animal experimentation has shown some embryotoxicity, therefore its use should be weighed against possible adverse effect on fetus. Animal experimentation has also shown some eye pathology, so periodic eye examinations are advised. This has not been shown in humans to date.	The dose of this drug should be reduced gradually over a period of 1 week. Abrupt stopping could cause rapid rise in blood pressure with such symptoms as nervousness, agitation and headache. Patients should be warned not to stop drug without consulting the doctor. Patients should also be warned about engaging in potentially hazardous activities because of possible sedative effect of the drug.
Guanethidine sulfate, U.S.P. (Ismelin).	10-50 mg. Dosage individually adjusted. Oral.	For treatment of moderate to severe and malignant hypertension and to treat peripheral vascular diseases. Is a strong hypotensive agent. Prior and concomitant use of a diuretic is recommended to give better therapeutic response.	Appears to interfere with the release of the chemical mediator (presumably norepinephrine) at the sympathetic neuroeffector junction. Hypotensive effect due to a reduction in cardiac output (due to reduced venous return and negative chronotropic and inotropic effects) and a fall in peripheral vascular resistance. Full	Orthostatic hypotension, bradycardia, diarrhea and retrograde ejaculation in males. Contraindicated in pheochromocytoma. Safe use during pregnancy has not been established. When used with amphetamine or other sympathetic agents such as ephedrine or methylphenidate, the effectiveness	Patients should be cautioned to avoid strenuous exercise or prolonged standing during administration for fear of severe hypotension. Dosage requirements may be reduced in patients with fever or impaired renal function and in hot weather. Caution patient about orthostatic hypotension, which is more severe during initiation of

			therapeutic effect delayed 2-7 days; excreted in urine. Tends to reduce orthostatic blood pressure more than recumbent blood pressure. Action long lasting.	of guanethidine in reducing blood pressure can be severely antagonized. The same effect takes place with desipramine and probably with imipramine, amitriptyline and nortriptyline.	therapy. Appears in breast milk but only in small amounts.
<u>Methyldopa</u>, U.S.P. (Aldomet) (Presinal, Sembrina [C]). <u>Methyldopa hydrochloride</u>, U.S.P. (Aldomet ester hydrochloride).	500 mg.- 2 Gm. Given daily in divided doses. Oral. 250-500 mg. q. 6 h. I.V.	Used in patients with sustained moderate to severe hypertension. Prior and concomitant use of a diuretic is recommended to give better therapeutic response.	Methyldopa or its metabolites are believed to cause antihypertensive effects by stimulation of central inhibitory alpha-adrenergic receptors or by acting as false neurotransmitters. Maximum lowering appears by second day. Half oral dose absorbed and excreted unchanged in urine and as its mono-o-sulfate. Therapeutic dose has maximal effect in 6-8 hours. Excreted in urine and feces.	Hemolytic anemia has occurred. Some patients develop a positive direct Coombs' test when on continued therapy. This disappears in weeks to months after discontinuing the drug. Sedation, anxiety, apprehension, dizziness, postural hypotension, diarrhea and impotence also occur. Reversible agranulocytosis and retroperitoneal fibrosis have been reported. Contraindicated in pregnancy, pheochromocytoma, acute hepatitis and active cirrhosis.	Liver and blood tests should be done during therapy. Orthostatic hypotension is an indication for dosage reduction. Patients should be advised to report such symptoms when they occur. Rebound hypertension has been reported rarely following abrupt withdrawal of oral methyldopa. Major toxic effect is drug-induced fever occurring within 21 days after initiation of therapy.

Name, Source, Synonyms, Preparations	Dosage and Administration	Uses	Action and Fate	Side Effects and Contraindications	Nursing Implications and Remarks
SYNTHETIC PREPARATIONS (Continued)					
Prazosin hydrochloride (Minipress).	Adjusted to patient's BP response. Initial dose 1 mg. t.i.d.; can increase slowly up to 20 mg./day. Higher doses do not usually bring better results but some patients have required up to 40 mg./day. At fixed dosage levels, 4-6 wks. of therapy is required before full effect of drug is achieved.	Treatment of hypertension. Generally more effective with concomitant use of diuretics.	Acts predominantly as a direct smooth muscle relaxant, but the exact mechanism is unknown. It does not appear to have alpha-adrenergic receptor blocking activity. Action is believed to be due to direct relaxation of peripheral arterioles and is associated with decreased total peripheral resistance. Widely distributed, highly bound to plasma protein, metabolized primarily in liver. About 6-10% excreted in urine, rest in feces via bile.	Most common: dizziness, 10.3%; HA, 7.8%; drowsiness, 7.6%; lack of energy, 6.9%; weakness, 6.5%; palpitations, 5.3%; and nausea, 4.9%. Other less frequent effects include vomiting, diarrhea, constipation, abdominal discomfort, edema, dyspnea, syncope, tachycardia, nervousness, vertigo, depression, paresthesia, rash, pruritus, frequency and impotence, blurred vision, reddened sclera, epistaxis, tinnitus, dry mouth and nasal congestion.	Increase dose slowly to help avoid syncope. Safety in pregnancy not established and no information for use in children. Advise patients of possibility of postural hypotension and of measures to follow if it develops.

BETA–ADRENERGIC BLOCKING AGENTS

These drugs produce a decrease in heart rate, reduction in cardiac output, reduction in resting stroke volume, reduction in oxygen consumption and increase in left ventricular and diastolic pressure.

Name, Source, Synonyms, Preparations	Dosage and Administration	Uses	Action and Fate	Side Effects and Contraindications	Nursing Implications and Remarks
Metropolol tartrate (Lopressor).	Dose individualized. Usual initial dose 50 mg. b.i.d., Maintenance dose 100-450 mg. per day.	Treatment of hypertension with or without diuretics.	Selective beta-adrenergic blocking agent of chiefly cardiac muscle; however, at higher doses, inhibits $beta_2$ adrenoreceptors located chiefly in bronchial and vascular musculature. Resultant effect is seen in reduction in heart rate and cardiac output at rest, reduction of systolic	Most adverse effects have been mild and transient and include tiredness, dizziness, depression, headache, nightmares, insomnia. Also reported have been: shortness of breath, bradycardia, cold extremities, Raynaud's disease, palpitation, congestive heart disease, wheezing,	Effects of metropolol may be reversed by administration of dobutamine or isoproterenol. Patients should be cautioned against interruption of treatment without physician's advice. Safe use in pregnancy and lactation has not been established.

			blood pressure during exercise, inhibition of isoproterenol-induced tachycardia and reduction of reflex orthostatic tachycardia. Absorbed rapidly and completely. Elimination is mainly by metabolism in the liver. Plasma half-life is 3-4 h.	diarrhea, nausea, heartburn, gastric pain, constipation, flatulence and pruritus. Contraindicated in sinus bradycardia, heart block greater than 1st degree, cardiogenic shock and overt cardiac failure. Use cautiously in patients with bronchospastic disease who cannot tolerate other antihypertensive therapy. Abrupt cessation of treatment with some beta-blocking agents has led to exacerbation of angina pectoris and at times myocardial infarction. The necessity of withdrawal of therapy before major surgery is controversial, but therapy may augment the risks of general anesthesia and surgery.	In general, the maximum effect of any given dosage level will be apparent after one week of therapy.
Propranolol hydrochloride, U.S.P. (Inderal). *Synthetic.*	Dose is individualized. Range: 160-480 mg./day in divided doses. Maximum: 640 mg./day. 40-320 mg. in divided doses daily. 10-30 mg. 3-4 times a day a.c. and h.s. 20-40 mg. 3-4 times a day a.c. and h.s. 60 mg. oral in divided doses for 3 days.	For hypertension (not for treatment of hypertensive emergencies). For angina pectoris. For cardiac arrhythmias. For hypertrophic subaortic stenosis. Preoperatively for pheochromocytoma. Used concomitantly with an alpha-adrenergic blocking agent for inoperable tumor.	This drug reduces pressor response to norepinephrine, potentiates that to epinephrine hydrochloride but has no effect on response to phenylephrine. It is widely distributed in the body, with the highest concentration in lungs, spleen and kidneys. After intravenous dose, the metabolic half-life is approximately 1 hour.	Side effects include nausea, vomiting, mild diarrhea, lightheadedness, mental depression, skin rash, paresthesia of hands, fever combined with sore throat, visual disturbances and hallucinations. Peyronie's disease has been reported with the use of propranolol. Contraindications: bronchial asthma, allergic rhinitis during hay fever season, sinus bradycardia and greater than second degree or total heart block,	Commercial brochure should be consulted before giving this drug. The arrhythmias that can be treated include: paroxysmal atrial tachycardia, sinus tachycardia and extra systoles (atrial and ventricular), atrial flutter and fibrillation, tachyarrhythmia of digitalis intoxication, ventricular tachycardias (when cardioversion technique is not available). Safe use during pregnancy has not been established. It appears in breast milk but

Name, Source, Synonyms, Preparations	Dosage and Administration	Uses	Action and Fate	Side Effects and Contraindications	Nursing Implications and Remarks
Propranolol *(continued)*	40-80 mg. in divided doses daily. 1-3 mg. I.V. given under ECG monitoring. Not to exceed 1 mg. per minute. Once an alteration is noted no more should be given until full effect is observed. A second dose may be given in 2 minutes but no additional for 4 hours. 160-240 mg. in divided doses (q.i.d.). Oral.	In overcoming or blocking some adrenergic symptoms associated with thyrotoxicosis. If excessive bradycardia occurs, atropine 0.5-1.0 mg. should be given I.V. Prevention of migraine.		cardiogenic shock, right ventricular failure secondary to pulmonary hypertension, congestive heart failure, in patients receiving anesthetic agents that produce myocardial depression, and in patients receiving adrenergic augmenting psychotropic drugs (including the monoamine oxidase inhibitors) and during the two week withdrawal period from such drugs. Propranolol can increase the acute central nervous system toxicity of hexobarbital. Propranolol and quinidine have synergistic effects and the dose of both drugs can be reduced when they are given concurrently.	in amounts probably too small to have an effect. When used for hypertension it is usually given in conjunction with a thiazide diuretic. When administered I.V., careful monitoring of ECG, blood pressure and central venous pressure should be made. Propranolol may mask typical signs of hypoglycemia. Patients on insulin and hypoglycemic agents should be advised of varying symptoms of hypoglycemia. With prolonged therapy the drug is withdrawn slowly and patient response is monitored.
Timolol maleate (Timoptic).	Gtt. i of 0.25% solution b.i.d. Adjusted to individual response.	Treatment of chronic open-angle glaucoma. Of value in aphakic glaucoma, secondary glaucoma, and ocular hypertension.	Mechanism of action not understood. Unlike other miotics, reduces intraocular pressure with little or no effect on pupil size or visual acuity and is long acting.	Usually well tolerated. Occasionally mild ocular irritation. Slight reduction in resting heart rate has been seen. Local hypersensitivity has occurred rarely. As with other miotics, tolerance may occur. However, after a 2 year study of 102 patients, no evidence of	Important to advise patients of the seriousness of glaucoma to ensure compliance with therapy and follow-up medical care.

				diminished responsiveness had been reported. Contraindicated in patients with hypersensitivity to any of its components. Use with caution in patients with known contraindications to systemic use of beta-adrenergic receptor blocking agents; also in patients with bronchial asthma and congestive heart failure. Patients receiving oral beta-adrenergic blockers should be observed for potential additive effects. Use in pregnancy has not been studied. Not recommended for children at this time.	

PARASYMPATHOMIMETICS (PARASYMPATHETIC STIMULANTS, CHOLINERGIC AGENTS)

Drugs that stimulate the parasympathetic divisions of the autonomic nervous system all to a greater or lesser degree decrease the rate of the heart, contract smooth muscle tissue, contract the pupils of the eye and increase the secretions of most of the glands. Since the two divisions of the autonomic nervous system work mainly in opposition to each other, the stimulation of one division will usually depress the other and vice versa. The drugs have been classified for their main therapeutic activity.

CHOLINE DERIVATIVES. *Synthetic.* Acetylcholine chloride (Miochol).	0.5 to 2 ml. (20 mg. per 2 ml.) instilled into the anterior chamber of the eye.	To obtain complete miosis in seconds. Used in cataract surgery or in iridectomies.	Rapid miotic. Deactivated by acetylcholine esterases and other esterases.	Note: in cataract surgery use only after delivery of the lens.	Prepare immediately before use and discard unused portion, as solutions are unstable.

Name, Source, Synonyms, Preparations	Dosage and Administration	Uses	Action and Fate	Side Effects and Contraindications	Nursing Implications and Remarks
CHOLINE DERIVATIVES (Continued)					
Bethanechol chloride, U.S.P. (Duvoid, Mictrol, Myotonachol, Urecholine, Urolax).	2.5-5 mg. t.i.d. or q.i.d. S.Q. 10-50 mg. t.i.d. or q.i.d. Oral.	For treatment of postoperative and postpartum nonobstructive urinary retention and for neurogenic atony of the urinary bladder with retention.	These preparations act in the body as does the endogenous acetylcholine, but are usually not inactivated as rapidly by cholinesterase. Poorly absorbed from G.I. tract. Distribution, metabolism and excretion have not been elucidated.	Can cause flushing, hyperhidrosis, salivation, nausea, vomiting, abdominal discomfort, headache, diarrhea, asthmatic attacks and hypotension. Contraindicated in mechanical intestinal or urinary tract obstruction, bronchial asthma, hyperthyroidism, peptic ulcer, severe heart disease, vasomotor instability, bradycardia, hypotension, vagotonia, pregnancy, epilepsy, parkinsonism and in patients receiving anticholinesterase agents.	Bethanechol chloride is not given intramuscularly or intravenously because severe effects including circulatory failure may result. Administer dose on an empty stomach to minimize nausea and vomiting.
Carbachol, U.S.P. (Carcholin, Carbamylcholine chloride) (IsoptoCarbachol, Carbamiotin [C]).	0.75-2.25% solution. q. 8-12 h. Topical in eyes.	Used in chronic open-angle and for emergency treatment of angle-closure glaucoma.	As above.	As above. Accommodative spasm, headache and conjunctival hyperemia. Systemic effects are rare but see under demecarium bromide. Contraindicated in asthma and hypertension.	Carbachol is not given systemically because of toxicity.
Carbachol (Miostat).	0.1% solution 0.5 ml. instilled into anterior chamber before or after securing sutures.	For intraocular pupillary miosis during surgery.	Miosis is usually maximal in 2 to 5 minutes.		

CHOLINESTERASE INHIBITORS. *Synthetic.*			These act by blocking the action of cholinesterase and thus prolong the action of acetylcholine. Some have an irreversible effect.	G.I. disturbances, sweating, excessive salivation, miosis, muscle weakness and urinary urgency.	The safety of use of the cholinesterase drugs during pregnancy has not been established, nor has the absence of adverse effects on the fetus or on the respiration of the neonate.
Ambenonium chloride, N.F. (Mytelase, Mysuran).	5-25 mg. t.i.d. or q.i.d. Oral.	A cholinesterase inhibitor used in myasthenia gravis.	Good oral absorption and longer duration of action than with neostigmine.	Similar to neostigmine bromide but is considered less toxic. First symptom of impending toxicity may be muscle weakness.	Dosage adjusted so patients take larger doses at times of greatest fatigue. Patients need to be cautioned not to increase their dose above the maximum response level. Patients should be taught to recognize muscarine side effects and modify their dose accordingly. Fewer muscarinic side effects when administered with milk or food.
Demecarium bromide (Humorsol).	0.25% solution. 1-2 gtt. q. 12-48 hours. Dosage individually adjusted. Topical.	A cholinesterase inhibitor used to treat chronic glaucoma if uncontrolled with short-acting miotics and epinephrine.	Long acting due to irreversible inactivation of cholinesterase.	In long-term use cataracts can occur, and also twitching of the eyelids, browache, headache, ocular pain, ciliary and conjunctival congestion, lacrimation and accommodation myopia. Symptoms of systemic toxicity include hypersalivation, sweating, nausea, vomiting, abdominal pain, diarrhea, bradycardia, hypotension and bronchoconstriction. Toxic doses can cause C.N.S. effects and muscular paralysis and result in death due to respiratory failure.	

Name, Source, Synonyms, Preparations	Dosage and Administration	Uses	Action and Fate	Side Effects and Contraindications	Nursing Implications and Remarks
CHOLINESTERASE INHIBITORS (Continued)					
Echothiophate iodide (Echodide, Phospholine iodide).	0.03-0.25% solution. 1-2 gtt. in eyes q. 12-48 hours. Individually adjusted. Topical.	As above.		As above. Use with extreme care in patients with history of retinal detachment or in closed-angle glaucoma.	
Isoflurophate, N.F. (D.F.P., Floropryl) (difluorophate, Dyflos [C]).	0.1% solution. Topical. 0.25% ophthalmic ointment.	As above.			
Neostigmine bromide, U.S.P. (Prostigmin bromide).	15 mg. Oral.	Used to increase urinary and intestinal peristalsis, and in the diagnosis and treatment of myasthenia gravis.	See ambenonium chloride. Oral dose, much is destroyed in intestines so much larger dose required. Metabolized in the liver and excreted in urine.	May cause hyperhidrosis, salivation, gastrointestinal distress, muscle cramps, weakness, fasciculation and, in overdose, can cause cholinergic crisis.	Side effects can be minimized by precise dosage adjustment. Atropine should be available as an antagonist for the muscarinic effects of neostigmine. Myasthenia patients may become refractory to neostigmine after prolonged therapy.
Neostigmine methylsulfate, U.S.P. (Prostigmin methylsulfate).	0.25-1 mg. Parenteral.	Used as an antidote for tubocurarines following surgery and to counteract the neuromuscular blockage seen when neomycin is given with tubocurarines and/or ether.		Contraindicated in mechanical intestinal or urinary blockage or in the presence of bradycardia. Should not be used with depolarizing neuromuscular blocking agents and choline esters. Use with caution in patients with bronchial asthma.	Responsiveness may be restored by decreasing the dosage or by withdrawing the drug for several days under medical supervision.
Pyridostigmine bromide, U.S.P. (Mestinon, Regonol).	600 mg.-1.5 Gm. daily in divided doses. Oral. 5 mg./ml. inj.	Main use in myasthenia gravis. Used as an antidote for tubocurarine-type muscle relaxants.	For action see ambenonium chloride. Fate in body is not known.	See above.	

OTHER CHOLINERGIC DRUGS				
DEXPANTHENOL. *Synthetic.* Dexpanthenol (D-pantothenyl alcohol, Intrapan, Tonestat) (dexpanthenol, panthenol [C]).	250-500 mg. I.M. or I.V. diluted and given slowly. q. 2-6 h.	Used to increase peristalsis in atony and paralysis of the lower bowel.	Alcoholic analog of D-pantothenic acid, which is converted in body to D-pantothenic acid; this is claimed to be a precursor of coenzyme A.	Toxicity apparently low. Is used in place of, but not with the prostigmine-like drugs. Should wait 12 hours after neostigmine and 1 hour after succinylcholine before starting dexpanthenol. Its use is contraindicated in hemophilia.
PHYSOSTIGMINE. *Physostigma venenosum* or *Calabar bean.* Physostigmine salicylate, U.S.P. (Antilirium, Eserine salicylate) (eserine, Isopto-Eserine [C]). Physostigmine sulfate (Eserine sulfate).	0.5-1 mg. S.Q. 0.2-1% solution. Topical in eyes. q. 4-6 h. 0.25% ointment in eyes at bedtime.	Used as a miotic in open-angle glaucoma and in the emergency treatment of angle-closure glaucoma. Stimulates respiration. Used as an antidote to the toxic effects of belladonna alkaloids and to reverse effects of atropine and scopolamine.	Postganglionic stimulant of parasympathetic system with direct action; causes miosis, bradycardia, increased intestinal motility. Rapidly absorbed from gastrointestinal tract, subcutaneous tissues and mucous membranes. Thought to be degraded in body by cholinesterase. After subcutaneous injection duration of effect approximately 2 hours.	Weak heart action, abdominal cramps, diarrhea, excessive perspiration, salivation, muscular twitching, pinpoint pupils, shock and collapse. Treatment: atropine and caffeine may be used. Treat for shock. Artificial respiration as indicated. Watch for asthmatic attack. Contraindicated in known asthmatic patients, gangrene, diabetes, cardiovascular disease, mechanical obstruction of the intestinal or urinary tract or in patients receiving neuromuscular blocking agents such as decamethonium or succinylcholine.

DRUGS AFFECTING THE AUTONOMIC NERVOUS SYSTEM (Continued)

PARASYMPATHOMIMETICS *(Continued)*

Name, Source, Synonyms, Preparations	Dosage and Administration	Uses	Action and Fate	Side Effects and Contraindications	Nursing Implications and Remarks
PILOCARPINE. *Pilocarpus jaborandi. Synthetic.* Pilocarpine hydrochloride, U.S.P. (Almocarpine, Isopto-Carpine, Miocarpine, Pilomiotin [C]).	0.25-10.0% solution. Up to q.i.d. Topical in eye.	Used mainly as a miotic in the treatment of primary open-angle glaucoma and most other chronic glaucomas. Also used for emergency treatment of acute angle-closure glaucoma.	Has direct action on cholinergic receptors and produces strong postganglionic and some ganglionic stimulation when acetylcholine is the mediator. Stimulates salivation and bronchial secretion, produces sweating and increases peristalsis. Improves drainage from anterior chamber of eye in glaucoma. After topical instillation miosis begins in 15-30 minutes and lasts 4-8 hours. Little is known of fate of pilocarpine in body. Some degradation but most is excreted in urine in combined form.	When used topically few side effects except ciliary spasm, local irritation and allergic reactions are seen. Systemic effects are uncommon but it can weaken and slow heart action, lower blood pressure, increase bronchial secretion, may produce pulmonary edema. Other symptoms include nausea, vomiting and muscular twitching. Treatment: atropine may be used. Treat for shock. Artificial respiration may be needed. Treat symptoms.	Action is similar to that of the choline derivatives..
Pilocarpine nitrate, U.S.P. (Carpine nitrate [C]).					
Pilocarpine nitrate solution, U.S.P.	0.5-6% solution. Up to q.i.d. Topical in eye.				

PARASYMPATHOLYTICS (PARASYMPATHETIC DEPRESSANTS, CHOLINERGIC BLOCKING AGENTS)

The general effects of these drugs are opposite to those of the parasympathetic stimulants but similar to those of the sympathetic stimulants. They produce mydriasis, cycloplegia, reduced secretion of certain glands, relaxation of smooth muscle tissue and increased heart action. Most of these drugs are derived from various plants of the Solanaceae family. Each plant yields all or most of the alkaloids. Many of the drugs have been synthesized, and many synthetic preparations similar to the natural alkaloids are available. These drugs are *contraindicated in glaucoma* and used with caution in patients with prostatic hypertrophy or pyloric obstruction. When used at high environmental temperatures, these drugs can precipitate heat prostration, due to fever and the decreased ability to sweat.

Name, Source, Synonyms, Preparations	Dosage and Administration	Uses	Action and Fate	Side Effects and Contraindications	Nursing Implications and Remarks
BELLADONNA. *(atropine, hyoscine, hyoscyamine). Atropa belladonna. Synthetic.* Atropine methylnitrate (Harvatrate, Metropine).	1 mg. a.c. and 2 mg. h.s. Oral. 1% solution. Topical.	Used in a wide variety of conditions; to decrease secretions, relax smooth muscle tissue, dilate pupils, increase heart rate, increase rate of respiration, for general cerebral stimulation, and	Atropine antagonizes the effects of acetylcholine at peripheral neuroeffector sites. It has no effect at autonomic ganglia (except in toxic doses) or at the neuromuscular junction of	Excessive dryness of mouth and throat, dysphagia, intense thirst, impaired vision, red and dry skin, delirium, convulsions, tachycardia and increased blood pressure. Treatment: symptomatic.	Preparations of mixtures of belladonna alkaloids are also available, such as Bellafoline.

Atropine sulfate, U.S.P. (Isopto-atropine [C]).	0.3-1.2 mg. q. 4-6 h. Oral or s.c. 0.5-1% ophthalmic ointment.	locally as an anodyne. Used with many other drugs in various combinations, as with phenobarbital in the treatment of gastrointestinal disorders.	skeletal muscle. It reduces the motility and secretory activity of the G.I. tract, reduces the tone of the ureter and bladder and has a slight inhibitory effect on the bile ducts and gallbladder. It inhibits the bradycardia induced by vagal stimulation. These compounds of the belladonna group interfere with transmission of postganglionic parasympathetic impulses, and this action is thought to be due to receptor site attachment. Most belladonna alkaloids are rapidly absorbed orally and can also enter circulation from mucosal surfaces. They are widely distributed in the body. The quaternary derivatives are only about one quarter absorbed and they do not cross the blood-brain barrier and so are lacking in central effects.	Parasympathetic stimulants such as pilocarpine are usually ordered, as are cardiac and respiratory stimulants. Use with caution in cardiovascular disease. Contraindicated with gastrointestinal or genitourinary obstruction, glaucoma, prostatic hypertrophy or during pregnancy.	Times of administration of these products vary with use and gravity of the situation.
Atropine sulfate solution (Atropisol).	0.5-2% solution. Topical.	As a mydriatic.			
Belladonna tincture, U.S.P. (Taladonna).	0.3-0.6 ml. Oral.	Also available as an extract for oral administration.			
Genatropine (Atropine-N-Oxide, X-tra) (hyoscine aminoxide [C]).	0.5-1 mg. two or three times a day. Oral.	See atropine.			

Name, Source, Synonyms, Preparations	Dosage and Administration	Uses	Action and Fate	Side Effects and Contraindications	Nursing Implications and Remarks
HYOSCYAMINE. *Active principle of Hyoscyamus niger.*		General uses same as those of belladonna.	Similar to belladonna but affects the peripheral organs more and the internal organs less than atropine.	Excessive dryness of mouth and throat, dysphagia, intense thirst, impaired vision, red and dry skin, delirium, convulsions, tachycardia and increased blood pressure. Treatment: symptomatic. Parasympathetic stimulants such as pilocarpine are usually ordered, as are cardiac and respiratory stimulants. For contraindications, see above.	See above.
Hyoscyamine hydrobromide, N.F. (Daturine).	0.25 mg. t. or q.i.d. Oral or parenteral.	Available also as extract, fluid extract and tincture.			
Hyoscyamine sulfate, N.F.	0.25 mg. q. 4-6 h. Oral or parenteral.				
Levohyoscyamine sulfate (Anaspaz, Levsin).	0.125-0.250 mg. q. 4-6h. daily. Oral.	Antispasmodic, antisecretory.			
SCOPOLAMINE *(Hyoscine* [C]). *Active principle of Scopolia atropoides. Synthetic.*		General uses same as those of belladonna.	Similar to belladonna. It exerts a depressant action on brain, heart and respiration	As above.	
Methscopolamine bromide, N.F. (Pamine, Scoline) (hyoscine methobromide, scopolamine methobromide [C]).	2.5-5 mg. t.i.d. and h.s. Oral.				
Methscopolamine nitrate (Epoxytropine tropate methylnitrate).	2-4 mg. t.i.d. and h.s. Also prepared for S.Q. and I.M. use and in delayed action tablets.				
Scopolamine aminoxide hydrobromide (Genoscopolamine) (hyoscine aminoxide [C]).	0.5 mg. Oral.				Scopolamine aminoxide hydrobromide is less apt to produce tolerance than scopolamine.
Scopolamine hydrobromide, U.S.P. (hyoscine hydrobromide) (Isopto-Hyoscine [C]).	0.2-0.5% solution. Topical. In eye. 0.3-0.6 mg. Oral or parenteral.			Tolerance may develop with prolonged use.	Scopolamine hydrobromide as a preoperative medication produces less tenacious sputum than atropine.
STRAMONIUM. *Datura stramonium.* Stramonium leaves.	None specified. Inhalation.	General uses same as those of belladonna. Used mainly in bronchial asthma.	Similar to belladonna.	Toxic symptoms rare but are the same as for atropine.	Leaves are burned and the smoke inhaled as a palliative treatment for asthma.

SYNTHETIC PARASYMPATHOLYTIC DRUGS

These drugs resemble the natural alkaloids in general structure or are simple bases with a trivalent nitrogen. They have a central nervous system effect as well as a ganglionic effect. These are all synthetic preparations. A number of drugs similar to atropine are listed here. Since lack of space prohibits inclusion of much detailed information, this list is not comprehensive. Almost all members of this group are available in combination with a barbiturate.

Alverine citrate (Spacolin).	120 mg. t.i.d. Oral.	Similar to atropine.	Similar to atropine.	Similar to atropine.	
Anisotropine methylbromide (Valpin 50).	50 mg. a.c. tablets or elixir. Oral.	Similar to atropine.	Similar to atropine.	Toxicity similar to that of atropine.	Safe use during pregnancy has not been established.
Clidinium bromide (Quarzan).	2.5-5 mg. t. or q.i.d. Individually adjusted (a.c. and h.s.). Oral.	Adjunct in peptic ulcer therapy.	As above.	As above.	
Dicyclomine hydrochloride, N.F. (Benacol, Bentyl, Dyspas) (dicycloverine, Bentylol [C]).	5-20 mg. t.i.d. or q.i.d. Individually adjusted. Oral. I.M.	General uses same as those of belladonna. Used mainly as an antispasmodic.	Similar to atropine, but it is not a secretory depressant.	Toxicity rare, but similar to that of atropine when it occurs.	
Oxybutynin chloride (Ditropan).	5 mg. b. or t.i.d. maximum: 5 mg. q.i.d.	Symptoms associated with voiding in patients with uninhibited neurogenic and reflex neurogenic bladder.	Has direct antispasmodic effect on smooth muscle and inhibits the muscarinic effect of acetylcholine on smooth muscle but has no blocking effects at skeletal neuromuscular junction or autonomic ganglia.	Similar to that of atropine.	
Oxyphencyclimine hydrochloride, N.F. (Daricon, Vio-Thene).	10 mg. Usually given b.i.d. Oral.	Anticholinergic used similarly to atropine.	Similar to atropine.	Toxicity similar to that of atropine.	
Piperidolate hydrochloride (Dactil).	50 mg. q.i.d. Oral.	Used as an antispasmodic, especially to control spasms of the stomach, upper intestinal tract and gall bladder. Not used to treat gastric ulcers.	Similar to the peripheral action of atropine. Depresses muscular action but not secretion.	Toxicity rare in therapeutic dosage.	

Name, Source, Synonyms, Preparations	Dosage and Administration	Uses	Action and Fate	Side Effects and Contraindications	Nursing Implications and Remarks
SYNTHETIC PARASYMPATHOLYTIC DRUGS (Continued)					
	This group contains a quaternary nitrogen and has lessened central nervous system effect and accentuated ganglionic effects, but absorption after oral use is usually incomplete. These are all synthetic preparations. Many members of this group are available in combination with a barbiturate.				
Diphemanil methylsulfate, N.F. (Prantal) (diphenmethanil [C]).	100-200 mg. q. 4-6 h. between meals. Oral. 2% cream, topical.	General uses same as those of belladonna. Used mainly as an anticholinergic agent to control peptic ulcers. Reduces pain, pyrosis and nausea. Also used to treat hyperhidrosis and as an antipruritic.	Similar to atropine.	Toxic symptoms rare, but similar to those of atropine when they occur.	The effects last longer than those of methantheline bromide.
Glycopyrrolate, N.F. (Robinul) (glycopyrronium bromide [C]).	1-2 mg. t.i.d. Oral. 0.2 mg./kg. S.Q., I.M., I.V. at 4 hour intervals t.i.d. or q.i.d.	An anticholinergic with uses and actions similar to those of others of this group; management of gastric and duodenal ulcers.	Similar to others of this group. G.I. absorption poor. Metabolic fate not known. Excreted in bile and urine.	Similar to others of this group. Safe use in pregnancy not established.	Parenteral administration may cause burning sensation at site of injection.
Hexocyclium methylsulfate (Tral).	25 mg. q.i.d. Oral. Also available as sustained release tablets given b.i.d.	As above.	As above.	Toxicity similar to that of atropine.	
Isopropamide iodide, N.F. (Darbid).	5 mg. Usually q. 12 h. Individually adjusted. Oral.	Used for gastric ulcers and for hypermotility of the gastrointestinal tract.	Similar to hyoscyamine but longer lasting. Inhibits gastric secretion and motility.	Toxicity similar to that of hyoscyamine.	
Mepenzolate methylbromide, N.F. (Cantil) (glycophenylate bromide [C]).	25 mg. Usually q.i.d. Individually adjusted. Oral.	Used mainly in conditions in which hypermotility of the lower bowel is a problem.	Similar to others of this group	Toxicity similar to that of atropine. Reduction of dosage is usually sufficient treatment.	

Methantheline bromide, N.F. (Banthine).	50-100 mg. q. 6 h. Individually adjusted. Oral or I.M.	General uses same as those of belladonna. Used mainly as an anticholinergic agent to control peptic ulcers and in urinary tract spasm.	Similar to belladonna. Reduces both motility and hyperacidity.	Rare, but similar to those of atropine when they occur. Occasionally, urinary retention in prostatic hypertrophy. Treatment: none usually required, but when needed is the same as for atropine.
Oxyphenonium bromide (Antrenyl).	10 mg. q.i.d. Oral.	Used in gastric ulcers and similar conditions, also in place of atropine or scopolamine in preoperative medications.	Similar to atropine.	Toxicity similar to that of atropine.
Pentapiperide methylsulfate.	10-20 mg. q.i.d. Oral. As much as 30 mg. q.i.d. may be used. Best given a.c. and h.s.	Used for the treatment of peptic ulcers.	Similar to atropine.	See atropine.
Penthienate bromide, N.F. (Monodral [C]).	5-10 mg. q.i.d. Oral.	Used mainly in the management of peptic ulcers.	Similar to atropine.	Usually mild, but similar to atropine.
Pipenzolate bromide (Piptal).	5-10 mg. q.i.d. Oral.	Similar to atropine and used for the same purposes.	Similar to atropine.	Toxicity lower than that of atropine.
Propantheline bromide, U.S.P. (Pro-Banthine) (Banlin, NeoBanex, Novopantheline [C]).	15 mg. q.i.d. Oral. 30 mg. p.r.n. I.M. or I.V.	General uses same as those of belladonna. Used mainly as an anticholinergic agent to control peptic ulcers. Reduces both motility and hyperacidity.	Similar to atropine.	Toxic symptoms rare but similar to those of atropine when they occur. Occasional urinary retention in prostatic hypertrophy. There are fewer side effects than with methantheline. Treatment: none usually required, but when needed is the same as for atropine.
Tridihexethyl chloride, N.F. (Pathilon).	25-75 mg. t.i.d. or q.i.d. Oral. 10-20 mg. q. 6 h. parenteral.	Similar to others of this group.	Similar to others of this group.	Toxicity similar to that of atropine.

Name, Source, Synonyms, Preparations	Dosage and Administration	Uses	Action and Fate	Side Effects and Contraindications	Nursing Implications and Remarks
SYNTHETIC PARASYMPATHOLYTIC DRUGS (Continued)					
Valethamate bromide, N.F. (Murel).	10-20 mg. t.i.d. or q.i.d. Oral, I.M. or I.V.	Similar to the atropine-scopolamine drugs.	An anticholinergic, musculotropic, ganglionic blocking agent.	Toxicity similar to that of atropine.	
Parasympatholytics primarily used in treatment of Parkinson's disease, acting mainly on central nervous system. Contain tertiary nitrogen instead of quaternary, and are well absorbed after oral administration.					
Benztropine mesylate, N.F. (Cogentin).	0.5-2 mg. Doses individually adjusted. Oral or parenteral.	Used in the treatment of parkinsonism. Also with phenothiazines to decrease extrapyramidal effects, but only for first 90 days of therapy.	Has both anticholinergic and antihistaminic action.	Toxicity usually low but drug has cumulative action. Side effects may be those of either the cholinergic or antihistaminic drugs.	Usually started with small dose h.s. and increased as required. Adjustment of dosage will usually overcome side effects. With severe reactions, drug should be withdrawn.
Biperiden, N.F. (Akineton).	1-2 mg. three to four times daily. Dosage individually adjusted. Oral. Occasionally given I.M.	Used in treatment of Parkinson's disease and certain forms of spasticity. Also with phenothiazines to decrease extrapyramidal effects, but only during first 90 days of therapy.	Claimed to have greater myospasmolytic effect and less drying effect on salivary glands than atropine.	Side effects include blurring of vision, drowsiness, nausea and vomiting. Reduce dose and treat symptoms. Contraindicated in all forms of epilepsy, and caution should be observed in patients with glaucoma.	
Cycrimine hydrochloride, N.F. (Pagitane hydrochloride).	1.25-2.5 mg. Dosage individually adjusted up to 15 mg. daily. Oral.	As above.	As above.	Avoid using in patients with glaucoma, urinary retention or tachycardia.	Epigastric distress may be avoided by giving the drug with meals.
Procyclidine hydrochloride (Kemadrin).	2-5 mg. three to four times daily. Oral.	Used mainly in the palliative treatment of Parkinson's syndrome.	Similar to atropine.	Toxicity similar to that of atropine.	Safe use during pregnancy or for children has not been established. If used with phenothiazines, see note under uses of biperiden.

Trihexyphenidyl hydrochloride, U.S.P. (Artane, Tremin) (benzhexol, Novohexidyl, Trinexy [C]).	2-5 mg. t.i.d. or q.i.d. Oral.	General uses same as those of belladonna. Used mainly as an antispasmodic in such conditions as parkinsonism.	Similar to others of this group. Rapidly absorbed from G.I. tract. Metabolic fate unknown. Excreted in urine, probably as unchanged drug.	Toxic symptoms are rare.	If sialorrhea is troublesome, the drug should be given a.c.; with the elderly, administer p.c.

Several antihistamine agents are also used in the treatment of Parkinson's disease, such as chlorphenoxamine hydrochloride (Histol, Phenoxene), ethopropazide hydrochloride (Parsidol) and orphenadrine hydrochloride (Disipal).

Anticholinergic drugs used primarily for local effects in the eye. These are synthetic or semisynthetic drugs.

Cyclopentolate hydrochloride, U.S.P. (Cyclogyl) (Mydplegic [C]).	0.5-2% solution. Topical.	Used as a cycloplegic and mydriatic.	Action is that of mydriatic and cycloplegic.	Nontoxic in topical use.	
Eucatropine hydrochloride, U.S.P. (Euphthalmine).	2% solution. Topical.	As a mydriatic.	Action is mydriatic.	Toxicity low.	Contraindicated in patients with glaucoma.
Homatropine hydrobromide, U.S.P. (Isopto Homatropine).	2-5% solution. Topical.	As a mydriatic.	Action is that of mydriatic and cycloplegic.	Toxicity similar to that of atropine is rare.	
Homatropine methylbromide, N.F. (Homapin, Malcotran, Mesopin, Novatropine, Sed-Tens Ty-Med) (Isopto-Homatropine [C]).	10 mg. Oral.	Similar to atropine. Used in gastric ulcers, colitis and as a mydriatic.	Action similar to that of atropine.		
Tropicamide, U.S.P. (Mydriacyl).	0.5-1% Solution. Topical for use in eyes.	Used as a mydriatic and cycloplegic.	As above.	None unless ingested.	As above.

Name, Source, Synonyms, Preparations	Dosage and Administration	Uses	Action and Fate	Side Effects and Contraindications	Nursing Implications and Remarks
STIMULANTS					
AMMONIA. *Chemical.* Aromatic ammonia spirits.	2 ml. Oral; also administered by inhalation.	Used as an emergency cardiac and respiratory stimulant, especially in fainting.	Acts as a reflex stimulant by irritation of nerve endings.	Rare in therapeutic dosage. Treatment: none usually needed.	Alcohol is also a reflex stimulant of nerve endings but is a depressant after absorption. Administer oral doses well diluted in water.
AMPHETAMINE. *Synthetic.* Amphetamine phosphate, U.S.P. (Acogesic, Biphetacel, Profetamine, Raphetamine).	10 mg. daily in divided doses. Oral or parenteral.	Used systemically to stimulate the nervous system in narcolepsy. Used in hyperkinetic behavior disorders and as an anorexic agent (see column 6).	Stimulates the cerebral cortex, and if respiratory depression is present, this will be improved. After an oral dose, the individual is more alert and better able to work, and has a general feeling of euphoria. After a large dose physical exertion may be much increased, but when it has worn off, there is greater fatigue and depression than before and a longer period of rest is required. Readily absorbed and widely distributed in body fluids. Some is excreted unchanged by the kidneys. Fate of remainder not well understood.	Restlessness and insomnia, with severe overstimulation, cardiac failure. Treatment: symptomatic, and includes rest, quiet and sedation. Contraindicated in hypertension. Used with caution in thyrotoxicosis, acute coronary disease, cardiac decompensation and pregnancy. Amphetamine should not be given concurrently with the monoamine oxidase inhibitors as it can cause a hypertensive crisis. The therapeutic effectiveness of guanethidine is antagonized by the concurrent use of the amphetamines. Amphetamines and chlorpromazine are antagonistic to their effects on noradrenergic and dopaminergic receptors. This can be used to advantage in poisoning of amphetamine-like drugs	In most cases should not be given after 4:00 P.M. to avoid insomnia. Although amphetamine causes central nervous stimulation it should not be used by normal individuals to induce capacity for extra work. Amphetamines have a significant potential for abuse. In view of their short-term anorectic effect and rapid development of tolerance, they should be used only for limited periods and with extreme caution in weight reduction programs. Abrupt withdrawal following prolonged use of high doses may result in psychotic manifestations and lethargy, which may persist for weeks. Safe use in pregnancy not established. Parenteral doses are discontinued when the patient regains consciousness.
Amphetamine sulfate, N.F. (Amphedrine, Benzedrine).	10-20 mg. daily in divided doses. Oral.	Analeptic, to counteract overdoses of depressant drugs such as barbiturates.			
Benzphetamine hydrochloride, N.F. (Didrex).	25-150 mg. daily in divided doses. Oral.	Anorexigenic agent.			
Dextroamphetamine phosphate, N.F. (Dextro-Profetamine)	5 mg. b.i.d. Oral.				
Dextroamphetamine sulfate, U.S.P. (Dexedrine) (dexamphetamine, d-amphetamine, Dexellets, Novamphene [C]),	5 mg. b.i.d. Oral.	Has stronger C.N.S. action and lesser action on peripheral nervous system than amphetamine.			
Dextroamphetamine tannate Obotan, Synatan).	17.5 mg. Oral.				
Levamphetamine (Ad-nil) (levanfetamine [C]).	5 mg. b.i.d. Oral.	More potent in cardiovascular effects.			

				but concurrent therapeutic use is not pharmaceutically sound.	
Methamphetamine hydrochloride, U.S.P. (Amphedroxin, Methedrine, Desoxyn, Neodrine [C]).	2.5-7.5 mg. b.i.d. or t.i.d. Oral or parenteral.	Mild stimulant and biochemical corrective for treating metabolic deficiencies of the brain. Used in chronic headaches of psychogenic origin and in control of obesity. See warning under amphetamine.	See amphetamine. Local vacoconstriction with topical application to mucous membranes and may be used as nasal decongestant.	See amphetamine.	As above.
CAFFEINE. *Active principle of Thea sinensis, Coffea arabica, kola nut, guarana and yerba. Other active principles: theobromine, theophylline.* Caffeine citrated, N.F. Caffeine and sodium benzoate, U.S.P.	 200-300 mg. p.r.n. Not over 2.5 Gm. daily. Oral. 500 mg. p.r.n., usually not over 2.5 Gm. daily. Oral or I.M.	Is a general cerebral stimulant and analeptic. Caffeine is a component of many over-the-counter "pepper-uppers." It is a diuretic and general body stimulant. Will help relieve certain types of headache.	Is a descending central nervous system stimulant. Small doses affect the cerebrum mainly; larger doses, the brainstem, including the medulla. Large doses increase heart action and cause peripheral vasodilation. Absorption of caffeine is erratic. Salts of caffeine are more readily absorbed. Rapidly distributed throughout body tissues, readily crossing the placenta and blood-brain barrier. Metabolized in the liver. Excreted by kidneys as 1-methy uric acid and 1-methyl xanthine, about 10% unchanged.	Rarely severe; mild symptoms include insomnia, restlessness, nervousness, palpitation, nausea, vomiting. Functional cardiac symptoms may occur. Treatment: stop drug and give evacuants and sedatives. Tolerance may develop to the diuretic, cardiovascular and C.N.S. effects.	Caffeine is one of the xanthine drugs. The others are theobromine and theophylline (refer to Diuretics). Since most people drink either coffee or tea they are used to receiving a daily dose of caffeine; hence, they have a tolerance for the drug and do not usually develop toxic symptoms from using it as a drug.

DRUGS AFFECTING THE CENTRAL NERVOUS SYSTEM (Continued)

STIMULANTS *(Continued)*

Name, Source, Synonyms, Preparations	Dosage and Administration	Uses	Action and Fate	Side Effects and Contraindications	Nursing Implications and Remarks
DEANOL. *Synthetic.* From acetylcholine. Deanol acetamidobenzoate (Deaner).	25-100 mg. q.i.d. Oral Adjusted to individual response.	Possibly effective in the following: to increase attention span and to improve behavior in children with various problems.	Exact mechanism not known, but claimed to enhance action of an acetylcholinic precursor and make it more readily available in the cortex.	Toxicity relatively low. Contraindicated in convulsive states, such as grand mal epilepsy. Safe use in pregnancy not established.	When administered to children with minimal brain dysfunction, deanol has a gradual onset of action with therapeutic effects not usually apparent for 2-3 weeks.
METHYLPHENIDATE HYDROCHLORIDE. *Synthetic.* Methylphenidate hydrochloride, U.S.P. (Ritalin hydrochloride).	5-20 mg. two or three times daily. Oral. Adjusted to individual response.	Used systemically to stimulate the nervous system in narcolepsy and postencephalitic parkinsonism. Also used in the treatment of hyperkinetic children.	Action somewhat like that of amphetamine and caffeine. Affects heart and blood pressure less. Does not affect appetite. Given I.V. it markedly stimulates depressed respiratory function. Well absorbed from G.I. tract, with effects persisting from 3-6 hr. Metabolites excreted in urine within 6 hr. to 24 hr. and 90 hr. respectively.	Side effects usually mild; not used alone in agitated patients. Anorexia, dizziness, nausea, headache, palpitation, drowsiness. Treatment: reduce dosage or discontinue. Rarely causes insomnia. May lower the convulsive threshold. Should be used with caution in patients with hypertension. For interactions see under amphetamines. Can raise serum levels of phenytoin, but this is rare. May affect warfarin levels when the last two are given together. Patients should be closely monitored for toxic side effects.	Methylphenidate can be abused and patients on long-term therapy must be closely monitored. Safe use during pregnancy and lactation has not been established. Abrupt withdrawal after prolonged therapy may unmask severe depression as well as effects of chronic overactivity. The patient should be monitored closely at this time.
NIKETHAMIDE. *Synthetic.* Nikethamide, N.F. (Coramine, Nikorin) (Cardiamine, Kardonyl, [C]).	1-5 mg. Oral or parenteral.	Used mainly as an analeptic with cautious parenteral dosage adjustment.	Main action is stimulation of the medullary centers. Causes increase in respiration, and peripheral vasoconstriction. There is some	Narrow margin of safety. Side effects include general weakness, feeling of fear, sneezing, coughing, nausea, vomiting, sweating, muscle	Safe use in pregnancy not established. Treat overdose convulsions with I.V. diazepam or barbiturates.

			cortical stimulation and usually a rise in blood pressure. Well absorbed, with metabolites excreted in urine.	twitching and slight increases in blood pressure, pulse and respiratory rates. Results of overdosage include tremors and generalized convulsions.	
NUX VOMICA. *Strychnos nux-vomica.* Strychnine, brucine. Nux vomica tincture Strychnine nitrate Strychnine phosphate (Anoro). Strychnine sulfate	 1 ml. Oral. 2 mg. Oral. 2 mg. Oral. 2 mg. Oral.	Used mainly to increase muscle tone in conditions such as gastrointestinal stasis, paralysis and debility.	An ascending stimulant affecting the spinal cord first and the cerebrum last. The margin between therapeutic and toxic action is narrow. Readily absorbed and widely distributed. Rapidly inactivated by kidneys, within 10 hours.	Stiffness of neck muscles, risus sardonicus, tetanic convulsions. Treatment: early—lavage, chemical antidotes (charcoal, potassium permanganate, tannic acid); later—hypnotics, sedatives (barbiturates), artificial respiration.	Strychnine is the active principle of nux vomica. Its therapeutic value has been questioned but it is still used, especially in many proprietary "tonics." These drugs have largely been replaced by less toxic drugs.
PENTYLENETETRAZOL. *Synthetic.* Pentylenetetrazol, N.F. (Metrazol, Pentrazol, Petrolone) (pentetrazol [C]).	 100-300 mg. three to four times daily. Oral or parenteral.	Used mainly as a respiratory and cardiac stimulant in shock and collapse, asphyxia neonatorum and as an antidote in depressant drug poisoning. Oral therapy advocated for treatment of psychoses, senility and mental depression associated with old age.	Stimulates cerebral medullary centers and increases spinal reflexes, especially if depressed. Does not appear to stimulate the myocardium or the blood vessels. Readily absorbed, widely and evenly distributed throughout body fluids. Inactivated by the liver and excreted by the kidneys. Exact form when excreted is not known.	Few if any side effects with oral dosage. Burning sensation in mouth, esophagus and stomach; salivation, nausea, vomiting, colic and diarrhea. Other symptoms that may occur include diaphoresis, pallor, headache, palpitation, shallow respirations, convulsions and lockjaw. Treatment: as for shock; convulsions treated with parenteral diazepam or barbiturates.	Was used to induce convulsions in treatment of psychoses; largely replaced by electric therapy. Narrow margin of safety with parenteral therapy.

Name, Source, Synonyms, Preparations	Dosage and Administration	Uses	Action and Fate	Side Effects and Contraindications	Nursing Implications and Remarks
		ANOREXIC DRUGS *These are all synthetic preparations.*			
Chlorphentermine hydrochloride (Pre-Sate).	65 mg. each morning after breakfast.	For the treatment of obesity.	Similar to amphetamine (page 100) but claimed to have little or no effect on blood pressure.	Mydriasis, nausea, constipation, dry mouth, nervousness, insomnia, drowsiness, sedation, headache, urticaria and dizziness may occur. Contraindicated in glaucoma, hyperthyroidism, hypertension, cardiovascular disease and in patients receiving monoamine oxidase inhibitors. Safety for use during pregnancy has not been established. Not recommended for use by lactating women.	The use of these drugs, as with the amphetamines, concurrently with the phenothiazines is not pharmaceutically sound as they are antagonistic relative to their effects on noradrenergic and dopaminergic receptors in the nervous system.
Clortermine hydrochloride (Voranil).	50 mg. daily midmorning. Oral.	Used in management of exogenous obesity, but only for short adjunct therapy (few weeks).	Action similar to amphetamines. It is a sympathomimetic. Readily absorbed from the G.I. tract with onset of action in 1-2 h. and duration of 4-6 hr. Widely distributed; crosses the placenta of laboratory mice. Excreted in urine.	Side effects: palpitation, tachycardia, elevated blood pressure, central nervous system stimulation, dryness of mouth, diarrhea or constipation, unpleasant taste, urticaria, impotence, changes in libido. Contraindications: hyperthyroidism, hypersensitivity to drug, glaucoma, agitated states; during or for 14 days following use of monoamine oxidase inhibitors or in patients with history of drug abuse.	Safe use during pregnancy or for children not established. Patients should be warned about driving a car or engaging in potentially hazardous occupations as their ability to do so safely may be questionable. Has potential for "drug abuse."
Diethylpropion hydrochloride, N.F. (Naterexic, Tenuate, Tepanil, Regenon) (amfepramone [C]).	25 mg. Usually given t.i.d. ½ hour before meals. Oral.	As above.	Similar to amphetamine but claimed to have less central nervous system stimulation.	Rare, but oral dryness and constipation have been reported. Reduce dosage.	

	75 mg. sustained release o.m.		Rapidly absorbed, with effects persisting for 4 hr.	Contraindicated in patients on monoamine oxidase inhibitors.	
Fenfluramine hydrochloride (Pondimin).	20-40 mg. t.i.d. a.c. Oral.	Short-term adjunct therapy for wieght control.	Sympathomimetic amine but appears to produce more central nervous system depression than stimulation. Rapidly absorbed. Duration of effects 4-6 hr. Widely distributed in almost all body tissues. Metabolites and unchanged drug excreted in the urine.	Side effects. Most common: drowsiness, diarrhea and dry mouth. Drug can impair the ability of the patient to engage in potentially hazardous activities such as operating machinery or driving a motor vehicle. Contraindications: glaucoma, during or for 14 days following the use of monoamine oxidase inhibitors. Interactions: this drug can cause diarrhea and central nervous system depression unlike most other anorexic drugs. Therefore, other central nervous system depressants should be used concurrently with caution, if at all. Fenfluramine can increase slightly the effect of antihypertensive drugs such as guanethidine, reserpine and methyldopa.	This drug is related chemically to the amphetamines and should be used cautiously, if at all, in persons with a history of drug abuse and tolerance. Safe use in pregnancy and in children under 12 years of age has not been established.
Mazindol (Sanorex).	1 mg. t.i.d. one hour a.c. or: 2 mg. before noon meal. Oral.	Used for short-term management of exogenous obesity.	Isoindole, with some amphetamine-like action including central nervous system stimulation. It is believed to exert its effect primarily on the limbic system. Readily absorbed, onset of action within 1 h. and duration of 8-15 h. Metabolites and unchanged drug excreted in urine.	Side effects and contraindications: see fenfluramine. Use with caution in patients with hypertension and/or arhythmias. Insulin requirements may need adjustment in diabetic patients receiving this drug.	

Name, Source, Synonyms, Preparations	Dosage and Administration	Uses	Action and Fate	Side Effects and Contraindications	Nursing Implications and Remarks
Phendimetrazine bitartrate (Pegine) (Dietrol [C]).	35 mg. Usually given b.i.d. or t.i.d. Oral.	As above.	Similar to amphetamine.	Occasional insomnia and nervousness. Rarely may cause dryness of mouth, nausea, blurred vision, dizziness, constipation and stomach pain. Treatment: reduce or interrupt dosage. Contraindicated in presence of coronary disease, hypertension, thyrotoxicosis. Use with caution in highly nervous or agitated patients.	Safe use in pregnancy has not been established.
Phenmetrazine hydrochloride, N.F. (Preludin) (Anorex, Metrabese, Neo-zine, Phenmetrazinal, Phentrol, Probese, Willpower [C]).	25 mg. b. or t.i.d. ½ hour a.c. Oral. 75 mg. Sustained release o.m.	Used mainly in obesity and as a euphoriant.	Similar to amphetamine.	Same as amphetamine but said to be less toxic and to have fewer side effects. Contraindicated in advanced arteriosclerosis, cardiovascular disease, hypertension, hyperthyroidism or known hypersensitivity to sympathomimetic amines or in glaucoma.	As above. Do not use in patients with history of drug abuse.
Phentermine (Adipex, Ionamine, Wilpo).	15-30 mg. o.m. Oral.	Anorexic agent used to treat obesity.	Similar to amphetamine.	Rare, but dryness of mouth, insomnia and mild central nervous system stimulation may occur. Adjust dosage.	

TRICYCLIC ANTIDEPRESSANTS

These are synthetic drugs. In overdosing with the tricyclic antidepressants, the slow I.V. injection of physostigmine salicylate has been reported to reverse the cardiovascular and central nervous system effects of these drugs. The physostigmine may have to be repeated at 30- to 60-minute intervals because of its short period of action.

Amitriptyline (Elavil, Elatrol, Levate, Mareline, Novotriptyn [C]).	10-50 mg. t.i.d. Oral 20-30 mg. q.i.d. I.M. 100-200 mg. h.s.	Antidepressant for depression resulting from psychoses or neuroses; also has a tranquillizing action.	Readily absorbed. Rapidly disappears from circulating blood. Probably metabolized or conjugated. Precise mechanism of action unclear, but the tricyclic antidepressants have been shown to block in varying degrees, the re-uptake of various neurotransmitters at the neuronal membranes. This may potentiate the effects of norepinephrine and serotonin. In addition, they exhibit strong anticholinergic activity. Most preparations are well absorbed from the G.I. tract. Their active metabolites are highly bound to plasma and tissue proteins. Distribution and metabolism varies with preparations. Primary route of excretion is urinary. Rate of excretion varies among drugs in this classification.	Frequent: atropine-like effects, hypotension, drowsiness, weight gain. Occasional: manic episodes, tremor, first-degree heart block, tachycardia and other arhythmias, rashes, facial sweating. Rare: cholestatic jaundice, bone marrow depression including agranulocytosis, epileptiform seizures, peripheral neuropathy, severe cardiovascular effects in patients with cardiac disease and photosensitization. Contraindication: glaucoma and urinary retention. Drug interactions: potentiation of sympathomimetic amines and C.N.S. depressants; antagonizes effects of guanethidine and causes convulsions and hypertensive crises with MAO inhibitors. (Atropine-like effects include dry mouth, mydriasis, cycloplegia, urinary retention, decreased G.I. motility, tachycardia and, in high doses, delirium.) Not recommended during acute recovery phase following myocardial infarction.	Most tricyclic antidepressants can be administered as a single dose either in the a.m. or h.s., depending on the side effects experienced by the patient. Administration of a single dose may increase compliance. Preparations are not terminated abruptly in patients who received large doses for prolonged periods. Maximum antidepressant effects from most tricyclics may not occur for 2 or more weeks after therapy is begun. Depressed patients are prone to suicidal tendencies. Appropriate supportive care should be initiated. Amitriptyline has been reported to increase plasma levels of dicumarol and increase prothrombin time in patients stabilized on warfarin. Safe use in pregnancy or lactation has not been established. Chlordiazepoxide, in combination with amitriptyline (Limbitrol 10-25 or 5-12.5) is also avilable. Same side effects and contraindications as amitriptyline.

Name, Source, Synonyms, Preparations	Dosage and Administration	Uses	Action and Fate	Side Effects and Contraindications	Nursing Implications and Remarks
TRICYCLIC ANTIDE-PRESSANTS (Continued)					
Desipramine hydrochloride, N.F. (Norpramin, Pertofrane) (desmethylimipramine [C]).	25-50 mg. t.i.d. Oral. (150 mg./day is maximum).	Main use is in depression of a psychogenic origin.	Relatively quick antidepressant that does not produce euphoria. Exact mode of action is not known. Absorption and excretion similar to amitriptyline.		Liver and blood tests should be done during prolonged therapy even though toxicity has not been observed in respect to liver and blood. Safe use during pregnancy has not been established.
Doxepin hydrochloride (Adapin, Sinequan).	75-300 mg. daily. Oral. Dosage individually adjusted.	Used for anxiety and depression such as occurs in alcoholism, psychotic disorders, involutional depression and manic-depressive reactions.	See tricyclic antidepressants. Well absorbed orally and rapidly metabolized.	Reported incidence of side effects is low. Apparently well tolerated by most geriatric patients.	See tricyclic antidepressants. Oral solutions should be well diluted with at least 120 ml. of water, milk, citrus or pineapple juice. The solution is physically incompatible with carbonated beverages.
Imipramine hydrochloride, N.F. (Presamine, Tofranil) (Chem-Ipramine, Imipramine, Impram, Impranil, Impril, Novopramine [C]).	Dosage should be determined for individual patient. Maintenance dose usually 50-150 mg. daily. Oral and parenteral.	Main use as an antidepressant in psychoses and non-psychotic conditions with depressed emotional tone. Used in the treatment of enuresis.	Mechanism of action is not known. See amitriptyline.	See tricyclics.	Caution: should not be given concurrently with or for 14 days after treatment with monoamine oxidase inhibitors. See tricyclics.
Nortriptyline hydrochloride, N.F. (Aventyl, Pamelor) (Acetexa, Avantyl [C]).	25 mg. t.i.d. Adjusted to suit patient's response. Oral.	Used in depression, anxiety and psychosomatic disorders.	Exact mode of action not well established. See amitriptyline.		
Protriptyline hydrochloride (Vivactil) (Triptil [C]).	15-40 mg. daily in divided doses t.i.d. or q.i.d. Oral.	Relief of symptoms of depression in the depressed patient who is under close medical supervision.	This drug is chemically related to amitriptyline. Rapid onset of antidepressant action usually without tranquilizing or sedative effects often within one week. Has autonomic	Side effects are very numerous (see commercial brochure for side effects and precautions). Some of the side effects are: tachycardia, postural hypotension, drowsiness	Exposure to sunlight should be avoided during treatment with protriptyline. See tricyclics.

			effects, including potentiation or prolonged effects of norepinephrine and by stimulation of sympathetic nerves. It reduces or blocks the effects of indirect sympathetic amines such as amphetamine, tyramine or phenethylamine. It antagonizes the prolonged depletion of tissue catecholamines by quanethidine and alpha-methylmetatyrosine. It has relatively weak anticholinergic properties. Well absorbed from G.I. tract and excreted in urine. Crosses the placenta.	(occasionally) and such things as bad taste, dry mouth, dystonia, tremors, fatique, weakness, blurring of vision, mental confusion and many others.	
MONOAMINE OXIDASE INHIBITORS					
Isocarboxazid, N.F. (Marplan).	Initially 30 mg. daily (10 mg. t.i.d.); then reduce to 10-20 mg. daily. Doses over 30 mg. daily are not recommended. Oral.	Used in moderate and severe depressive states in adults.	This is a monoamine oxidase inhibitor and raises both the serotonin and norepinephrine levels. Readily absorbed. Thought to be rather rapidly excreted, but it takes some time for enzyme to be reactivated. Exact fate not known. Action is cumulative; it may take a few days to several months for effects of the drug to be recognized. Effects may persist for up to 3 weeks after discontinuing.	Frequent: hypotension, restlessness, insomnia, dry mouth, nausea, dizziness, constipation and anorexia. Occasional: flushing, urinary retention, tremors, impotence, paresthesias. Rare: skin rash, hepatitis, tinnitus, muscle spasm and mania. Contraindicated in patients with severe impairment of liver or renal function, cardiovascular disease, pheochromocytoma, epilepsy or pregnancy.	Interactions that may occur up to 2 weeks after last dose of drug include hypertensive crises in patients receiving a sympathomimetic amine concurrently with MAO inhibitors, or if food containing tyramine or other amines such as ripe cheeses, fava beans, avocado, pickled herring, chicken livers, fermented bologna, salami, canned figs, chocolate, beer, sherry, chianti and so on is eaten. When given with tricyclics, convulsions and hypertensive crises have been observed.

Name, Source, Synonyms, Preparations	Dosage and Administration	Uses	Action and Fate	Side Effects and Contraindications	Nursing Implications and Remarks
MONOAMINE OXIDASE INHIBITORS (Continued)					
Phenelzine dihydrogen sulfate (Nardil).	15 mg. t.i.d. for treatment; maintenance dose 15 mg. once dailv. Oral.	Use and action similar to those of isocarboxazid.	Monoamine oxidase inhibitor. See isocarboxazid for absorption data.	As above.	Meperidine should not be used for patients on the monoamine oxidase inhibitors since the combination can have catastrophic results.
Tranylcypromine sulfate, N.F. (Parnate).	20 mg. given 10 mg. twice daily to start. May increase to a total of 30 mg. per day. Oral.	Used to treat various states of depression.	Monoamine oxidase inhibitor. See isocarboxazid for absorption data.	As above, but many contraindications; see manufacturer's pamphlet before using this drug.	Caution: Use only in hospitalized patients or patients in whom all other drugs have been ineffective; do not use in patients over 60 or those with a history of hypertension.
OTHER ANTIDEPRESSANTS					
Pipradrol hydrochloride, N.F. (Meratran).	1-2.5 mg. morning and noon. Oral.	Used mainly to counteract depression.	A mild cerebral stimulant producing elevation of mood, increased ability to work and to concentrate and increased confidence. Has little effect on pulse, blood pressure or respirations.	Side effects rare and mild. May produce insomnia, excitability and anorexia.	
			DEPRESSANTS		
INTOXICANTS					
ALCOHOL. *Synthetic*					
Alcohol, dehydrated, N.F. (Absolute Alcohol).	99% by volume Rarely used.	Used for temporary reflex stimulation in certain cases of shock or fainting.	Initial effects: increased heart and respiratory rate, superficial vasodilation, rise in blood pressure, increase in flow of digestive juices.	Alcohol can interact with a large number of compounds. These include the following. With the tricyclic antidepressants, there is an	Nongrain alcohols such as methyl, denatured, isopropyl, butyl, etc., are never used for internal administration because
Alcohol, U.S.P. (ethyl alcohol, ethanol).	95% by volume. Rarely used.	Used to increase appetite and as nerve block.			

	5% alcohol in 5-10% dextrose solution. I.V.	Antifoaming agent in the treatment of acute pulmonary edema secondary to left heart failure, and to retard premature labor in selected cases. Analgesia and sedation when narcotics contraindicated.	Later effect: depression. Many authorities feel no effective stimulation is secured from alcohol. Absorption from the stomach varies with the amount of food it contains. Rapid if empty. From the intestines absorption is rapid with or without food. Widely distributed throughout the body and crosses the placenta. Most is oxidized by liver or other tissues. About 2-10% is excreted unchanged by the kidney. Progressive descending depression starting with the higher cerebral centers, gradually descending to the brainstem medulla and in large doses to the spinal cord.	impairment of motor function, especially in the first few days of antidepressant therapy. Alcohol can accentuate occult blood loss and damage to gastric mucosa induced by aspirin. This is important clinically in patients taking 2 to 3 Gm. of aspirin daily. With the barbiturates or chloral hydrate, the depressant action of each drug is increased over its action if taken alone. This can be very serious. With chlordiazepoxide, there is some enhancement. With diazepam or meprobamate, the potential for central nervous system depression is in proportion to the alcoholic intake. With the monoamine oxidase inhibitors, there is a possible interaction with alcohol other than the reaction with the high tyramine beverages, wine and beer. Patients treated with tolbutamide and who regularly consume considerable alcohol will metabolize the tolbutamide at a much more rapid rate than is usual. The half-life may be reduced 50% of the expected time.	of toxicity. When administered I.V., the patient should be observed frequently and if signs of inebriation appear, the rate of flow should be decreased. Contraindicated in pregnancy especially during the first trimester.
Brandy (spiritus vini vitis). Diluted alcohol.	51% by volume. Oral. 49% by volume. Rarely used.				Brandy and whiskey must be aged in wood at least 4 years.
Whiskey (spiritus frumenti).	50% by volume. Oral.				
Wines.	Concentration varies. Oral.	Sometimes ordered for relaxation and vasodilation, especially h.s. for the elderly patient.			Many types and strengths of wines are used medicinally, especially to increase appetite.

Name, Source, Synonyms, Preparations	Dosage and Administration	Uses	Action and Fate	Side Effects and Contraindications	Nursing Implications and Remarks
ANALGESICS					
NARCOTICS, OPIUM.					
OPIUM. *(Morphine, codeine, thebaine, narcotine, papaverine). Papaver somniferum.*		Used to relieve pain, to induce sleep (especially when sleep is prevented by pain), to check peristalsis, to suppress cough, to relieve dyspnea. Also used as preoperative medication, to check diarrhea and reduce excitement and convulsions. Morphine, codeine and thebaine affect the cerebral cortex mainly. Morphine relieves pain, and codeine reduces cough; thebaine has same effect but to a minor degree. Papaverine relaxes muscle tissue, especially smooth muscles. Narcotine (noscopine, nectadon) also relaxes smooth muscle tissue and reduces cough.	The exact method of action is not known, but it depresses the cerebral cortex and probably the thalami. Opium (morphine) produces mood elevation, euphoria, and relief of fear and apprehension. Slows both mental and physical activity. It is a strong respiratory depressant, but affects heart and blood pressure to only a minor degree. The cough center is depressed and gastrointestinal motility decreased. Other effects include increase in perspiration, contraction of pupils and relaxation of muscle tissues. The fate of the different alkaloids varies. Morphine is absorbed from the gastrointestinal tract, but the rate and amount are unpredictable. Morphine is widely distributed throughout the body and though its main effect is in the central nervous system, most of the drug is not concentrated in	Acute poisoning. Early symptoms include mental stimulation, physical ease, rapid pulse. Later symptoms are dizziness, nausea, languor, slow weak pulse, pinpoint pupils, slow respirations, cyanosis. Terminally there is Cheyne-Stokes respiration, coma and death. Treatment: naloxone (Narcan) given parenterally, lavage, colon flush, purgation, central nervous stimulants. A respirator and intravenous drugs such as nikethamide or doxapram (Dopram) may be ordered. Chemotherapeutic drugs and antibiotics may be used to combat pneumonia. Undesirable side effects of opium and particularly of morphine are common and include constipation, nausea, vomiting, itching, diaphoresis.	Heroin, morphine and propoxyphene have been shown to appear in breast milk.
Opium powdered, U.S.P.	60 mg. p.r.n. for pain. Oral or rectal.				
Opium tincture (laudanum).	0.6 ml. p.r.n. for pain or diarrhea. Oral.				
Paregoric, U.S.P. (opium camphorated tincture).	2-10 ml. Oral. p.r.n. for diarrhea and dysmenorrhea.				

Pantopium hydrochloride (Pantopon).	5-20 mg. q. 3-4 h. p.r.n. for pain. Oral or parenteral.		the cerebrospinal fluid. It is taken up mainly by the spleen, liver, lungs and kidneys and crosses the placenta. Morphine is conjugated with glucuronic acid and exreted mainly in conjugated form by the kidneys. About 90% is excreted in 24 hours after usual dose. Other alkaloids such as codeine, heroin and the morphine surrogates are metabolized by the liver and excreted by the kidneys.		Pantopon is a mixture of the purified alkaloids of opium in the same proportions as in crude opium.
ANTISPASMODIC PREPARATIONS DERIVED FROM OPIUM					
Ethaverine hydrochloride (Ethaquin, Harverine, Neopavrin A, Papertherine, Verina) (ethylpapaverine [C]).	100-200 mg. t.i.d. Oral. 15-100 mg. I.V.	An antispasmodic similar to but more effective than papaverine. Used in peripheral or cerebral vascular insufficiency associated with arterial spasm.	The tetraethyl analog of papaverine.	Toxicity similar to that of papaverine but not as severe. Use with caution in glaucoma. Its use is contraindicated in complete arterioventricular dissociation.	Not a narcotic drug.
Papaverine hydrochloride, N.F. (Pavabid).	30-60 mg. I.M. or slowly I.V. 100-200 mg. three to five times daily. Oral.				Papaverine is an antispasmodic and not an analgesic. See under spasmolytics.

Name, Source, Synonyms, Preparations	Dosage and Administration	Uses	Action and Fate	Side Effects and Contraindications	Nursing Implications and Remarks
ANTISPASMODIC PREPARATIONS DERIVED FROM OPIUM (Continued)	*Preparations from or similar to opium. Morphine and morphine type: some derived directly from opium, some semisynthetic, others entirely synthetic.*				
Apomorphine. See under Emetics.					
Morphine sulfate, U.S.P.	8-15 mg. q. 3 h. p.r.n. Oral or parenteral.	Analgesia.	Morphine crosses the placenta and can cause neonatal addiction, respiratory depression and has been responsible for some neonatal deaths.	See opium.	Absorption from the G.I. tract is erratic; thus the parenteral route is preferred.
Codeine phosphate, U.S.P.	15-30-60 mg. q. 3-4 h. p.r.n. Oral or parenteral.	For pain and is found in many cough preparations.			
Codeine sulfate, N.F.	15-30-60 mg. q. 3-4 h. p.r.n. Oral or parenteral.				
Dextromethorphan hydrobromide, N.F. (Romilar, Tussade).	5-15 mg. p.r.n. for cough. Oral.	A morphine derivative used mainly in the control of cough.	Depresses the cough center mainly. Does not have analgesic property.	Similar to other narcotics. Toxicity low.	
Diamorphine hydrochloride (diacetyl-morphine, heroin).		See opium.	See opium.	See opium.	Heroin is not legally available in the United States or Canada.
Ethylmorphine hydrochloride, N.F. (Dionin).	16 mg. p.r.n. Oral or I.M. 1-5% solution. Topical.	As an expectorant. As an anodyne for ophthalmic use.			
Fentanyl (Sublimaze).	Given I.M. or I.V. Brochure should be consulted for specific dosage, which varies from 0.025-0.1 mg.	Narcotic analgesic; main use is in anesthesia.	With I.V. use, full effect in 3-5 minutes, lasts 30-60 minutes. With I.M. onset in 7-8 minutes, duration 1-2 hours. For further action see narcotic analgesics.	Contraindicated in children under 2 or women during pregnancy as safety has not been demonstrated. Main toxic effect is respiratory depression. Not recommended for use with monoamine oxidase inhibitors. When used with other depressants dose should be reduced. For further information see narcotic analgesics.	Drug also available in combination with droperidol (Innovar).
Hydrocodone bitartrate, N.F. (Dicodid, Mercodinone) (dihydrocodeinone bitartrate, Hycodan [C]).	5-15 mg. p.r.n. Oral or parenteral.	Uses and action similar to those of codeine.	Similar to codeine.	Similar to codeine.	

Hydromorphone hydrochloride, N.F. (Dilaudid, Hymorphan) (dihydromorphinone hydrochloride [C]).	2.0-3.0 mg. p.r.n. Oral or parenteral.	For pain.	Similar to morphine.	Similar to morphine.	
Levorphanol tartrate, N.F. (Levo-Dromoran) (levorphan [C]). Methorphinan (Dromoran).	2-3 mg. q. 3-4 h. p.r.n. Oral or parenteral. 2.5-5 mg. q. 3-4 h. p.r.n. Oral or parenteral.	Use is similar to that of morphine when given parenterally and to methadone when administered orally.	Analgesic action similar to that of morphine. Has less effect on smooth muscle tissue than morphine.	Same as for morphine, but much less severe. Treatment same as for morphine. Can cross placenta and cause neonatal respiratory depression.	Tolerance is developed with long usage.
Metopon hydrochloride.	3 mg. p.r.n. Oral.	Used mainly in cancer, as it relieves pain when taken orally.	Similar to morphine.	Rare in therapeutic dosage. Treatment: none usually required. Has few side effects.	Does not produce tolerance quickly.
Oxycodone (available in combination products: Percodan (aspirin, phenacetin and caffeine), Percobarb (hexobarbital, homatropine, aspirin, phenacetin and caffeine), Tylox (acetaminophen).	1 tab q. 6 h. p.c. or with meals. Oral.	Analgesic for mild-moderate pain.	Similar to hydrocodone. Well absorbed. Detoxified in liver and kidney. Primarily excreted in urine.	Milder than morphine but usual precautions should be initiated. Addiction is possible.	Cautions of combination product ingredients must be observed.
Oxymorphone, N.F. (Numorphan).	1-15 mg. q. 4-6 h. I.M or S.Q. 5 mg. q. 4-6 h. Rectal.	A potent analgesic.	Similar to morphine in analgesic effect but with less respiratory depression, nausea and constipation.	Relatively low, but respiratory depression, nausea and constipation may occur. Treatment: symptomatic.	May be habit forming.
Phenazocine (Prinadol) (Xenagol [C]).	2 mg. q. 4-6 h. p.r.n. I.M.	A synthetic narcotic used as adjunct to anesthesia, for postoperative pain, obstetrics and acute and chronic pain of all kinds, including cancer.	Synthetic molecule similar to morphine; claimed to have fewer sedative and hypotensive effects.	Watch for respiratory depression, which can be corrected with levallorphan or nalorphine. Contraindications: hepatic disorders, coma, increased intracranial pressure, convulsions, acute alcoholism, myxedema.	

Name, Source, Synonyms, Preparations	Dosage and Administration	Uses	Action and Fate	Side Effects and Contraindications	Nursing Implications and Remarks
ANALGESICS (Continued)					
MEPERIDINE GROUP. *Synthetic narcotic preparations.* Meperidine hydrochloride, N.F. (Demerol, Dolosal) (isonipecaine, pethidine, Phytadon [C]).	25-100 mg. q. 3-4 h. p.r.n. Oral or parenteral.	Widely used as an analgesic and sedative. Used to produce analgesia in obstetrics.	A descending central nervous system depressant. It is analgesic and sedative, but does not cause constipation or pupillary constriction as does morphine. May produce temporary euphoria. Respiratory depression occurs only with very high dosage. These drugs are readily absorbed from most routes. They are demethylated and conjugated by the liver and excreted by the kidneys. Very little is excreted unchanged. Appears in mother's milk.	Lowering of blood pressure, bradycardia, shock, vasodilation (nitritoid reaction), dizziness, nausea, vomiting, Treatment: symptomatic. Meperidine should not be given to patients taking monoamine oxidase inhibitors because of possible catastrophic results, including convulsions, excitation, hypertension and, less often, hypotension and hallucinations.	Can be given orally but is less effective. May cause habituation or addiction. Is available as an oral syrup, which should be administered with 120 ml. water, since undiluted syrup may produce slight topical anesthesia on mucous membrane. Local tissue irritation and induration may occur with frequent S.Q. injection.
Alphaprodine hydrochloride, N.F. (Nisentil).	40-60 mg. q. 3-4 h. p.r.n. for pain. S.Q. or I.V.	Used for quick short-duration analgesia.	Produces mild euphoria, sedation, dizziness, itching and sweating. Has little or no cumulative action. Duration of action less than meperidine.	Rare in therapeutic dosage. Treatment: none usually required. Can cross placenta and cause neonatal respiratory depression, if given late in labor.	Tolerance may develop. Addiction is rare.
Anileridine, N.F. (Leritine).	25-50 mg. q. 3-4 h. p.r.n. for pain. Oral or parenteral.	Uses much like those of other synthetic narcotics, especially meperidine.	Similar to meperidine.	Similar to other synthetic narcotics.	The drug comes as several salts: phosphate salt for oral use, hydrochloride for parenteral.
Ethoheptazine citrate, N.F. (Zactane).	75 mg., 1-2 tablets three to four times daily. Oral.	Uses similar to those of aspirin.	The analgesic action is similar to that of synthetic analgesics of the meperidine group but it is much less potent and is said not to have the addiction property.	Side effects similar to meperidine, but usually are less severe and occur less often.	
METHADONE GROUP Methadone hydrochloride, U.S.P. (Adanon, Dolophine, Miadone, Polamidon).	5-10 mg. q. 3-4 h. p.r.n. Parenteral. 5-10 mg. q. 3-4 h. p.r.n. Oral.	Used to relieve pain in trauma, myalgia, dysmenorrhea, and cancer. Also used in opium withdrawal and in	Similar to morphine. Less euphoria occurs. Respiratory depression occurs except in low dosage. Does not	Nausea, vomiting, dizziness, and drowsiness may occur. Treatment: symptomatic. Drug crosses placenta and	

	Dose for maintenance and withdrawal is quite variable.	maintenance programs.	cause constipation. Readily absorbed. Concentrated mainly in liver, spleen, lungs and kidneys. Degraded mainly by the liver and excreted by the kidneys. Excretion is relatively slow. Less than 10% is excreted unchanged.	can cause respiratory depression in fetus and also dependence if mother is dependent.	
MISCELLANEOUS ANALGESICS					
Synthetic.					
Butorphanol tartrate (Stadol).	1-4 mg. I.M. or 0.5-2 mg. I.V. q. 3-4 h.	Analgesia in moderate to severe pain.	Induces analgesia similar to morphine, meperidine or pentazocine with duration of action 3-4 h. Has narcotic antagonist activity comparable to nalorphine. Low physical dependence.	Sedation, nausea, clammy sweating, headache, vertigo, dizziness, confusion, lightheadedness as well as other C.N. S. effects. Respiratory depression similar to morphine. Increases workload of heart and is contraindicated in coronary patients. Because of its narcotic antagonist action is contraindicated for narcotic addicts lest it precipitate withdrawal symptoms.	Safe use in pregnancy not established. Exercise precautions in administering to patients with emotional instability, history of drug misuse, asthma or coronary disease.
Mefenamic acid (Ponstel) (Ponstan [C]).	250 mg. Oral. p.r.n.	Relief of pain when therapy will not exceed one week.	For complete action see commercial brochure. Action differs in quality from the anti-inflammatory effects of the glucocorticoids. It is independent of the pituitary adrenal system and is not associated with depression of general growth. Absorbed slowly with high percentage bound to plasma proteins. Analgesic effects may last up to 6 h. Metabol-	Contraindicated in intestinal ulceration, children and women of child-bearing potential. Used with caution in inflammatory diseases of the gastrointestinal tract, known asthma and renal dysfunction. If rash or diarrhea occurs, drug should be stopped.	Low order of toxicity, with most frequent side effects involving G.I. and neurological systems. Margin of safety reduced at higher doses and longer administration.

Name, Source, Synonyms, Preparations	Dosage and Administration	Uses	Action and Fate	Side Effects and Contraindications	Nursing Implications and Remarks
MISCELLANEOUS ANALGESICS (Continued)			ized in part by liver, excreted in urine, bile and feces.		
Methotrimeprazine, N.F. (Levoprome) (levomepromazine, Nozinan [C]).	5-40 mg. at intervals of q. 1-24 h. Usual dosage 10-20 mg. q. 4-6 h. Deep I.M.	Relief of pain in chronic illness. For obstetric and pre- and postoperative analgesia.	Analgesia. 10-20 mg. said to be as effective as 10-15 mg. morphine or 50-100 mg. meperidine. This is a phenothiazine derivative and has antiemetic and tranquilizing action. Actively metabolized and largely excreted in urine as such. Elimination into urine usually continues for several days after the drug is discontinued.	Contraindications: addiction to drugs, coma, overt or incipient uropathy, hypotension, severe cardiac or renal disease. Side effects: main side effect is orthostatic hypotension, which usually clears after a few doses. Other side effects: amnesia, disorientation, dizziness, drowsiness, weakness, slurring of speech, gastrointestinal disturbances, nasal congestion, chills, difficulty in urination, uterine inertia. Pain may occur at site of injection. With prolonged use jaundice and agranulocytosis may occur.	Do not give I.V. or subcutaneously. Has been shown to have additive effect and dosage should be reduced with antihypertensive drugs, barbiturates, atropine, reserpine and meprobamate. If a vasopressor is required, phenylephrine is preferred. Epinephrine may cause a paradoxical lowering of the blood pressure. Has not been shown to be addictive. Do not give to children under 14 years of age. Ambulation should be supervised for at least 6 h. following administration of the drug because of the orthostatic hypotension, dizziness and possible fainting that may occur.
Pentazocine, N.F. (Talwin).	30-60 mg. S.Q., I.M. or I.V. q. 3-4 h. 50-100 mg. q. 3-4 h. Oral.	Supposedly nonaddicting, narcotic type analgesic. However, special care must be exercised in prescribing this drug for emotionally unstable patients and those with a history of drug abuse, since there have been cases of psychological and physiological dependence in such patients.	Congeners similar to nalorphine and levallorphan. Analgesia usually occurs within 15-20 minutes after I.M. or subcutaneous injection, 2-3 minutes after I.V. and 30-60 minutes after an oral dose. Pentazocine has about 1/50 of the effect of nalorphine as an antagonist. Not as well absorbed from G.I. tract as from parenteral	Drowsiness, vertigo, hyperhidrosis, respiratory depression, nausea, vomiting, tachycardia, palpitation, hypertension and increased psychomimetic effects. Epileptiform abnormalities and grand mal convulsions have been seen (very rare) after large I.V. doses. Should be used with caution in patients with impaired renal or hepatic function,	30 mg. of drug is said to be as effective as 10 mg. morphine or 75 to 100 mg. of meperidine. Duration of action may be less than morphine. In case of overdosing, use the narcotic antagonist naloxone (Narcan) only. The others are not effective and can increase respiratory depression. Do not mix in syringe with soluble barbiturates as a precipitate will

			sites. Widely distributed, crosses the placenta. Appears to be metabolized in liver. Excreted in urine as unchanged drug and metabolites.	in treating pain of myocardial infarction when nausea and vomiting are present, if respiration is depressed or in patients about to have surgery of the biliary tract. Pentazocine can increase intracranial pressure and is contraindicated in most cases if increased cranial pressure, head injury or other intracranial lesions are present. Additive or may potentiate effects of other CNS depressants.	occur. Can be used for those patients taking oral anticoagulant drugs and needing short-term analgesic therapy. Should not be administered to children under 12 and use with caution during pregnancy and labor.
Propoxyphene, N.F. (Darvon, Dolene, Propoxychel) (dextropropoxyphene, Depronal, Levodal, Neo-Mal, Progesic, Proxyphene [C]).	30-60 mg. q. 4-6 h. p.r.n. Oral.	A non-narcotic analgesic used in all mild to moderate pain. Not useful in severe pain.	Similar to codeine. Does not suppress cough. Has little effect on the gastrointestinal tract.	Dizziness, headache, sedation, somnolence, paradoxical excitement, insomnia, skin rashes and G.I. disturbances. Acute toxicity as with narcotic analgesics. Tolerance and dependence as well as abuse have been reported.	Claimed to be devoid of any antipyretic activity. Often combined with other analgesic drugs. The levoisomer is claimed to have antitussive effect. Safe use in pregnancy not established.
Propoxyphene napsylate, N.F. (Darvon-N).	100 mg. q. 4-6 h. p.r.n. Oral.				
NARCOTIC ANTAGONISTS					
Synthetic or *Semisynthetic.*					
Levallorphan tartrate (Lorfan).	0.3-1.2 mg. Parenteral.	Used to lessen respiratory depression occurring from narcotic drugs.	Like nalorphine.	Like nalorphine.	

Name, Source, Synonyms, Preparations	Dosage and Administration	Uses	Action and Fate	Side Effects and Contraindications	Nursing Implications and Remarks
NARCOTIC ANTAGONISTS (Continued)					
Nalorphine hydrochloride, U.S.P. (Lethidrone). Synthetic from morphine.	Adult 5-10 mg. Parenteral. Infant, 0.2 mg. Parenteral.	Used as a narcotic antidote and to combat extreme narcosis. It is not used in drug addiction but only in acute poisoning. It is also a powerful emergency respiratory stimulant when cause of depression is the narcotic analogs. Addicts may be detected by rapid appearance of withdrawal symptoms following its administration.	Acts as an antagonist of morphine and similar drugs. Is a powerful respiratory stimulant when cause of depression is the narcotic analogs. In patients who have not received narcotics, produces effects similar to morphine: analgesia, respiratory depression, sedation, etc., but produces psychic effects that make it unsuitable for analgesic use. Readily absorbed after subcutaneous injection but poorly absorbed from gastrointestinal tract. Crosses the placenta. It is inactivated by the liver. Excreted in urine.	Large doses cause lethargy, drowsiness, sweating and dysphoria. In morphine addicts rapid withdrawal symptoms occur.	Is not effective in treating barbiturate poisoning.
Naloxone (Narcan).	0.4 mg. I.V., I.M. or S.C., repeat in 2-3 minutes x 3. If no improvement, probably condition will not respond to this drug. Neonates: 0.01 mg./kg. I.M., I.V. or S.Q. Postoperative: 0.1-0.2 mg. I.V. at 2-3 minute intervals. Repeat doses for all	Used to reverse the respiratory depression induced by natural or synthetic narcotics or by pentazocine.	A pure narcotic antagonist, it does not possess any morphine characteristics, as do other antagonists. Does not produce respiratory depression, psychotomimetic effects or pupillary constriction. In absence of narcotic drugs, exhibits no respiratory stimulation activity. Will produce withdrawal	Side effects: in rare instances nausea and vomiting have been reported in postoperative patients after receiving higher than recommended doses. Contraindications: caution. This drug is not effective when respiratory depression is caused by nonnarcotic drugs. Not recommended for use	

	conditions may be required in 1 to 2 hours depending on length of action of drug causing the respiratory depression.		symptoms in those who are physically dependent upon narcotics. Onset of action given I.V. is about 2 minutes. Rapidly inactivated with oral dosage. Rapidly metabolized by liver. Readily crosses placenta.	during pregnancy except during labor.	
COMPOUNDS USED TO POTENTIATE ANALGESIA					
Synthetic preparations.					
Promethazine hydrochloride, U.S.P. (Ganphen, Phenergan) (Histaritil [C]).	25-50 mg. q. 3-4 h. p.r.n. I.M. or I.V.	See page 180 for other uses.	Readily absorbed, inactivated by liver and excreted by kidneys.	See Antihistamines, pages 176, 177, and 180.	See under Antihistamines.
Propiomazine hydrochloride, N.F. (Largon).	10-30 mg. q. 3-4 h. p.r.n. I.M. or I.V.	For pre- and postoperative sedation and to potentiate analgesic and hypnotic action in obstetric and surgical patients.	Phenothiazine derivative with antihistamine and sedative properties that enhance the action of analgesic.	Causes irritation if extravasation occurs. Contraindications as for other phenothiazine antihistamines.	Doses of hypnotics should be reduced by one-half and narcotics by one-fourth or one-half.
ANTIPYRETICS					
SYNTHETIC PHENOL DERIVATIVES.					
Acetaminophen, N.F. (Anapap, Apamide, Datril, Febrolin, Fendon, Nasprin, Nebs, Pyrapap, Sk-Apap, Tempra, Tylenol, Valadol) (APAP, NAPAP, Atasol, Chem-Cetaphen, Dymadon, Paracetamol, Paralgin [C]).	300-600 mg. p.r.n. Oral or rectal.	Used as an analgesic for relief of headache, myalgia and arthralgia and to reduce fever.	Similar to acetanilid but less toxic in the therapeutic dosage range.	Toxicity apparently low, but on ingestion of overdose hepatotoxicity is seen. This can also occur with chronic use of very high doses. Very little gastric irritation and does not affect prothrombin time. It can be used for patients on anticoagulants and those patients who are allergic to aspirin.	Also prepared in flavored liquid for children. Available in combination with oxycodone and with codeine.

Name, Source, Synonyms, Preparations	Dosage and Administration	Uses	Action and Fate	Side Effects and Contraindications	Nursing Implications and Remarks
SYNTHETIC PHENOL DERIVATIVES (Continued)					
Acetanilid (Acetylaniline, Antifebrin).	200 mg. q. 4 h. p.r.n. Oral.	Used for the relief of pains such as headache, neuralgia, dysmenorrhea, etc. Also used to reduce fever.	Decreases activity of brain. Relieves various pains and nervous irritability. If fever is present, it will be reduced owing to peripheral vasodilation and perhaps action on hypothalami. Sweating is increased. Readily and almost completely absorbed from gastrointestinal tract. Peak plasma level reached in ½-2 hours. Rapidly diffused throughout tissue. Degraded by liver and excreted by kidneys about 30 minutes later.	Acute: cyanosis, weakness, sweating, weak pulse and respirations, dyspnea, delirium, convulsions. Treatment: lavage, evacuants, central nervous system stimulants. Chronic: weakness, palpitation, anorexia, dizziness, nausea, numbness of extremities, anemia, renal damage. Withdraw drug, substitute barbiturates, aspirin or codeine if needed. Antianemia treatment is indicated.	Habituation may occur.
Phenacetin, U.S.P. (Acetophenetidin).	300 mg. q. 4 h. p.r.n. Oral.	Used for the relief of pains such as headache, neuralgia, dysmenorrhea, etc. Also used to reduce fever.	Similar to acetanilid. Somewhat less analgesic but less toxic.	Similar to acetanilid but is less toxic. Skin eruptions occasionally occur. Treatment: same as for acetanilid, and symptomatic.	Same as for acetanilid. Has been implicated in some blood dyscrasias and may be harmful to the kidneys on long-term use.
SYNTHETIC PYRAZOLONE DERIVATIVES.					
Aminopyrine (Amidofebrin, Amidopyrazoline, Novamidon, Pyradone).	300 mg. q. 4 h. p.r.n. Oral.	Used mainly as an analgesic but is also antipyretic and antispasmodic. Acts slowly, but longer-lasting than antipyrine.	Action similar to acetanilid. The pyrazolones are readily and almost completely absorbed. Peak blood levels in 1-2 hours. Slowly metabolized mainly by the liver and excreted by kidneys. About 2-5% excreted unchanged.	Same as antipyrine but is more apt to cause toxic symptoms. Drug is said to cause granulocytopenia. Treatment: same as antipyrine, and symptomatic.	Habituation may occur. Formerly a common ingredient in many "headache" remedies in combination with other drugs. This is now prohibited by law without a prescription.

Antipyrine, N.F. (Analgesine).	300 mg. q. 4 h. p.r.n. Oral.	Used mainly as an antipyretic but has analgesic and antispasmodic action.	Similar to others of this group, but more antipyretic and less analgesic.	Depression, rapid pulse, collapse, cyanosis, diaphoresis, fall in temperature. Convulsions and delirium may occur. Treatment: lavage, evacuants, central nervous system stimulants, artificial respiration.	An ingredient of some analgesic ear drops.
Dipyrone (Dimethone, Divarine, Mypron, Narone, Pyralgin, Pyro). (Methampyrone [C]).	300-600 mg. t.i.d.-q.i.d. Oral. 500 mg.-1 Gm. q. 3 h. p.r.n. Parenteral.	An analgesic and antipyretic, used to moderate serious or life-threatening fevers when salicylates and other measures are known to be ineffective or not tolerated.	Similar to others of this group.	Skin rashes, dizziness, chills have been reported. This drug should not be given in large doses for prolonged periods unless leukocyte and differential counts are done frequently. Most serious toxic effect is blood dyscrasias.	An aminopyrine derivative, and has been reported to cause agranulocytosis. Use should be as brief as possible.
SALICYLIC ACID. *Synthetic from willow and poplar.*		Used as an analgesic, antirheumatic, diaphoretic, antiseptic and cholagogue. Some derivatives have anodyne action and some are anthelmintics.	Tends to raise blood pressure. Most of these drugs given in correct dosage will reduce pain and swelling in arthritis. They do not remove the cause. Exact mode of action is not clearly understood. Antipyretic in patients with fever. Acts on hypothalamus to increase heat dissipation as a result of vasodilation and increased peripheral blood flow. Locally, salicylic acid is irritating to skin and mucous membranes. It loosens the outer horny layers of skin and is keratolytic.	Toxic symptoms – severe (relatively uncommon): heart depression, polyuria, impairment of hearing and vision and skin eruptions. Stop drug and treat symptoms.	Patients should be cautioned against too high a dosage as well as indiscriminate use of these drugs. Salicylates should not be given to pregnant women during the last month of pregnancy.

Name, Source, Synonyms, Preparations	Dosage and Administration	Uses	Action and Fate	Side Effects and Contraindications	Nursing Implications and Remarks
SALICYLIC ACID (Continued)					
Aspirin, U.S.P. (acetylsalicylic acid, A.S.A.) (Acetal, Acetophen, Acetyl-Sal, Ancasol, Cetasal, Ecotrin, Empirin, Entrophen, Measurin, Monasalyl, Neopirine, Novo-Phase, Novasen, Rhonal, Supasa, Tolerin [C]).	300-600 mg. q. 3-4 h. p.r.n. (not more than 3 Gm. in 24 hours). Oral.	An extremely common analgesic and antirheumatic drug alone and in many combinations.	Readily and almost completely absorbed from gastrointestinal tract. Peak blood levels in 1-2 hours. Widely distributed throughout body with lowest concentration in brain. Aspirin is rapidly hydrolyzed to salicylic acid, mainly in liver. Excreted by the kidneys as salicylates and salicyluric acid. Salicylates cross the placental barrier and have been associated with neonatal bleeding.	As above. Aspirin and other salicylates in large doses (6 Gm. or more) daily, may significantly increase prothrombin time and, in lower doses (1-3 Gm.), can cause gastric blood loss and prolonged bleeding time.	Aspirin with a buffering agent (buffered aspirin) is available from various mfgs. under a variety of trade names. The buffer is said to decrease the gastric irritation that is seen with aspirin.
Aluminum aspirin, N.F. (aluminum acetylsalicylate).	670 mg. q. 4 h. p.r.n. Oral.	As above.			
Methyl salicylate (oil of wintergreen).	Dosage varies. Topical.	As an anodyne in lotions or ointments in arthritis.			
Salicylamide, N.F. (Amid-Sal, Liquiprin, Salicim. (Chem-Sal [C]).	300 mg.-2 Gm. q. 3-4 h. p.r.n. (not more than 3 Gm. in 24 hours). Oral.	Uses are similar to those of aspirin.			
Salicylic acid, U.S.P. (psoriacide [C]).	Dosage varies. Topical.	As an anodyne in lotions or ointments in arthritis. Also is keratolytic.			
Sodium salicylate, U.S.P.	300 mg.-1 Gm. q. 4 h. Oral. 6-8 Gm. Rectal.	Mainly used as an antirheumatic.			
Ammonium salicylate (Armyl).	1 Gm. Oral.	Antirheumatic.			
Calcium acetylsalicylic carbamide (Calurin).	300 mg. Oral.	Antirheumatic.			
Choline magnesium trisalicylate (Trilisate).	500-1000 mg. b.i.d. Oral.	Symptomatic relief for acute and long-term treatment of rheumatoid arthritis, osteoarthritis and other arthritides.	Anti-inflammatory, analgesic and antipyretic activity. Mechanism of action unknown.	Well tolerated at recommended dosage levels. With extended therapy or large doses, salicylism and/or	Some patients may need 2-3 weeks of therapy for optimum effects. Patients hypersensitive to

			Absorbed rapidly, excreted by kidneys.	salicylate intoxication may occur. Reduce dose if tinnitus occurs. Use with caution in chronic renal insufficiency, active erosive gastric or peptic ulcer. Risk of ulceration increased with concomitant administration of steriods, butazones, or alcohol. Use with caution in patients requiring coumarin, indandione anticoagulants or heparin.	salicylates should not receive this drug. Exercise care in giving drug during pregnancy. Because of possibility of prostaglandin inhibition with high doses of salicylates, it is not recommended before parturition. Not recommended for children under 12 years of age.
Choline salicylate (Actasal, Arthropan).	870 mg. Oral.	Antirheumatic.			
Ethylsalicylate (Sal-Ethyl Carbonate).	300-600 mg. Oral.	Antirheumatic.			
Gensalate sodium.	500 mg. Oral	Antirheumatic.			
Salicylsalicylic acid.	300 mg. Oral.	Antirheumatic.			
ANTIRHEUMATICS	*See also miscellaneous analgesics, and the preceding group of salicylates especially.*				
CINCHOPHEN. *Synthetic.* Neocinchophen (Novatophan).	300 mg. t.i.d. Oral.	Used in the treatment of gout, arthritis and similar conditions. Acts as an analgesic, antipyretic and cholagogue.	Analgesic, antipyretic and uricosuric. Causes a marked increase in quantity of uric acid secreted by kidneys. Adequately absorbed from gastrointestinal tract. Widely distributed mainly in the extracellular fluid. Almost completely metabolized. Only about 2% excreted unchanged by the kidneys.	Anorexia, nausea, vomiting, skin eruptions; liver damage may occur. Stop drug, force fluid (oral and I.V.) and treat symptoms.	Neocinchophen is less effective and also less toxic than cinchophen.

Name, Source, Synonyms, Preparations	Dosage and Administration	Uses	Action and Fate	Side Effects and Contraindications	Nursing Implications and Remarks
ANALGESICS—ANTIRHEUMATICS (Continued)					
COLCHICUM. *Meadow saffron, Colchicine.*					
Colchicine, U.S.P. (Novocolchine [C]).	0.5-0.6 mg. Oral.	Used in the treatment of gout, arthritis and similar conditions. Action is mainly analgesic.	Action not well understood. It relieves the pain of gouty arthritis, but does not reduce the level of uric acid. It is thought, however, to decrease lactic acid production by leukocytes and thereby decrease depositing of urate crystal and subsequent inflammatory response. It also arrests cell division by preventing spindle formation in metaphase in numerous plant and animal cells. Readily absorbed. Transported to liver, excreted in bile and some is reabsorbed. Concentrated in kidneys, liver, spleen and intestines. Some is deacetylated by the liver. In normal persons 28% of a given dose is excreted as colchicine and 8% as metabolites within 48 hours. In patients with gout the percentages are 3.5 and 12. Reason for this difference is not known.	Nausea, vomiting, diarrhea, abdominal pain, diaphoresis, rapid thready pulse, slow shallow respirations. Treatment: lavage or emetics, external heat, stimulants, and symptomatically. Prolonged administration may cause bone marrow depression with agranulocytosis, thrombocytopenia, and/or aplastic anemia.	Considered very toxic; watch carefully. Times and dosage individually adjusted.
Colchicine inj.	0.5-1.0 mg. I.V. 1-2 mg. I.V. followed by 0.5-1.0 mg. q. 3 h. until satisfactory response is obtained.				May enhance response to sympathomimetic and CNS depressant drugs.
SYNTHETIC PREPARATIONS					
Ibuprofen (Motrin).	300-400 mg. t.i.d. or q.i.d. Oral. Dosage not to exceed	Used for symptomatic treatment of rheumatoid arthritis or osteoarthritis.	Mode of action unknown. Analgesic, anti-inflammatory and antipyretic.	Gastric distress, cramps, pain, indigestion, heartburn, bloating, flatulence, nausea,	Not advised during pregnancy, as it inhibits prostaglandin synthesis and release, or for

	2.4 Gm. per day.		Rapidly absorbed after oral administration. Peak blood level reached within an hour, decreasing to about ½ that amount in 4 hours. Excreted by kidneys unchanged or as inactive oxidative metabolites. Excretion usually complete 24 hours after last dose.	vomiting, constipation, and/or diarrhea. Rarely: ulceration, some complicated by bleeding or perforation; skin rashes; dizziness; amblyopia. Contraindications: sensitivity to drug, patients with nasal polyps, angioedema, bronchospastic reactivity to aspirin. Prolongs bleeding time.	children under 14 years of age. A nonsteroid anti-inflammatory agent with action about equal to that of aspirin. Aspirin given concurrently with ibuprofen causes net decrease in anti-inflammatory activity. Patients should report to their physicians untoward gastrointestinal symptoms, any skin rash or eye disorder.
<u>Fenoprofen calcium</u> (Nalfon).	600 mg. q.i.d. 30 minutes before or 2 hours after meals. If there are G.I. complaints, give with meals or milk. Doses over 3200 mg. are not recommended.	Relief of signs and symptoms of rheumatoid arthritis. (Safety and effectiveness in Class IV arthritics has not been established.)	Mode of action is unknown, but anti-inflammatory effects are not mediated through the adrenal gland. It reduces the joint swelling, pain and duration of morning stiffness. Inhibits prostaglandin synthetase in *in vitro* studies. Well absorbed under fasting conditions. Food decreases rate and extent of absorption. Approximately 90% of a single dose is excreted in the urine in 24 hours. It is highly bound to albumin. The co-administration of aspirin decreases the metabolic half-life of fenoprofen.	Fenoprofen can cause peptic ulceration and G.I. bleeding. Other G.I. symptoms include skin rash, sweating, urticaria, dizziness, tremor, confusion, insomnia, tinnitus, blurred vision, decreased hearing, tachycardia, headache, nervousness, asthenia, dyspnea, peripheral edema, fatigue, anemia, dysuria and increase in alkaline phosphatase, LDH and SGOT. Contraindicated in patients who are sensitive to aspirin or other nonsteroidal anti-inflammatory drugs.	Give drug with caution to patients with renal impairment as it has caused glomerulonephritis, renal papillary necrosis and hepatocellular hypertrophy in rats. Safety in pregnancy and lactation has not been established. Because of protein binding, possible interactions with other serum-bound drugs may occur.

Name, Source, Synonyms, Preparations	Dosage and Administration	Uses	Action and Fate	Side Effects and Contraindications	Nursing Implications and Remarks
ANALGESICS–ANTIRHEUMATICS (Continued)					
Naproxen (Naprosyn).	250 mg. b.i.d. (morning and evening). Doses above 750 mg./day are not recommended.	Anti-inflammatory and analgesic used in symptomatic treatment of acute and chronic rheumatoid arthritis.	See above.	See above. Rare: angioneurotic edema, thrombocytopenia, agranulocytoses and jaundice. No elevation of SGOT, LDH or alkaline phosphatase reported. An elevation in the BUN has occurred. For interactions see Fenoprofen.	Safety in pregnancy and lactating mothers has not been established, but 1% of plasma level found in milk of lactating women. Readily crosses the placenta. Warning: use with caution in patients with renal problems, PUD or hepatic problems. Naproxen may give increase in urinary value for 17-ketosteroid if *m*-dinitrobenzene is used in the assay.
Sunlindac (Clinoril).	150-200 mg. b.i.d. Oral with food. Maximum recommended dose is 400 mg. daily.	Symptomatic relief in rheumatoid arthritis, osteoarthritis, acute gouty arthritis, acute shoulder pain.	Nonsteroidal anti-inflammatory agent with analgesic and antipyretic action. About 90% absorbed following oral dose. Half-life 7-8 h. and for sulfide, 16 h.	Mild G.I. reactions; rash, headache, dizziness, tinnitus, edema. Exercise caution in patients on anticoagulants or with history of G.I. bleeding or ulcer.	Administer sulindac with meals to minimize G.I. effects.
Tolmetin sodium (Tolectin).	600-1800 mg. in divided doses 3 or 4 times a day including a dose on rising and on retiring.	Relief of signs and symptoms of rheumatoid arthritis and in the treatment of acute flare-ups and the long-term management of the chronic disease. (Safety and effectiveness in Class IV arthritics has not been established.)	Animal studies demonstrate anti-inflammatory, analgesic and antipyretic activity. Exact mode of action is not known but tolmetin inhibits prostaglandin synthetase in vitro and lowers the prostaglandin E plasma levels in man. It is rapidly and almost completely absorbed after an oral dose and essentially all is recovered in the urine in 24 hours, either as an inactive oxidative metabolite or as conjugates.	Most prevalent side effects include epigastric or abdominal pain, 1:6; nausea, 1:25; vomiting, 1:30; to a lesser extent indigestion, heartburn, constipation. Peptic ulcer occurred in 1:50 persons tested but some had a history of PUD. Significant G.I. bleeding without evidence of ulceration has been reported in about 1:250. Other side effects include dizziness, nervousness, drowsiness, rash, urticaria, pruritus, tinnitus,	Use with caution in patients with history of PUD and only after other forms of therapy such as gold are tried. It is not recommended for use in pregnancy and it is not known whether it is secreted in the milk of nursing mothers. Caution if used in patients with eye problems, renal problems or compromised cardiac function. Tolmetin will give false positive proteinuria tests when the tests rely on acid precipitation as their end point. With

				mild edema and small and transient decrease in hemoglobin and hematocrit not associated with G.I. bleeding. Granulocytopenia has also been seen.	dye-impregnated strips there is no interference.
Oxyphenbutazone, N.F. (Oxalid, Tandearil).	100 mg. Oral. Usually given 300-600 mg./day in divided doses with reduction to minimum required for maintenance.	Uses, action and precautions similar to those of phenylbutazone.	Similar to phenylbutazone.	Similar to phenylbutazone. Same interactions as under phenylbutazone.	Similar to phenylbutazone.
Phenylbutazone, N.F. (Azolid, Butazolidin) (Anevral, Butagesic, Eributazone, Intrabutazone, Malgesic, Nadozone, Nedozone, Phenbutazol, Tazone [C]).	100-200 mg. Usually t.i.d. Individually adjusted. Give with meals or glass of milk. Oral.	Used in the treatment of gout, arthritis and similar inflammatory conditions. This drug should not be considered a simple analgesic. Each patient should be carefully evaluated before therapy and be under close supervision of a physician. In persons over 60 the drug should be restricted to short-term periods only (if possible one week maximum.)	Acts as analgesic, antipyretic, anti-inflammatory agent. In gout, uric acid is reduced in blood. Renal excretion of sodium and chloride occurs. Rapid and complete absorption. Slowly metabolized by the liver, some to oxyphenbutazone. Slowly excreted in the urine. Appears in breast milk.	Gastrointestinal irritation, edema, rash, anemia. Has caused agranulocytosis. Reduce or stop drug and treat symptoms. Contraindicated in edema, renal, cardiac or hepatic damage; also in marked hypertension or in patient who has peptic ulcers. This drug can potentiate the effect of the warfarin type anticoagulants. When used in patients taking these drugs, care should be taken to adjust the dose of the anticoagulant. Phenylbutazone enhances the hypoglycemic effects of acetohexamide, and the dose of acetohexamide should be adjusted downward. The other sulfonureas may give the same reaction and should be closely watched. Phenylbutazone may diminish the effects of the steroids by enzyme induction.	Low sodium diet is often recommended. Sodium free antacid aids in preventing gastric irritation. Use with caution during pregnancy, especially in the 1st trimester, weighing possible risks against benefits. This drug can cross the placental barrier and has been implicated in neonatal goiter.

Name, Source, Synonyms, Preparations	Dosage and Administration	Uses	Action and Fate	Side Effects and Contraindications	Nursing Implications and Remarks
ANALGESICS–ANTIRHEUMATICS (Continued)					
OTHER SYNTHETIC PREPARATIONS.					
Indomethacin, N.F. (Indocin) (Indocid [C]).	As adverse reactions appear to correlate with size of dose it is best to determine the smallest effective dose for the individual patient. 25 mg. two or three times a day. If necessary, dose may be increased to 200 mg. in divided doses daily. Larger doses than this probably will not be more effective. Oral.	Used to treat moderate to severe rheumatoid arthritis, rheumatoid spondylitis, degenerative joint disease of the hip (osteoarthritis) and to relieve pain, reduce fever, swelling and tenderness in acute gouty arthritis. This drug should not be considered a simple analgesic and should be used only in those conditions recommended.	Anti-inflammatory agent with antipyretic and analgesic properties unlike the corticosteroids, as it has no effect on pituitary or adrenal function. Well absorbed orally. Peak plasma levels in about 2 hours. About 90% is bound to plasma proteins. Metabolized in liver and kidneys. Eliminated by kidneys as the glucuronide. Appears in milk of nursing mothers.	May mask the signs and symptoms of peptic ulcer, or cause single or multiple ulceration including perforation and/or hemorrhage of the gastrointestinal tract. Should not be given to patients with active peptic ulcer, gastritis or ulcerative colitis for this reason. Side effects include dizziness and lightheadedness; feeling of detachment; gastrointestinal disturbances such as nausea, vomiting, epigastric distress, abdominal pain and diarrhea. Psychic disturbances, depersonalization, depression, mental confusion have been reported. Aspirin and other salicylates decrease and delay the gastrointestinal absorption of indomethacin. When indomethacin is given concurrently with probenecid, it can cause a rise in serum level, since excretion is blocked. Dose of indomethacin should be adjusted.	Renal function should be checked in individuals receiving long-term therapy. Manufacturer does not recommend use in pediatric age groups, pregnancy or nursing mothers until indications for use and dosage have been established for these groups. Caution patients performing hazardous tasks requiring mental alertness or physical coordination about side effects of dizziness and lightheadedness. Give after meals, or with food or antacids to minimize G.I. effects.

				Indomethacin may potentiate the effects of warfarin-type anticoagulants. A few cases of psychic disturbances, blurred vision, stomatitis, pruritus, urticaria, angioneurotic edema, skin rashes and edema have been reported. Contraindicated in patients under 14 years of age.

SEDATIVES–HYPNOTICS

Most of the drugs in this group either potentiate or act in an additive fashion with other CNS depressants. Many of them cause development of tolerance during prolonged use and may also be addictive, causing psychic or physical dependence.

See also General Anesthetics. *Synthetic.*				
Acetylcarbromal (Acetyl adalin, Abasin, Sedamyl).	250 mg. 1 or 2 tablets t.i.d. Oral.	Used mainly for daytime sedation.	Relieves tension and anxiety with little effect on perception and alertness.	Does not have undesirable side effects. Toxicity rare in therapeutic dosage. Contraindicated in patients with bromide hypersensitivity.
Carbromal.	300 mg. 1 or 2 tablets h.s.	Used as a sedative-hypnotic.	Fate of these drugs is similar to that of bromide, which they liberate.	Carbromal can decrease the duration of activity of dexamethasone by liver enzyme induction.

Name, Source, Synonyms, Preparations	Dosage and Administration	Uses	Action and Fate	Side Effects and Contraindications	Nursing Implications and Remarks
SEDATIVES–HYPNOTICS (Continued)					
BARBITURATES. Salts and derivatives of barbituric acid. *Long Duration – Slow Action.* Barbital (Veronal, Barbitone). Barbital sodium (Medinal) (barbitone sodium [C]).	- 300 mg. Oral. 300 mg. Oral	Used for sedation, hypnosis, suppression of convulsion, partial and complete anesthesia, amnesia and analgesia (especially in obstetrics); for analgesia in migraine headaches, neuritis, and neuralgia and to reduce peristalsis. These drugs have a wide and expanding field of effectiveness. Barbiturates are often added to analgesic drugs to produce sedation as well as relief of pain. Various combinations with amphetamine derivatives have been used for their euphoric effect.	Depression of the central nervous system, beginning usually with the diencephalon; certain preparations affect the motor centers mainly. Therapeutic doses have little effect on the visceral organs, but heavy doses cause respiratory and cardiac depression. Most of the barbiturates tend to lower blood pressure. Barbiturates are well absorbed and are rapidly distributed to all tissues and fluids, and they cross the placenta. After initial distribution, they are concentrated in	Acute: mental confusion, drowsiness, fall in blood pressure, coma, rapid pulse, moist skin, pulmonary edema, collapse. Treatment: lavage, oxygen, cardiac stimulants, intravenous glucose. Chronic: habituation is easily acquired. Anorexia, headache, weakness, psychoses, visual disturbances, anemia, renal damage, amnesia. Stop drug and treat symptoms. The barbiturates, especially the short acting ones such as pentobarbital and secobarbital, may cause de-	Residual sedation or "hang-over" with subtle distortion of mood occurs commonly with hypnotic doses. Act slowly (30-60 minutes), but effects are of relatively long duration (6-8 hours). Tablet preparations are given orally. Ampule preparations (sodium salts) may be administered parenterally. Dosage given is for one dose. Repeated dosage is individually adjusted. The use of barbiturates with any alcohol should be avoided since these drugs reinforce each other with serious, even fatal, results.
Mephobarbital, N.F. (Mebaral) (methylphenobarbital [C]).	30-200 mg. Oral. Up to 600 mg. daily in divided doses. Oral.	Used as a sedative in neuroses and in treating epilepsy.	certain tissues, depending upon which compound is used and the time elapsed after administration. Three	pendency. If this occurs, withdrawal may have serious effects.	
Metharbital (Gemonil).	100 mg. Oral. Up to 800 mg. daily if needed.	For epilepsy.	factors affecting distribution and fate are lipid solubility, protein binding and extent of ionization.	The barbiturates significantly reduce the effectiveness of the oral anticoagulants. Phenobarbital and possibly other barbiturates will	
Phenobarbital, U.S.P. (Barbipil, Barbita, Eskabarb, Lixophen, Luminal) (phenobarbitone, Epilol, Epsylone, Fenosed, Gardenal, Hypnotone, Novo-Pheno, Novo-Rectal, Phenocaps, Phen Bar, Sedabar, Sedlyn [C]).	15-100 mg. Oral.	Relatively nontoxic. May be given over a long period of time. Widely used for many purposes.	The ultra short acting have the greatest lipid solubility, then progressively less from short to long acting compounds. The barbiturates are redistributed in the body. The oxybarbiturates are metabolically	significantly reduce the effectiveness of griseofulvin. The monoamine oxidase inhibitors and the sulfonylureas enhance the central nervous system effects of the barbiturates. Antacids may decrease the	

Phenobarbital elixir, U.S.P.	5 ml. (5 ml. contains 20 mg.) Oral.		degraded by the enzymes of the liver. The thiobarbiturates are degraded mainly by the liver and to a small degree by the enzymes in the kidneys and brain. They are excreted by the kidneys.	absorption of the barbiturates by raising the pH of the gastric contents and by reducing their solubility. The barbiturates can reduce or shorten the effect of cortisone derivatives by enzyme induction.	
Phenobarbital sodium, U.S.P. (Luminal sodium).	15-100 mg. Oral or parenteral.				
Intermediate					
Amobarbital, U.S.P. (Amospan, Amytal) (amylbarbitone, Isonal [C]).	50-300 mg. in divided doses daily. 65-200 mg. h.s.	As a sedative. As a hypnotic.		Concurrent use of the antihistamines with the barbiturates can give additive central nervous system depression. They can increase the orthostatic hypotension which occurs with the phenothiazines. The barbiturates can cross the placental barrier and can depress neonatal respiration.	Action and duration of moderate effect. Administer I.M. doses deeply into muscle to decrease possibility of sterile abscess or sloughs.
Amobarbital sodium, U.S.P. (Amytal sodium) (amylbarbitone sodium, Novomobarb [C]).	60-100 mg. Oral. 250-500 mg. Parenteral.				
Aprobarbital, N.F. (Alurate).	60 mg. Oral.	As a hypnotic.			
Aprobarbital sodium (Alurate sodium).	10 mg. Oral.	As a sedative.			
Butabarbital sodium (Bubartal, Butak, Butazem, Butisol, Buta-Barb, Interbarb, Neo-Barb, Neurosidine [C]).	15-60 mg. 6-8 h. Oral. 45-100 mg. h.s. Oral.	As a sedative. As a hypnotic.			
Butethal (butobarbital, butobarbitone, Soneryl [C]).	50-100 mg. Oral	Often given in small doses over several hours for sedation.			
Cyclopentyl allylbarbituric acid (Cyclopal).	50-100 mg. Oral.	As a quick-acting sedative.			
Diallylbarbituric acid (Diadol) (allobarbitone, Analgyl [C]).	100-300 mg. Oral.	Sedative effects last 18-24 hours.			
Probarbital calcium (Ipral calcium).	100-200 mg. Oral.	Sedative effects often last into second night.			

Name, Source, Synonyms, Preparations	Dosage and Administration	Uses	Action and Fate	Side Effects and Contraindications	Nursing Implications and Remarks
BARBITURATES (Continued)					
Short Acting					
Cyclobarbital calcium (Phanodorn).	200 mg. Oral.	Mainly used for hypnosis.	As above.		Short acting. Acts quite rapidly, but effects not prolonged.
Hexethal sodium (Ortal).	200-400 mg. Oral.	As above.		Absolute contraindications: latent or manifest porphyria or a familial history of intermittent porphyria. Relative contraindication: impaired hepatic or renal function.	
Hexobarbital sodium (Sombucaps).	250-500 mg. Oral. p.r.n.	Pre- and postanesthesia sedation, hypnosis.			
	3-6 ml. of a 10% solution I.V.	For induction or short anesthesia.			
Pentobarbital sodium, U.S.P. (Nembutal, Penta) (pentobarbitone sodium, Butylova, Hypnotal, Hypnol, Ibalal, Novopentobarb, Pentanca, Pentogen, Somnotol [C]).	100-200 mg. h.s. Oral, rectal or parenteral. 30 mg. t. or q.i.d. Oral.	Hypnotic sedative.			
Secobarbital sodium, U.S.P. (Seconal) (quinalbarbitone, Secolone, Hyptrol, Secogen, Secobal, Notrium, Secotal, Secotabs [C]).	As above.	As above.			
Talbutal (Lotusate).	30-120 mg. Oral.	As above.			
Vinbarbital sodium.	100-200 mg. Oral or parenteral.	As above.			
Very Short Acting					
Methitural sodium (Neraval).	3-6 ml. I.V.	Used for induction anesthesia and for short anesthesia.	As above.	Respiratory depression and laryngospasm may occur. May cause hypotension and tachycardia.	Very short acting: quick acting but effects of short duration. Dose is repeated as is deemed advisable. All dosages subject to individual patient's reaction.
Methohexital sodium (Brevital) (methohexitone, Brietal [C]).	5-12 ml. of a 1% solution. I.V.	As above.		There are many contraindications. See manufacturer's pamphlets for details.	
Thiamylal sodium, N.F. (Surital).	3-6 ml. of a 2.5% solution. I.V.	As above.			
Thiopental sodium, U.S.P. (Pentothal sodium).	2.3-3 ml. I.V.	As above.			

BROMIDES. *Synthetic* from bromine.		Used for sedation and hypnosis; as an antiemetic, aphrodisiac, and anticonvulsant; in some cases in pyelography.	Depress the central nervous system, including the spinal cord, but have little or no effect on the medullary centers. Produce drowsiness, some loss of muscle coordination and reflexes, decreased reception of sensory stimuli. Do not markedly affect cardiac, respiratory or gastrointestinal activity. Hypnotic action is indirect, owing to lessened sensations and mental activity. Readily absorbed and widely distributed in extracellular fluid. The distribution of the bromide ion is dependent upon the concentration of the chloride ion as they are somewhat interchangeable. Excreted by the kidneys slowly. Biologic half-life is about 12 days in patients with normal chloride intake. Maximum accumulation does not occur for approximately 2 mos.	Acute: sweet odor to breath, coated tongue, slurred speech, ataxia, dilated pupils, tachycardia and sometimes acute bromoderma. Stop drug, force fluids (I.V. if necessary), give sodium chloride. Chronic: mental depression, foul breath, coated tongue, slow pulse, slow speech, skin lesions and ataxia. Stop drug, give sodium chloride and vitamin B (niacinamide). Bromides cross the placental barrier and have caused neonatal skin eruptions. Also found in mother's milk.	Individual tolerance to bromides varies greatly.
Ammonium bromide, N.F.	1 Gm. t.i.d. Oral.				
Bromide 5 elixir.	4 ml. h.s. Also available as tablets. Oral.				Bromide 5 contains ammonium, sodium, calcium, lithium, potassium bromide.
Bromide 3 elixir.	4 ml. As above. Oral.				Bromide 3 contains ammonium, sodium, potassium bromide. For hypnosis, bromide is given in one dose h.s. For sedation and as an anticonvulsant, usually t.i.d. or q.i.d. Little use today except as OTC preps.
Calcium bromide.	1 Gm. t.i.d. Oral.				
Lithium bromide.	1 Gm. t.i.d. Oral.				
Potassium bromide.	1 Gm. t.i.d. Oral.				
Sodium bromide.	300 mg.-1 Gm. t.i.d. Oral.	Sodium bromide preferred because it is less irritating to G.I. tract.			
Sodium bromide elixir, N.F.	4 ml. h.s. Oral.				
Syrup of bromides.	4 ml. h.s. Oral.				

Name, Source, Synonyms, Preparations	Dosage and Administration	Uses	Action and Fate	Side Effects and Contraindications	Nursing Implications and Remarks
SEDATIVES (Continued)					
CHLORAL HYDRATE. *Synthetic.* Chloral hydrate, U.S.P. (Aquachloral, Felsules, Noctec, Rectules, Somnos) (Cloralixir, Cloratol, Chloralvan, Novochlorhydrate [C]).	250-600 mg. h.s. Available as liquid and capsules. Oral or rectal.	Used as sedative, hypnotic, analgesic and antispasmodic. Chloral derivatives are used locally as antipruritics.	Depresses central nervous system and decreases the reception of sensory stimuli. Therapeutic doses produce little effect on cardiovascular or respiratory action. Blood absorption and distribution. Degraded by the liver mainly to trichloroethanol and other products. Degraded products excreted by the kidneys and in bile and in breast milk.	Gastric irritation. "Hangover" or residual sedation with hypnotic doses occurs occasionally. Coma, muscle relaxation, cold extremities, low blood pressure, convulsions, delirium. Treatment: lavage, oxygen, artificial respiration, central nervous system stimulants. When given to patients on oral anticoagulants, chloral hydrate can cause transient potentiation of hypoprothrombinemia. Concurrent ingestion of chloral hydrate and alcohol results in greater central nervous system depression than when either is taken alone. Use with caution in severe cardiac disease, mental depression and in patients with suicidal tendencies or history of drug abuse.	Usually given one dose, h.s., but may be given in smaller dose t.i.d. May be habit forming. Do not give with alcohol. Chloral hydrate can cross the placental barrier and in large doses can cause death of the fetus. Contraindicated in patients with marked hepatic or impaired renal function.
Chloral betaine, N.F. (Beta Chlor).	440-870 mg. 1 or 2 tablets h.s. (Equals 250-500 mg. chloral hydrate). Oral.	Sedative.	Same as choral hydrate but said to cause less gastric distress.		
Chlorobutanol, U.S.P. (Chloretone).	600 mg. Oral.	Can be given subcutaneously; preserves injectables. Mild local anesthetic (dentistry).			
Triclofos sodium (Triclos).	1.5 Gm. h.s. Oral.	Used to induce sleep.	Rapidly absorbed. Triclofos is dephosphorylated in the gut, mainly yielding trichlorethanol, which is the same active metabolite of chloral hydrate. Peak serum levels reached in one	Side effects: headache, "hangover," drowsiness, gastrointestinal disturbances (gas, flatulence, nausea, vomiting, bad taste), staggering gait, ataxia, ketonuria, relative eosinophilia,	Caution: may be habit forming. Safety for use during pregnancy and lactation has not been established. Should be used with caution in patients with cardiac

			hour. Has a half-life in the body of about 11 hours. Crosses the placenta. Excreted in bile and feces, with small amount in breast milk. C.N.S. depression similar to chloral hydrate.	urticaria, lightheadesness, vertigo, nightmares, malaise and reduction in total white blood cell count. Contraindications: in renal or hepatic impairment and in patients known to be sensitive to chloral hydrate. Triclofos will increase the effects of other central nervous system depressants such as alcohol and the tranquilizers.	arrhythmias or any severe cardiac disease.
OTHER SYNTHETIC PREPARATIONS.					
<u>Ectylurea</u> (Nostyn).	150-300 mg. t.i.d. Oral.	As a sedative in mild anxiety-tension states.	Produces mild depression of central nervous system. Hypnosis occurs only with very high doses.	Skin rashes, cholestatic jaundice, dizziness, nausea, vomiting and headache.	Is said to be of little value in overexcited or over-agitated patients.
<u>Ethchlorvynol,</u> N.F. (Placidyl).	500-750 mg. Hypnotic h.s.; sedative 100-500 mg. two to three times daily. Oral.	A nonbarbiturate sedative hypnotic.	Central nervous system depressant producing sedation and hypnosis if pain is not a factor. Is not analgesic. Acts quickly, within 15-30 minutes. Effects last 5-6 hours. Readily absorbed orally, but in first 24 hours after 1 oral dose less than 0.1% is excreted in the urine. It has been shown to be highly localized in body lipids and to cross the placenta.	Low toxicity, though it may cause drowsiness, fatigue and some "hang-over." Overdose gives symptoms similar to those of barbiturates. Not recommended during the 1st and 2nd trimesters of pregnancy or in children. Can reduce the effectiveness of the oral anticoagulants. Additive C.N.S. depression when administered concomitantly with other C.N.S. depressants, such as barbiturates or alcohol as well as with monoamine oxidase inhibitors.	Use with caution in patients with impaired hepatic or renal function.

Name, Source, Synonyms, Preparations	Dosage and Administration	Uses	Action and Fate	Side Effects and Contraindications	Nursing Implications and Remarks
SEDATIVES (Continued)					
Ethinamate, N.F. (Valmid).	500 mg.-2 Gm. h.s. Oral.	A mild sedative hypnotic which is effective when deep hypnosis is not needed.	Central nervous system depression with mild sedation and light hypnosis. Acts quickly, within 15-30 minutes. Lasts 4-5 hours. Good absorption. Believed to be inactivated by the liver and excreted in the urine.	Safe use during pregnancy has not been established. Rare cases of thrombocytopenia, purpura and oral idiosyncrasies with fever have been reported. Mild gastrointestinal disturbances and skin rashes have occurred. Concurrent use of alcohol, especially in overdosage, can increase potential hazards.	Habituation, addiction, and tolerance have been reported.
Flurazepam (Dalmane).	15-30 mg. h.s. Oral.	Used for insomnia.	This drug is a benzodiazepine and the exact mode of action is not known. However, animal studies indicate it reduces the pressor response to electrical stimulation of the hypothalamus and increases the arousal threshold to stimulation of the amygdala and the hypothalamus. It is rapidly absorbed from the gastrointestinal tract and rapidly metabolized.	Side effects most commonly seen include dizziness, drowsiness, lightheadedness, staggering, ataxia and falling. These latter have occurred mostly in elderly or debilitated patients. For other side effects, toxicity, etc., see brochure. Contraindications: sensitivity to the drug. This drug has similar interactions to chlordiazepoxide (page 162). This drug does not appear to interact with the oral anticoagulants.	Use during pregnancy is not recommended. The drug is not recommended for children under 15 years, as studies have not been carried out for this age group. Additive C.N.S. depression may occur when given concomitantly with other C.N.S. depressants such as alcohol or barbiturates.
Glutethimide, N.F. (Doriden) (Somide [C]).	250-500 mg. h.s. Oral.	Used for insomnia and in first stages of labor.	Central nervous system depression producing sedation or hypnosis according to dosage. Also has anticholinergic activity.	Rare in therapeutic doses, but nausea and skin rashes have occurred. Stop drug; use evacuants, if indicated, and treat symptoms.	Use with caution in patients with prostatic hypertrophy, stenosing peptic ulcer, glaucoma or cardiac arrhythmias.

			Poor and irregular oral absorption. Well distributed throughout body. Degraded by the liver, excreted in bile. Some reabsorbed. Some excreted by the kidneys. Crosses the placenta with small amounts appearing in milk.	Glutethimide interacts with the oral anticoagulants to decrease their effectiveness. Additive with other C.N.S. depressants.	
Methaqualone (Quaalude, Parest, Sopor) (Hyptor, Mequelon, Pexaqualone, Rouqualone, Somnafac, Tiqualoine, Tualone [C]).	75 mg. p.c. and h.s. 150-400 mg. h.s. Oral.	For sedation and sleep.	C.N.S. depression similar to barbiturates. Induces liver microsomal enzymes and may alter metabolism of other drugs. Rapidly absorbed. Onset of action rapid (within 30 min. and lasting 5-8 h. with hypnotic dose). Well distributed and localized in adipose tissue. Excreted in urine.	Used with caution in impaired hepatic function and the anxiety states, especially if there is evidence of impending depression or when suicidal tendencies exist. Most frequent side effects include headache, dizziness, torpor, fatigue and residual sedation or "hangover." Tolerance and dependence develop with prolonged use.	
Methyprylon, N.F. (Noludar).	50-400 mg. h.s. for insomnia. Oral.	Hypnotic used for insomnia.	Action similar to that of the barbiturates but it is unrelated chemically. Produces less respiratory depression.	Rare; occasional vertigo, nausea and vomiting occur. Morning drowsiness, dizziness, headache and skin rash.	Additive with other C.N.S. depressants. Safe use in pregnancy or lactation not established.
PARALDEHYDE. *Synthetic. Ethane derivative.* Paraldehyde, U.S.P. (Paral)	4 ml. Oral. 32 ml. Rectal. 4 ml. I.M. (maximum dose by injection should not exceed 0.2 ml./kg.). 1 ml. I.V.	Used for sedation, hypnosis and as an anticonvulsant. It has antiseptic properties. Mainly used in status epilepticus, delirium tremens and tetanus.	Depresses central nervous system, but not the medullary centers (in therapeutic dosage). Produces sleep in 10-15 minutes which lasts 6-8 hours. It is not an analgesic. Rapid absorption from gastrointestinal tract or parenteral site. Some excreted unchanged by lungs. Remainder metabolized, probably by liver. End products believed to be carbon dioxide and water.	Nausea, headache, dizziness and unconsciousness may occur. Fatalities are rare. Treatment: lavage, external heat, central nervous system stimulants. Contraindicated in lung congestion. Paraldehyde crosses the placental barrier and, in large doses, can depress neonatal respiration.	Give ice cold or with cold fruit drink. May be habit forming. Gives bad odor to breath.

Name, Source, Synonyms, Preparations	Dosage and Administration	Uses	Action and Fate	Side Effects and Contraindications	Nursing Implications and Remarks
ANTISPASMODICS					
ANTICONVULSANTS					
HYDANTOIN DERIVATIVES					

Warning: Abrupt withdrawal of these agents should be avoided as this has been known to precipitate the condition being treated or, in some cases, status epilepticus. Gradual reduction in dosage is recommended when the clinician desires to reduce the dose, discontinue the drug or substitute another agent. Recent studies have implicated this group of drugs in a higher incidence of birth defects in children born to mothers on anticonvulsant therapy. The studies are not conclusive, and it has not been determined whether more harm would be done by taking the person off the therapy or by leaving him on.

Interactions: Phenytoin can diminish the effect of dexamethasone and may impair therapeutic response. When it is given to patients who are genetically slow inactivators of isoniazid, phenytoin toxicity can occur. Methylphenidate may raise the sensitivity levels of phenytoin. It is not common, but if ataxia appears, the dose of phenytoin should be lowered. Phenobarbital can affect the blood levels of phenytoin in any of three ways–increase, decrease or cause no change. Probably this is not clinically significant with the usual dosage used for anticonvulsive therapy. Phenytoin may be expected to cause some elevation in glucose tolerance, especially in the older age groups, owing to suppression of endogenous insulin secretion. Phenytoin can potentiate the effect of oral anticoagulants, probably because of displacement of the anticoagulant from protein binding sites in the plasma. The possiblity that all hydantoin derivatives can react as does phenytoin should be considered.

Name, Source, Synonyms, Preparations	Dosage and Administration	Uses	Action and Fate	Side Effects and Contraindications	Nursing Implications and Remarks
Phenytoin, U.S.P., N.F. (Dantoin, Dilantin, Diphenlyn) (phenyltoin, Divulsan, Novodiphenyl [C]). Phenytoin, U.S.P. (Denyl sodium, Dilantin sodium, Diphentoin, Diphenylan sodium, Kessodanten) (See above [C]).	30-400 mg. Oral. Individually adjusted. As above. Dosage regulated to suit patient. Available in flavored tablets and suspension for children. Oral, I.M. or I.V. Do not exceed 50 mg./min. I.V.	Used mainly as an anticonvulsant in epilepsy. Its action is highly selective, affecting only motor centers and not the remainder of the cerebral cortex.	Action is through selective depression of motor center in brain. Has little or no sedative or hypnotic action. Readily but slowly absorbed. The sodium salts are rapidly absorbed, widely distributed, slowly detoxified by the liver and excreted in the urine. Exhibits antiarrhythmic properties similar to quinidine and procainamide.	Tremors, ataxia, blurring of vision, loss of taste, insomnia, irritability, gastric irritation, gingivitis and hyperplasia of the gingiva, nystagmus, hirsutism, dysarthia, morbilliform rash. Reports of phenytoin causing peripheral neuropathy, L.E. syndrome, hepatitis, lymphadenopathy, ricketts and osteomalacia. Can depress serum folate and vitamin K levels.	Safe use of the antispasmodic anticonvulsant drugs during pregnancy has not been established. When tolerated, the total daily dose may be given at one time.
Ethotoin (Peganone).	500 mg.-3 Gm. Dosage individually adjusted. Oral.	Similar to phenytoin. Used alone or with other drugs to treat grand mal epilepsy.	Same as above.	Toxicity is low but is similar to that of phenytoin.	Somewhat slower acting, but fewer side effects than with other similar drugs.

Mephenytoin (Mesantoin) (methoin [C]).	200-600 mg. Dosage regulated to suit patient. Oral.	Used mainly as an anticonvulsant in grand mal epilepsy and in psychomotor equivalent. Also used in chorea.	Similar to phenytoin. Somewhat less potent and more sedative than phenytoin.	Rare, but may cause morbilliform rash and pruritus. Stop drug and treat symptoms. Some patients develop tolerance or blood damage.	
SUCCINAMIDE DERIVATIVES					
Ethosuximide (Zarontin).	250 mg.-1 Gm. Dosage individually adjusted. Oral.	For treatment of absence seizures (petit mal epilepsy).	Elevates seizure threshold in the cortex and basal ganglia and reduces synaptic response to low frequency repetitive stimulation. Suppresses the wave pattern of the EEG which is common in absence seizures. Absorbed from G.I. tract. Excreted slowly in urine.	Similar to other drugs of this type. Most common side effects include anorexia, weight loss, nausea, vomiting and epigastric distress and dyskinesias.	4-7 days of therapy required to achieve steady state plasma concentration.
Methsuximide, N.F. (Celontin) (mesuximide [C]).	150-300 mg. Dosage individually adjusted. Oral.	Used for absence seizures (petit mal) and psychomotor attacks.	As above.	See above.	
Phensuximide, N.F. (Milontin).	250-500 mg. Dosage individually adjusted. Oral.	Used to treat absence seizures (petit mal epilepsy).	As above.	Drowsiness, nausea, vertigo occur. Adjust dosage.	
OXAZOLIDINEDIONE DERIVATIVES					
Paramethadione, U.S.P. (Paradione).	300-900 mg. Dosage regulated to suit patient. Oral.	Used mainly as an anticonvulsant in absence seizures (petit mal), myoclonic and akinetic epilepsy refractory to other drugs. It is also used with other drugs in grand mal epilepsy and as a sedative.	As above. Changed mainly by the liver, but other tissues may aid in its degradation. Excreted in the urine.	Drowsiness is the most frequent side effect; mistiness of vision, skin rash, dermatitis, gastric disturbances. Aplastic anemia has been reported after its use. Much less toxic than trimethadione. Contraindicated in severe renal or hepatic disorders.	

Name, Source, Synonyms, Preparations	Dosage and Administration	Uses	Action and Fate	Side Effects and Contraindications	Nursing Implications and Remarks
ANTISPASMODICS (Continued)					
Trimethadione, U.S.P. (Tridione) (troxidone, Trimedone [C]).	100-300 mg. Dosage regulated to suit patient. Oral.	Used mainly as an anticonvulsant in absence seizures (petit mal), myoclonic and akinetic epilepsy refractory to other drugs. It is also used with other drugs in grand mal epilepsy and as a sedative.	Similar to paramethadione. Readily absorbed, widely distributed.	Drowsiness, mistiness of vision, skin rash, gastric disturbances. Aplastic anemia has been reported after its use. Stop drug and treat symptoms.	
BARBITURATES		**(Refer to page 132 for information concerning these drugs.)*			
Mephobarbital*					
Metharbital*					
Phenobarbital*					
OTHERS					
Carbamazepine, U.S.P. (Tegretol).	100-200 mg. b.i.d. Oral. Dose adjusted to individual.	For control of seizures when other antiepilepsy agents ineffective. For symptomatic relief of pain with true trigeminal neuralgia.	Has action similar to hydantoin derivatives. Provides pain relief in trigeminal neuralgia by reducing synaptic transmission within the trigeminal nucleus. Has demonstrated sedative, antidepressant, muscle relaxation, anti-arrhythmic, anti-diuretic and neuromuscular transmission-inhibitory actions. Slowly absorbed from G.I. tract. Relatively long plasma half-life of 8-72 h. Widely distributed, crosses the	May produce dangerous side effects such as hemopoietic, cardiovascular, hepatic and renal disturbances. Shares the toxic potentials of hydantoin derivative antiepilepsy drugs. Patients should be under close medical supervision during treatment. Neurological and sensory side effects occur and include: headache, dizziness, vertigo, drowsiness, fatigue, ataxia, confusion, nystagmus, sensory disturbances and involuntary movements.	Should not be administered to pregnant women or nursing mothers. May take 2-4 days of therapy to achieve steady-state plasma levels. Carbamazepine should be withdrawn slowly to avoid precipitating seizures or status epilepticus.

			placenta. Metabolic fate unknown. Appears in breast milk, excreted in urine.	G.I. and dermatological side effects may also occur.	
Clonazepam (Clonipin).	Adult: initial daily dose 1.5 mg./day, increase by 0.5-1.0 mg./day to a maximum of 20 mg./day or until seizure controlled. Children: 0.01-0.05 mg./kg./day. Increase every 3rd day to a maximum maintenance dose of 0.1 to 0.2 mg./kg./day or seizure control.	Absence seizures (petit mal). infantile spasms, myoclonic seizures, infantile atypical absence, and akinetic seizures.	Exact mechanism is unknown. Benzodiazepines are known to enhance polysynaptic inhibition at all CNS levels. Clonazepam limits spread of EEG discharge but doesn't suppress the primary focus. After oral dose it reaches a peak serum level in about 2 hours. It has a ½ life between 20 and 30 hours. Effective serum levels are said to be between 5 and 50 nanograms/ml. Metabolized in the liver, excreted via kidneys.	Rare but serious side effects include: aplastic anemia, Stevens-Johnson syndrome, hepatitis, inappropriate antidiuretic hormone secretion and lupus erythematosus syndrome. Adverse effects seen most often are drowsiness, which may decrease with continued therapy, ataxia and behavioral disturbances, especially in children. May increase salivation and cause some respiratory depression so use with caution in patients with chronic respiratory disease. See hydantoin derivatives for warning.	For drug interactions see chlordiazepoxide. With patients on long-term therapy, periodic blood and liver tests are recommended. Mothers should not breast feed while taking clonazepam. Concurrent administration with valproic acid is not recommended.
Magnesium sulfate, U.S.P.	1-2 Gm. in 10-20% solution with flow rate not exceeding 1.5 ml./min. I.V. 1-2 Gm. in 25-50% solution I.M.	Anticonvulsant primarily for prevention and control of seizures in severe pre-eclampsia or in eclampsia. Also in conditions of hypomagnesemia.	Exhibits anticonvulsant activity when given parenterally. Depresses C.N.S. and blocks neuromuscular transmission, producing anti-convulsant effects. Exact mechanism unknown; however, excessive magnesium appears to decrease the amount of acetylcholine liberated by motor nerve impulse. Also acts peripherally, producing vasodilation.	Side effects due to magnesium intoxication include flushing, sweating, hypotension, reflex depression, depression of cardiac function and C.N.S. depression. Can proceed to fatal respiratory paralysis. Administer with caution to patients with impaired renal function because of danger of magnesium intoxication. Parenteral administration	Patients on parenteral therapy should have serum magnesium closely monitored to avoid overdosage. Disappearance of patellar reflex is a useful sign for detection of onset of magnesium intoxication. Check this reflex before each dose to determine if additional doses should be given. Check urinary output.

Name, Source, Synonyms, Preparations	Dosage and Administration	Uses	Action and Fate	Side Effects and Contraindications	Nursing Implications and Remarks
ANTISPASMODICS (Continued)			Moderate doses produce sweating. Larger doses lower blood pressure. Action of hypermagnesemia can be antagonized by administration of excess calcium. Excreted by the kidneys.	contraindicated in patients with myocardial damage or heart block. When given concomitantly with C.N.S. depressants, dosage must be readjusted because of additive depressant effects. Excessive neuromuscular blockade has occurred in patients receiving parenteral magnesium sulfate and a neuromuscular blocking agent. Give with caution to digitalized patients.	Discontinue if output is less than 100 ml. during the preceding 4 h. period. A parenteral calcium preparation should be available to counteract the potential hazard of magnesium intoxication.
Phenacemide (Phenurone) (phenacetylcarbamide [C]).	500 mg. Dosage individually adjusted. Oral.	Used mainly as an anticonvulsant in petit mal, myoclonic and akinetic epilepsy. It is also used to treat grand mal epilepsy and as a sedative. Used to control severe epilepsy, particularly mixed forms of psychomotor seizures refractory to other drugs.	Exact mechanism is not known, but it is thought to act similarly to the hydantoins, and is effective against psychic and psychomotor types of epilepsy. Well absorbed orally, slowly changed by liver. Little if any excreted unchanged.	Highly toxic. Personality changes, signs of hepatic disorder, depression of blood count and drug rash may occur. Stop drug and treat symptoms.	Used only when other anticonvulsants are ineffective.
Primidone, U.S.P. (Mysoline).	50-250 mg. Dosage individually adjusted. Oral. Up to 2 Gm. daily may be required.	Used mainly in grand mal epilepsy and psychomotor equivalent.	Pyrimidine derivative similar to phenobarbital. Absorbed from gastrointestinal tract. Exact fate unknown, but it is thought that both liver and kidneys act to metabolize it. Primidone is converted to two active metabolites, phenobarbital	Toxicity may cause nausea, vomiting, drowsiness, headache, ataxia, lethargy and malaise. Adjustment of dosage usually suffices. Emotional disturbances, skin rash and megaloblastic anemia have been reported infrequently.	Blood picture should be checked with prolonged use.

			and phenylethylmalonamide (PEMA). The plasma half-life varies widely with different individuals (3-24 hours). Excreted in urine.		
Valproate sodium (Depakene syrup) Valproic acid (Depakene)	5-10 mg./kg./day initially with dose adjusted weekly until seizures controlled. 30 mg./kg./day maximum. Oral.	Alone or with other agents in prophylactic management of absence (petit mal) seizures. Some success in management of psychomotor, myoclonic and akinetic epilepsy and seizures precipitated by photic stimuli.	Mechanism of action not known. Effects may be related to increased brain levels of inhibitory neurotransmitter, gamma-aminobutyric acid. Valproate sodium is converted to the acid after oral administration. Valproic acid is rapidly and almost completely absorbed from G.I. tract. Peak plasma levels usually attained in 1-4 h. Onset of effects occurs in several days to more than 1 week following initiation of therapy. Rapidly distributed, crosses placenta of animals. Metabolized primarily in the liver and excreted in urine with small amounts in feces and expired air.	Most frequent side effects are nausea, vomiting and indigestion. These are usually transient and can be minimized by giving with meals or by beginning therapy with low doses and gradually increasing. Hypersalivation, anorexia, weight loss, increased appetite and weight gain, abdominal cramps, diarrhea and constipation also reported. Leukopenia and hair loss possible. Sedation and drowsiness may occur if patient receiving other antiepileptic drug. May prolong bleeding time. Drug should not be given to women who are or may become pregnant unless possible benefits outweigh potential risks. Since effects in nursing infants are unknown, should not be given to nursing mothers.	May produce false positive results in tests for urine ketones. Valproic acid capsules should be swallowed and not chewed to prevent irritation to mouth and throat. Valproate sodium syrup should not be given in carbonated drinks to prevent release of the acid, which causes an unpleasant taste and local irritation. Daily doses exceeding 250 mg. should be divided. Warn patient against concurrent use of alcohol and depressant drugs as well as hazardous activities until drug's sedative effect is determined. Additive C.N.S. depression when given with other C.N.S. depressants, including phenobarbital, primidone and alcohol as well as with monoamine oxidase (MAO) inhibitors.

Name, Source, Synonyms, Preparations	Dosage and Administration	Uses	Action and Fate	Side Effects and Contraindications	Nursing Implications and Remarks
SKELETAL MUSCLE RELAXANTS. (Also see diazepam and chlordiazepoxide.)					
All of the following may cause drowsiness and the patient should be cautioned about driving a car or operating machinery during therapy.					
SYNTHETIC PREPARATIONS					
Baclofen (Lioresal)	Requires individual titration, 5-20 mg. t.i.d. with maximum of 20 mg. q.i.d. Oral.	Alleviation of spasticity resulting from multiple sclerosis, particularly for relief of flexor spasms and accompanying pain, clonus and muscular rigidity. Also used in patients with spinal cord injuries.	Precise mechanism of action not known. Capable of inhibiting both monosynaptic and polysynaptic reflexes at the spinal level. It is shown to have C.N.S. depressant properties in studies with animals. Rapidly and extensively absorbed. Excreted primarily in urine in unchanged form. Absorption may be dose dependent and may decrease with increasing doses.	Most common side effects are transient drowsiness, dizziness, weakness and fatigue. Other effects include: confusion, headache, insomnia, hypotension, nausea, constipation, urinary frequency, rash, pruritus, ankle edema, excessive perspiration, weight gain and nasal congestion. Overdosage: vomiting, muscular hypotonia, drowsiness, accommodation disorders, coma, respiratory depression and seizures. Hallucinations have occurred with abrupt withdrawal. Use with caution in patients with impaired renal function. Use in pregnancy, lactation, and children under 12 years of age is not recommended. C.N.S. effects may be additive to those of other C.N.S. depressants, including alcohol.	Use with caution in patients in whom spasticity is utilized to sustain upright posture and balance in locomotion or whenever spasticity is used to obtain increased function. In epileptic patients the clinical state and EEG should be monitored regularly because deterioration in seizure control and EEG has been reported occasionally. Abnormal lab tests found in a few patients and include increased SGOT, alkaline phosphatase and blood sugar.

Carisoprodol (Rela, Soma) (isomeprobamate [C]).	350 mg. Usually given q.i.d. Oral.	Muscle relaxant and analgesic for back pain, sprains and traumatic injuries.	Similar to meprobamate but said to have a greater skeletal muscle relaxant effect. Carisprodol is metabolized by the liver and excreted by the kidneys. Crosses the placenta and may appear in breast milk.	May cause drowsiness and other central nervous system effects or skin rashes of the allergic-reaction type. See meprobamate for interactions.	Safe use in pregnancy and lactation not established.
Chlormezanone (Chlormethazanone, Trancopal).	100-200 mg. Usually given q.i.d. Oral.	Treatment of mild anxiety and tension states.	Exact mechanism is not known, but does not appear to have specific effect on spasticity or difficulties associated with organic neuro disorders.	May cause drug rash, dizziness, flushing, nausea, weakness, anorexia, voiding difficulties and jaundice.	As above.
Chlorphenesin carbamate (Maolate).	400 mg. q.i.d. to 800 mg. t.i.d. Oral.	As an adjunct in short-term therapy of inflammatory and traumatic conditions of skeletal muscles when relief of discomfort is desired.	Said to have selective internuncial blocking action. It antagonizes the convulsions produced by strychnine or electroshock, but not those produced by pentylenetetrazol. Structurally and pharmacologically related to mephenesin.	Drowsiness, dizziness, nausea, insomnia, increased nervousness and headache. If skin rash or other signs of sensitivity occur the drug should be stopped. Chlorphenesin is not recommended for patients with hepatic dysfunction.	Safety for use during pregnancy and lactation or for children has not been established. Patients should be cautioned about driving a motor vehicle or using dangerous mechanical apparatus.
Chlorzoxazone (Paraflex).	250 mg. Usually given three to four times daily. Oral.	Uses as for carisoprodol.	Similar to mephenesin in ability to interrupt nervous impulses in polysynaptic pathways of spinal cord.	Anorexia, headache, weakness, drowsiness and skin rash. Impaired liver function and jaundice have been reported.	Use with caution in patients with history of liver disease. Safe use in pregnancy not established.

Name, Source, Synonyms, Preparations	Dosage and Administration	Uses	Action and Fate	Side Effects and Contraindications	Nursing Implications and Remarks
SKELETAL MUSCLE RELAXANTS (Continued)					
Cyclobenzaprine hydrochloride (Flexeril).	20-40 mg./day in 2-4 divided doses. Should not be administered for more than 2-3 weeks.	Relief of discomfort associated with acute painful musculo-skeletal conditions.	Parmacologically related to tricyclic antidepressants. C.N.S. depressant with sedative and skeletal muscle relaxant effects. Potentiates effect of norepinephrine and has anticholinergic effect. Almost completely absorbed from G.I. tract. Metabolized by liver and excreted as metabolite in urine and feces via bile.	Shares toxic potential of tricyclic antidepressants and usual precautions should prevail. Most frequent side effects are drowsiness, dry mouth and dizziness. Occasional side effects include G.I. discomfort, unpleasant taste, weakness, blurred vision, paresthesia and insomnia. Use with caution in patients with history of urinary retention, narrow angle glaucoma or increased intraocular pressure. Contraindicated in patients with hyperthyroidism, congestive heart failure, arrhythmias, heart block or conduction disorders.	Safe use in pregnancy and lactation and in children under 15 years not established. Patient should be warned that the drug may impair ability to perform hazardous activities requiring alertness or physical coordination.
Dantrolene sodium (Dantrium).	25 mg. t.i.d. to 200 mg. q.i.d. Oral.	Used to control spasticity (where reversible) from chronic disorders such as spinal cord injury, cerebrovascular accident, cerebral palsy, multiple sclerosis.	Acts directly on muscles to cause skeletal muscle relaxation without affecting coordination or neuromuscular transmission effect, probably by interfering with the release of activator from the sarcoplasmic reticulum. Absorption is slow and incomplete but consistent. Dose-related blood levels are obtained. Duration and intensity of skeletal muscle	Drowsiness, dizziness, fatigue weakness, diarrhea, malaise and more. It is potentially hepatotoxic and liver function must be closely monitored, especially in patients receiving the drug for more than 60 days, and in women over 35 receiving concurrent estrogen therapy. Contraindication where spasticity is utilized to maintain upright position or increased	Patients should be warned about driving a car or participating in any hazardous occupation while taking this drug. Concomitant use of tranquilizing agents should be avoided, if possible. Carcinogenicity cannot be fully excluded so this should be weighed against benefits in long-term use. Safe use in

			reaction is related to blood level obtained. Mean biologic half-life is 7-8 hours after a 100 mg dose.	function. Drug may evoke photosensitivity. Used with caution in patients with obstructive pulmonary disease, impaired pulmonary function and decreased cardiac function due to myocardial disease.	pregnancy or for children under 5 years of age not established.
Mephenesin (Daserol, Myanesin, Romeph, Tolsil) (Tolserol [C]).	1-3 Gm. Individually adjusted. Oral.	See carisoprodol.	Depresses the basal ganglia, brainstem and synaptic connections in the spinal cord. Some sedation also occurs. Good absorption and distribution by all routes. Higher concentration found in brain than in plasma. Metabolic degradation occurs in liver, products of which are excreted in urine.	Rare in therapeutic dosage. Treatment: none usually required. Lassitude occasionally occurs, and leukopenia has been reported but rarely.	
Meprobamate, N.F. (Equanil, Meprospan, Meprotabs, Miltown, Vio-Bamate)(Gene-Bamata, LanDol, Meditran, Mep-E, Meprox-400, Novomepro, Neo-Tran, Probasan, Quietal, Tranquate, Tranquiline, Trelmar, Wescomep [C]).	400 mg. t.i.d. or q.i.d. Oral and I.M.	Used in treatment of neuroses and as a muscle relaxant. Especially valuable in emotional disturbances. Used as a tranquilizer alone and in various combinations. The only indication for intramuscular meprobamate is in tetanus.	Acts as a skeletal muscle relaxant and ataractic. It is said to block interneural synaptic passage of impulse and to reduce sensitivity of the thalami. Good oral absorption and uniform distribution throughout body. Some excreted unchanged but most as hydroxymeprobamate and as the glucuronide. Crosses the placenta. Excreted in urine, and in milk of nursing mothers.	Drowsiness and allergic reactions have been reported. Dosage adjustment, antihistamine or both usually suffice. When taken concurrently, meprobamate and alcohol give an additive or synergistic increase in central nervous system depression. Meprobamate is capable of inducing hepatic microsomal enzymes which metabolize warfarin, but it has been shown in animals only, not in man.	Dependence can occur after long-term use at high doses (1.6-2.4 Gm. per day). Should not be used during pregnancy or lactation. Pain, induration, nodules or sterile abscesses may occur at I.M. injection sites.

Name, Source, Synonyms, Preparations	Dosage and Administration	Uses	Action and Fate	Side Effects and Contraindications	Nursing Implications and Remarks
SKELETAL MUSCLE RELAXANTS (Continued)					
Metaxalone (Skelaxin).	400-800 mg. q.i.d. Oral.	A skeletal muscle relaxant for treatment of acute muscle spasms caused by traumatic injuries.	Drug blocks synaptic pathways in the spinal cord. Good oral absorption. Metabolized in liver and excreted in urine. Not known whether it crosses the placenta or appears in milk.	Nausea, vomiting, dizziness, headache, nervousness and skin rash. Blood changes may occur in some patients. Contraindicated during pregnancy or in patients with a tendency to drug-induced leukemia or anemia.	Should not be given longer than 10 days. Additive C.N.S. depression when administered along with other C.N.S. depressants such as alcohol. May cause false positive for glucose in tests using cupric sulfate (Benedict's, Clinitest, etc.).
Methocarbamol, N.F. (Robamol, Robaxin) (glyceryl guaiacolate carbamate, [C]).	500 mg.-2 Gm. Usually given q.i.d. Oral. 1 Gm. I.V. or I.M.	Uses as for carisoprodol. Low therapeutic index.	Similar to mephenesin. Rapidly absorbed from G.I. tract. Widely distributed, crossing the placenta. Metabolized in liver, excreted primarily in urine.	May cause lightheadedness, drowsiness, mental confusion and skin eruptions. Nausea, flushing, dizziness, hypotension and bradycardia have been reported with I.V. administration.	Safety for use in pregnancy or lactation not established.
Orphenadrine citrate, N.F. (Norflex).	100 mg. b.i.d. or t.i.d. Oral.	Used for acute spasm of voluntary muscles, regardless of location. Especially for post-traumatic, discogenic and tension spasms.	Mechanism of action unknown, but may be due to analgesic properties.	Side effects are due mainly to anticholinergic action of drug. Orphenadrine can cause lightheadedness and syncope and may impair ability of patient to engage in potentially hazardous activities. It should not be used in patients with glaucoma, pyloric or duodenal ulcer, prostatic hypertrophy, obstruction of bladder neck or myasthenia gravis.	Safe use in pregnancy has not been established.

MUSCLE RELAXANTS. (Strong, Surgical Adjunct Drugs)					
Hexafluorenium bromide (Mylaxen) (hexaflurenium bromide [C]).	Adjusted according to amount of succinylcholine administered. See package insert. Parenteral.	Used to prolong and potentiate the relaxing action of succinylcholine during surgery.	Neuromuscular blocking agent with action similar to that of curare, when given to an anesthetized subject.	When used in conjunction with succinylcholine, it shares the toxic potentials of the neuromuscular blocking agents. Usual precautions should be followed. Use with caution in patients with bronchial asthma. Contraindicated in patients hypersensitive to bromides.	A synthetic preparation.
CURARE. *Species of Strychnos and synthetic.*					

INTERACTIONS: The use of quinidine in the immediate postoperative period following use of tubocurare can result in recurarization and can lead to respiratory paralysis. Tubocurare, when used concurrently with the following antibiotics–neomycin, streptomycin, kanamycin, polymyxin-B, bacitracin, viomycin, colistin and gentamicin–can result in a significant incidence of prolonged respiratory failure. The neuromuscular block of tubocurare can be augmented, in both magnitude and duration, by the concurrent use of propranolol. The action of all nondepolarizing muscle relaxants may be enhanced by the thiazide diuretics, chlorthalidone, furosemide and ethacrynic acid.

Dimethyl tubocurarine iodide, N.F. (Metubine). Tubocurarine chloride, U.S.P. (Delacurarine) (Tubarine [C]).	1.5-6 mg. I.V. 6-9 mg. I.V.	Used to relax the skeletal muscles in surgery, tetanus, encephalitis, poliomyelitis and in any condition in which a strong muscle relaxant is needed. Used also to lessen the convulsions in shock therapy.	Blocks passage of nerve impulse at the myoneural junctions. Action starts in muscles of eye, finger and toes and then spreads. Respiratory muscles are affected last. A less pronounced action is the blocking of the impulse in the autonomic ganglia. Widely distributed with concentrations at neuromuscular junction. After intravenous administration, effects begin to wear off in 20 minutes, with residual effect for 2 to 4 hours.	Respiratory and cardiac paralysis may occur. Treatment: artificial respiration. Neostigmine (Prostigmin) and edrophonium are the physiologic antidotes.	Dosage of curare or curare-like drugs varies with individual cases.

Name, Source, Synonyms, Preparations	Dosage and Administration	Uses	Action and Fate	Side Effects and Contraindications	Nursing Implications and Remarks
MUSCLE RELAXANTS (Continued)			Approximately half is excreted unchanged by the kidneys; remainder probably metabolized by the liver. Dimethyl tubocurarine has a shorter duration of action.		
Pancuronium bromide (Pavulon).	Individualized. Adults usually 0.04 to 0.1 mg./kg. initially. For endotracheal intubation 0.06 to 0.1 mg./kg. I.V.	Used to induce skeletal muscle relaxation during surgery or for endotracheal intubation.	Has all the characteristics of curare-like drugs on the myoneural junctions. Approximately 5 times as potent as *d*-tubocurarine chloride, mg. for mg. basis. Major portion is excreted unchanged in the urine.	Side effects: Main side effect is duration of action that is longer than usually required for surgery, and can leave skeletal muscle weakness for prolonged periods, resulting in respiratory insufficiency or apnea. Also, there is inadequate reversal by anticholinesterase agents, requiring manual or mechanical ventilation until the dose wears off. Slight increase in pulse rate, salivation and a transient rash have been seen.	Caution: Should be used only by physicians thoroughly prepared to handle this type of medication and having facilities to deal with any complication. Safe use in pregnancy has not been established. Patients with a history of myasthenia gravis can suffer profound effects from very small doses of the drug.
Decamethonium bromide (Syncurine).	2-25 mg. I.V.	As above.	Decamethonium bromide and succinylcholine chloride act by persistent depolarization of the motor end plate. Decamethonium and gallamine are excreted by the kidneys unchanged. Succinylcholine is rapidly hydrolized by the pseudocholinesterases to succinic acid and choline which are naturally occurring body constituents. About 10% excreted unchanged by the kidneys.	Decamethonium bromide or succinylcholine chloride is never counteracted with neostigmine or edrophonium, as either of these will enhance the depolarizing effect of the drugs.	The action resulting from the use of decamethonium bromide and gallamine iodide is similar to that of curare. However, gallamine is a nondepolarizing type of muscle relaxant. Succinylcholine chloride is similar to curare and does not have cumulative action.
Gallamine triethiodide, U.S.P. (Flaxedil).	1 mg./kg. of body weight. I.V.	As above.			
Succinylcholine chloride, U.S.P. (Anectine, Quelicin, Sucostrin, Suxinyl) (suxamethonium chloride, Scoline, Sux-Cert [C]).	10-30 mg. I.V.	As above.			

TRANQUILIZERS AND SIMILAR DRUGS

(Refer also to antiemetics, antihistamines, antihypertensives, skeletal muscle relaxants and central nervous system depressants.) With many of these drugs, drowsiness or delayed reflexes may occur. Patients should be cautioned on initiation of drug about driving or operating machinery. These are all synthetic preparations unless otherwise noted.

INTERACTIONS OF PHENOTHIAZINES, BUTYROPHENONES AND THIOTHIXENES: The phenothiazines and the barbiturates interact in a number of ways. The phenothiazines can potentiate the central nervous system depressant effect of the barbiturates. The barbiturates can increase the risk of orthostatic hypotension, especially when given intravenously. When barbiturates are given concurrently with the phenothiazines, both in large doses, the barbiturates can cause an increase in metabolic inactivation of the phenothiazines.

Adrenergic blocking agents such as propranolol and phentolamine should be used in lower dosage when given concurrently with the phenothiazines.

Phenothiazines can enhance the hypotensive effects of some antihypertensive drugs, but with guanethidine the opposite appears to be true.

Concurrent use of phenothiazines and amphetamines, except in amphetamine overdosage, is not pharmacologically sound owing to their antagonistic effects. The reverse may also be true.

Epinephrine should not be given to patients who are taking phenothiazines, since it may result in a fall in blood pressure. However, levarterenol and phenylephrine can be used.

Haloperidol may reduce the prothrombin time when given concurrently with phenindiones or indandiones.

The phenothiazine derivatives all have similar actions, but vary as to degree. All exert a depressant action on selective portions of the brain, probably the hypothalamus. They tend to make patients more cooperative, less anxious, etc. They all are to some extent antiemetic, antihistaminic, weak beta-adrenergic blockers, antispasmodic, hypotensive and hypothermic. These drugs all potentiate other depressant drugs, but amount of depression varies.

Name, Source, Synonyms, Preparations	Dosage and Administration	Uses	Action and Fate	Side Effects and Contraindications	Nursing Implications and Remarks
PHENOTHIAZINE DERIVATIVES *Aliphatic Type* Acepromazine (Atravet, Plegicil).	10-30 mg. Oral. 150-200 mg. Oral.	Indications for phenothiazines, butyrophenones and thioxanthenes: acute and chronic schizophrenia, may be used as an adjunct to anesthesia, as antiemetics, for motion sickness and the treatment of amphetamine psychosis. They are indicated for patients with non-psychotic excitement, anxiety or severe tension syndromes when other agents are ineffective.	Readily absorbed from gastrointestinal tract and parenteral sites. Widely and rapidly distributed with highest concentration in lungs and in following organs in decreasing order: liver, adrenal glands, spleen, brain and plasma. Metabolic degradation occurs in the liver. Metabolites excreted	Side effects of aliphatic phenothiazines: Frequent—drowsiness, hypotension and atropine-like effects. Various skin problems may occur, often with marked photosensitivity. Occasional—parkinsonism, dystonia, galactorrhea, photosensitivity, menstrual changes, cholestatic	Periodic blood checks are advised.
Promazine hydrochloride, N.F. (Sparine) (Atarzine, Intrazine, Promagen, Promanyl, Promwill, Promazettes, Premezerine [C]).	25-100 mg. q. 4-6 h. Oral and parenteral.		by kidneys. Unchanged drug found about equally in urine and stools. Excretion is relatively slow. Some found in body for days or weeks. Acts primarily at subcortical levels on the	jaundice, rashes, convulsions and ECG changes. Rare—lenticular deposits and opacities (after long-term use at high doses) and blood dyscrasias.	
Chlorpromazine hydrochloride, U.S.P. (Promapar, Thorazine) (Chlor-Promanyl, Chlorpromazine, Chlorprom, Chlorprom-Ez-Ets, Elmarine, Largactil, Onazine, Promosol [C]).	10-200 mg. t.i.d. Oral or I.M., depending on condition being treated.		reticular formation, hypothalamus, and limbic system. No significant cortical depression. Produces sedation without hypnosis, analgesia, blockade of conditioned		If patient is ambulatory, watch for signs of over-depression; with prolonged therapy, watch for jaundice.
Methoxypromazine maleate (Tentone).	10-50 mg. t.i.d. Dosage individually adjusted to a total of 30-500 mg./day in divided doses. Oral.		avoidance behavior, alterations of temperature regulation and skeletal muscle tone, antiemetic and antipruritic effects, facilitation of seizure		
Triflupromazine hydrochloride, N.F. (Vesprin).	10-50 mg. t.i.d. to q.i.d. Oral. 2-20 mg. t.i.d. to q.i.d. Parenteral. 35-70 mg. One b.i.d. Suppository.		discharge and endocrine alteration. Action on autonomic nervous system results in effects from: cholinergic blocking, alpha-adrenergic potentiating, antiserotonin,		

			and prevention of uptake of biological amines. Also results in antihistamine effects.		
Piperazine Type					
Acetophenazine maleate, N.F. (Tindal).	20-40 mg. t.i.d. Oral.	Treatment of anxiety, tension, agitation, and hyper-excitability in ambulatory patients.	As above.	Side effects of piperazine-type phenothiazines: Frequent–parkinsonism, akathisia, dystonic reactions, atropine-like effects. Occasional–photosensitivity reactions, galactorrhea, menstrual changes, drowsiness, postural hypotension, anorexia and rashes. Rare–cholestatic jaundice, blood dyscrasias, lenticular deposits and opacities (with long-term use at high doses), ECG abnormalities, decreased libido and convulsions.	Contraindicated in comatose patients, especially those whose depression is due to drugs, in the presence of circulatory collapse and bone marrow depression, in patients with a history of jaundice, blood dyscrasias or hypersensitivity to phenothiazines.
Butaperazine (Repoise).	Up to 100 mg. per day. Start with 5-10 mg. t.i.d. and increase as indicated.	Treatment of chronic schizophrenia.			
Carphenazine maleate, N.F. (Proketazine).	12.5-50 mg. Dosage individually adjusted. Oral.	An ataractic and tranquilizing agent used to treat certain schizophrenic reactions in hospitalized patients.	Similar to other phenothiazine drugs.	Alteration in cephalin flocculation; contraindicated in excessive psychomotor agitation, in comatose states and during pregnancy. Used with caution if central nervous system depressants are being used.	

Name, Source, Synonyms, Preparations	Dosage and Administration	Uses	Action and Fate	Side Effects and Contraindications	Nursing Implications and Remarks
PHENOTHIAZINE DERIVATIVES (Continued)					
Fluphenazine enanthate (Prolixin enanthate).	25 mg. every 2 weeks. I.M. or S.Q.	Treatment of acute and chronic schizophrenia.	As other phenothiazine derivatives. Distribution and metabolism not known.	As with phenothiazines.	When given I.M., the fluphenazine decanoate or enanthate in sesame oil allows for onset of action within 24-72 h., with duration of 1-6 weeks (and an average of 2 weeks).
Fluphenazine hydrochloride, N.F. (Permitil, Prolixin, Trancin) (Moditen [C]).	0.25-5 mg. three times daily. Dosage individually adjusted. Oral, I.M.				
Fluphenazine decanoate (Prolixin Decanoate Inj.).	Dosage individually adjusted. Usually 25-50 mg. every 2 or 3 weeks. I.M. or subcutaneously.			See phenothiazines, p. 154.	Usual phenothiazine precautions.
Perphenazine, N.F. (Trilafon).	2-16 mg. t.i.d. Oral. 5 mg. I.M. Repeat in 6 hours if required. Dosage should be individually adjusted.	Uses similar to those of others of this group.	As above.		The oral concentrate should not be mixed with Coca Cola, black coffee, tea, grape or apple juices.
Prochlorperazine, N.F. (Compazine) (Stemetil [C]).	5-25 mg. three to four times a day. Rectal.	As above.	As above.	As above.	
Prochlorperazine edisylate, U.S.P. (Compazine edisylate).	5-10 mg. Oral or I.M.	As above.	As above.	As above.	
Prochlorperazine maleate, U.S.P. (Compazine dimaleate).	10-75 mg. b.i.d. Sustained-release capsules. Oral. 5-25 mg. three to four times a day. Dosage should be individually adjusted. Oral.	As above.	As above.	As above.	
Trifluoperazine (Stelazine) (Chem-Flurazine, Clinazine, Fluazine, Novoflurazine, Pentazine, Solazine, Triflurin, Terfluzine, Trifluoper-Ez-Ets [C]).	1-10 mg. three to four times daily. Dose individually adjusted. Oral or I.M.		See beginning of phenothiazine group.	Contraindicated in patients with impaired cardiovascular systems.	Maximum therapeutic response achieved within 2-3 weeks after therapy initiated.

Thiopropazate dihydrochloride, N.F. (Dartal [C]).	5-10 mg. three to four times daily. Oral.		This is said to be hydrolyzed to perphenazine.	Apparently low.	
Piperidine Type					
Mesoridazine besylate (Serentil).	10-400 mg. daily. Oral or I.M. Dosage individually adjusted.		Action as with others of this group. Well absorbed orally; biological half-life between 24 and 48 hours; excreted mainly in urine, but there is some via biliary tract.	Side effects of piperidine-type phenothiazines: Frequent–drowsiness, hypotension, atropine-like effects, weight gain, inhibition of ejaculation. Occasional–parkinsonism, akathisia, menstrual changes, photosensitivity reactions, ECG abnormalities and galactorrhea. Rare–pigmentary retinopathy (after long-term at high doses), cholestatic jaundice, blood dyscrasias, dystonic reactions, convulsions and rashes.	As with others of this group. Safe use of this drug during pregnancy or for children under 12 years of age has not been established.
Piperacetazine (Quide).	10-160 mg. daily. Oral. Dosage individually adjusted. Starting dose not to exceed 40 mg./day.		See phenothiazines, p. 154.		Safe use during pregnancy or for children has not been established.
Thioridazine (Mellaril) (Novoridazine, Thioril [C]).	10-200 mg. three to four times daily. Oral.				
BUTYROPHENONE DERIVATIVES					
Droperidol (Inapsine).	2.5-10 mg. I.M. or I.V. 30-60 minutes prior to induction. 2.5 mg./20-25 lb., usually I.V. 1.25-2.5 mg. I.V. 1.0-1.5 mg./20-25 lb. for children 2-12 years of age.	As premedication, before surgery. For induction anesthesia. Maintenance of anesthesia. Drug is sedative, tranquilizer, has antianxiety activity and will reduce nausea and vomiting.	See haloperidol.	Side effects of butyrophenones: Frequent–parkinsonism, akathisia, dystonia (especially in children). Occasional–blood dyscrasias, postural hypotension, sedation, menstrual changes and galactorrhea. Rare–cholestatic jaundice, photosensitivity, rashes, weight gain, convulsions, impotence and neurotoxicity in hyperthyroid patients.	Use with caution in patients with liver or kidney dysfunction and those with parkinsonism. Safe use during pregnancy has not been established.

Name, Source, Synonyms, Preparations	Dosage and Administration	Uses	Action and Fate	Side Effects and Contraindications	Nursing Implications and Remarks
BUTYROPHENONE DERIVATIVES (Continued)					
Haloperidol, N.F. (Haldol).	Initial 1-5 mg. b.i.d. Adjust individually. Oral, I.M.	Acute or chronic psychosis.	This is a butyrophenone with chemical structure similar to meperidine but with action similar to the piperazine-substituted phenothiazines. Well absorbed from G.I. tract. Appears to be detoxified in liver. Excreted slowly in urine and feces, human milk. Small amounts excreted for about 28 days following oral administration.	Contraindications: Comatose patients, those depressed by alcohol or other centrally acting agents, patients with parkinsonism, those under 12 years of age and during pregnancy. Use with caution in patients receiving anticoagulant therapy.	Appears to have very narrow range between effective therapeutic dose in acute psychoses and that causing extrapyramidal symptoms.
THIOXANTHENES					
Chlorprothixene, N.F. (Taractan) (Tarasan [C]).	10-100 mg. daily. Oral. 25-50 mg. I.M. Dosage individually adjusted.	See Phenothiazine Derivatives, page 154.	Is a thioxanthene derivative and has action similar to that of the phenothiazines. Partially absorbed from G.I. tract. With I.M. injection, exerts effects within 10-30 min. Presumably metabolized by liver and excreted in urine and feces.	Side effects of thioxanthenes: Chlorprothixene: Frequent–drowsiness, hypotension, atropine-like effects. Occasional–parkinsonism, dystonic reactions, galactorrhea, photosensitivity reactions, menstrual changes, cholestatic jaundice, rashes, convulsions, ECG abnomalities and weight gain. Rare–lenticular deposits and opacities (with long-term use at high doses) and blood dyscrasias.	Hematologic studies advised with prolonged use. Oral liquid preparation can be made more palatable by mixing the concentrate with milk, water, fruit juices, coffee or carbonated beverages.

Thiothixene (Navane).	Initial 5 mg. b.i.d., then adjust to suit response. Maximum 60 mg. daily. Oral. Up to 30 mg. daily I.M. Usually 2 to 4 mg. q.i.d.	See Phenothiazine Derivatives.	Similar to phenothiazine. Well absorbed and widely distributed. May remain in body for several weeks following administration. Metabolized by the liver and excreted primarily in bile and feces.	Frequent–parkinsonism, akathisia, dystonic reactions and atropine-like effects. Occasional–photosensitivity reactions, galactorrhea, menstrual changes, drowsiness, postural hypotension, anorexia and rashes. Rare–cholestatic jaundice, blood dyscrasias, lenticular deposits and opacities (with long-term use at high doses), ECG abnormalities, decreased libido and convulsions.	Contraindications: patients with respiratory collapse, comatose states, central nervous system depression due to any cause, blood dyscrasias. Not recommended for children under 12 years of age.
DIBENZOXAZEPINE DERIVATIVE (Closely related to phenothiazines).					
Loxapine succinate (Loxitane).	20-100 mg. daily divided in 2-4 doses.	To treat schizophrenia.	Exact mechanism has not been determined. Well absorbed orally and distributed to all tissues. Approximately 17% is distributed to the brain. It is metabolized extensively and excreted as conjugates in the urine and in the feces in unconjugated form.	Contraindicated in narrow angle glaucoma, epilepsy, urinary retention and cardiovascular disease. Side effects: Frequent–parkinsonism, akathisia, oculogyric crises, drowsiness. Occasional–dystonic reactions, hypotension, hypertension, convulsions and atropine-like effects. Rare–rashes, edema, hyperpyrexia and paresthesias.	Tardive dyskinesia may occur with prolonged high dose therapy. Safe use in pregnancy, lactation and children under 16 years of age not established.

Name, Source, Synonyms, Preparations	Dosage and Administration	Uses	Action and Fate	Side Effects and Contraindications	Nursing Implications and Remarks
OTHERS					
Molindone hydrochloride (Moban).	5 mg. t.i.d. or q.i.d. Doses up to 225 mg. per day may be used in severe cases. Oral.	Used in the management of schizophrenia.	Action resembles that of major tranquilizers causing reduced spontaneous locomotion and aggressiveness, suppression of conditioned response and bizarre stereotyped behavior and hyperactivity induced by amphetamines. Based on EEG studies, drug is believed to exert its effect on one ascending activating system. Rapidly absorbed. Drug reaches peak level an hour after oral administration. Duration of action following single dose is 36 h. Widely distributed; probably metabolized in liver. Excreted in urine and feces with small amounts via lungs.	Frequent—drowsiness, parkinsonism, akathisia, atropine-like effects. Occasional—dystonic reactions, menstrual changes, postural hypotension, anorexia and rashes. Rare—leukopenia and ECG abnormalities. Contraindications: severe central nervous system depression or comatose states and hypersensitivity to this drug.	Safe use during pregnancy or for children under 12 years not established. Patient should be warned of possible drowsiness and advised about avoiding activities requiring mental alertness. Appears to be a narrow range between effective therapeutic dose and dose causing extrapyramidal symptoms.
RAUWOLFIA DERIVATIVES					

INTERACTIONS: Concurrent use of rauwolfia alkaloids and cardiac glycosides can increase the likelihood of cardiac arrhythmias, even though in most cases they can be used without adverse effects. Patients on long-term rauwolfia (reserpine) therapy may require larger than normal pressor doses of ephedrine and related drugs. In patients on rauwolfia (reserpine) therapy, the dose of quinidine used to convert atrial fibrillation to normal sinus rhythm should be considerably decreased or, if given together, the initial dose of quinidine should be lower than normal. The use of rauwolfia (reserpine) with the tricyclic antidepressants has been effective in tricyclic-refractory endogenous depression, but the hazard of reserpine reversal and resultant mania that can be produced suggests caution in using this combination.

RAUWOLFIA SERPENTINA *Rauwolfia.* Alseroxylon (Koglucoid, Raudolfin, Rautensin, Rauwiloid, Vio-Serpine). Deserpidine (Harmonyl). Rauwolfia serpentina, N.F. (Raudixin, Rauserpa, Rautina) (Novoralfia, Raufonol, Rausenal-S1, Rautabs [C]), Rescinnamine, N.F. (Moderil) (Anaprel-500 [C]).	2-4 mg. 0.1-1 mg. 50-300 mg. 0.25-0.5 mg. These are all given orally two to four times daily according to conditions being treated and response of patient.	Used as an antihypertensive agent in essential hypertension and rarely for its tranquilizing effect.	Has a calming action, probably owing to depression of central nervous system at the hypothalamic level. It releases serotonin and tends to suppress the sympathetic branch of the autonomic system centrally, thus allowing the parasympathetic system to predominate. Results include calming without analgesia or true sedation, lowering of blood pressure, increased motility and secretions of the gastrointestinal tract, slowing of the heart rate and constriction of the pupils. It does not potentiate other central nervous system depressants. Rapid absorption from gastrointestinal tract or parenteral site. Widely distributed in body. Crosses the blood-brain barrier and placenta. Exact method of degradation and excretion not known but many metabolites have been identified. Excreted slowly in urine, feces and breast milk.	Sedation, nasal congestion, weight gain and varied gastrointestinal symptoms. It can cause paradoxical anxiety, nervousness, nightmares, extrapyramidal tract symptoms, pruritus, rash, thrombocytopenic purpura and edema. Ophthalmic symptoms seen include glaucoma, uveitis, optic atrophy and conjunctival injection. Reduce dosage or stop drug and treat symptoms. Safety of the rauwolfia preparations for use during pregnancy has not been established; therefore, these drugs should be used only when in the judgment of the doctor their use is essential for the welfare of the patient.	*Rauwolfia serpentina* contains the whole root with all the alkaloids. Studies have shown possible carcinogenic effects.
Reserpine, U.S.P. (Lemiserp, Rau-Sed, Reserpoid, Sandril, Serpanray, Serpasil, Sertina, Vio-Serpine) (Alserin, Ebserpine, Eskaserp, Neo-Serp, Resercine, Reserpanca, Serpone, Sertens [C]).	0.25-1 mg. b.i.d. to q.i.d. Oral or parenteral. 0.1-0.5 mg. Daily. Oral.	To lower blood pressure.			Reserpine was one of the first tranquilizers to be used. Full effects of fixed oral doses are usually delayed for at least 2-3 weeks.
Syrosingopine, N.F. (Singoserp).	0.5-1 mg. two to three times daily. Oral.				Syrosingopine is partially synthetic. It is derived from reserpine.

Name, Source, Synonyms, Preparations	Dosage and Administration	Uses	Action and Fate	Side Effects and Contraindications	Nursing Implications and Remarks
BENZODIAZEPINES *Synthetic*					
Chlordiazepoxide HCl, U.S.P. (A-poxide, Librium) (Chem-Dipoxide, Corax, C-Tran, Diapox, Gene-Poxide, Medilium, Nack, Novopoxide, Protensin, Quiecil, Solium, Sterium, Via-Quil [C]).	5-10 – 25 mg. t.i.d. or q.i.d. Oral. 100 mg. q. 4-6 h. I.M. or I.V. Dosage individually adjusted.	Used to reduce tension, fears, and anxiety in simple and severe forms. For alcoholism and acute anxiety.	Sedative-tranquilizer with muscle relaxant properties. Acts by unknown mechanism. It is slowly absorbed. Does not reach peak blood levels for several hours and is excreted slowly. Plasma levels may last several days after discontinuance of the drug. Readily crosses the placenta. The drug is metabolized in the liver, slowly excreted in urine and feces. Because of slow excretion, a cumulative effect may be observed the first several days of therapy.	Occasional nausea, constipation, skin rashes or ataxia may occur. Reduce dosage. Withdrawal symptoms have been seen 7-8 days following high doses (300 to 600 mg. daily). Can enhance central nervous system depression, seen with alcohol and barbiturates. With the monoamine oxidase inhibitors an additive effect may occur, both depressive and excitatory. With the phenothiazines, the central nervous depression can be potentiated and an atropine-like effect can result. Safety for use during pregnancy has not been established.	Injections should be prepared immediately before administration and unused solutions should be discarded.
Chlordiazepoxide, N.F. (Libritabs).	As above.	As above.			
Clorazepate dipotassium (Tranxene).	15-30 mg. daily in divided doses. Elderly or debilitated start with 7.5-15 mg.	Anxiety associated with neuroses or psychoneuroses when anxiety is a prominent symptom. In any disease	Similar to other benzodiazepines. Primary metabolite nordiazepam. Peak blood level in about	Side effects: drowsiness most common. Others: dizziness, gastrointestinal disturbances, dry mouth,	Caution: due to drowsiness, operating machinery or driving should not be done.

	daily in divided doses. Oral.	state in which anxiety is manifested.	1 hour. Plasma half-life about 24 hours. Metabolized in liver; excreted mainly in urine. Crosses the placenta and is probably excreted in human milk.	blurred vision, nervousness, headache and mental confusion. Contraindications: narrow angle glaucoma, nursing mother, pregnancy.	Concurrent use of alcohol or central nervous system depressants should only be under direct medical supervision. Use for children under 18 years of age not advised.
Clorazepate monopotassium, (Azene).	13-52 mg./day in divided doses. Adjusted to patient response. Oral.	Symptomatic relief of anxiety and acute alcohol withdrawal. Not used longer than 4 mos.	As above.	As above.	As above.
Diazepam, U.S.P. (Valium). (Vivol [C]).	2.5-10 mg. t.i.d. or q.i.d. Oral. 2-10 mg. I.M. or I.V. q. 3-4 h. I.V. rate should not exceed 5 mg./min.	Used as a skeletal muscle relaxant, anticonvulsant, antianxiety agent, as an adjunct to anesthesia and in alcoholic withdrawal.	See chlordiazepoxide.	Fatigue, drowsiness, ataxia, following cessation of drug after very large doses. Withdrawal symptoms have been observed for long periods. Safe use during pregnancy or lactation has not been established.	Do not mix or dilute injectable Valium with other solutions or drugs. Do not add to I.V. fluids or use small veins for injection sites.
Flurazepam (Dalmane).	15-30 mg. h.s. Oral.	Used for insomnia.	This drug is a benzodiazepine and the exact mode of action is not known. However, animal studies indicate it reduces the pressor response to electrical stimulation of the hypothalamus and increases the arousal threshold to stimulation of the amygdala and the hypothalamus. It is rapidly absorbed from the gastrointestinal tract and rapidly metabolized.	Side effects most commonly seen include: dizziness, drowsiness, lightheadedness, staggering, ataxia and falling. These latter have occurred mostly in elderly or debilitated patients. For other side effects, toxicity, etc., see brochure. Contraindications: sensitivity to the drug. This drug has similar interactions to chlordiazepoxide (page 162). This drug does not appear to interact with the oral anticoagulants.	Use during pregnancy is not recommended. The drug is not recommended for children under 15 years as studies have not been carried out for this age group.

Name, Source, Synonyms, Preparations	Dosage and Administration	Uses	Action and Fate	Side Effects and Contraindications	Nursing Implications and Remarks
BENZODIAZEPINES (Continued)					
Lorazepam (Ativan).	1-10 mg./day in divided doses with largest dose h.s. Oral.	Symptomatic relief of anxiety, tension, agitation, irritability and insomnia associated with anxiety neuroses and transient situational disturbances.	Tranquilizing effect on C.N.S. No appreciable effect on cardiovascular or respiratory centers. Readily absorbed. At clinically relevant concentrations, about 85% bound to plasma proteins. Rapidly conjugated and excreted in urine. No evidence of accumulation up to 6 mos.	Most frequent side effects are dizziness, weakness, and unsteadiness. Tolerance develops to these effects with continued therapy. Other effects reported: depression, disorientation, G.I. symptoms, headache, skin symptoms and eye disturbances. Contraindicated in patients with known sensitivity to the drug or with acute narrow angle glaucoma. Not recommended in primary depression disorders or psychosis. Withdrawal symptoms have occurred with abrupt discontinuance of benzodiazepines; thus Lorazepam should be terminated gradually. Additive C.N.S. depression when given along with other C.N.S. depressants.	In patients with depression accompanying anxiety, the possiblity of suicide should be considered and safety precautions initiated. Use of Lorazepam during first trimester of pregnancy or while breast feeding should be avoided. Safety for use in children under 12 years not established. Some patients have developed leukopenia or had elevations of LDH. Periodic blood counts and liver tests recommended during long-term therapy.
Oxazepam, N.F. (Serax).	10-30 mg. three or four times daily. Oral.	See chlordiazepoxide.	See chlordiazepoxide. Can be used in patients with impaired liver function.	Drowsiness, dizziness, vertigo, headache and syncope have been reported. Instances of minor diffuse skin rashes (morbilliform, urticarial and maculopapular) have occurred. Nausea, lethargy, edema, slurred speech, tremors, altered libido and	Caution: Administer with caution to patients in whom a drop in blood pressure might lead to cardiac complications. Safety for use during pregnancy has not been established. During prolonged therapy

				ataxia have been reported, but rarely. When excessive dosage is continued for weeks or months, dosage should be reduced gradually rather than abruptly. Patients should be told that they may have a lowered tolerance to alcohol.	periodic blood counts and liver function tests are advisable.
Prazepam (Verstran).	20-60 mg./day in divided doses adjusted to patient response. Oral.	Symptomatic relief of anxiety associated with anxiety neuroses and other psychoneuroses.	C.N.S. depressant. Normal subjects achieve peak blood levels 6 h. after administration, with significant amounts present after 48 h. Slowly absorbed over prolonged period with rather constant blood levels. Excretion prolonged.	Most frequent side effects are fatigue, weakness, drowsiness, light-headedness and ataxia. Others include headache, confusion, tremor, slurred speech, palpitation, stimulation, dry mouth, diaphoresis and various G.I. complaints. Other findings comparable with benzodiazepine drugs.	See lorazepam.
VARIED. *Synthetic preparations.* Buclizine hydrochloride.	50 mg. t.i.d. Oral.	Used to treat mild anxiety states, tension, and for sedation.	An antihistamine with prominent sedative powers.	Said to be relatively non-toxic, but excessive drowsiness may occur.	Available as ingredient in combination products. (Ex. Bucladin).
Hydroxyzine hydrochloride, N.F. (Atarax, Vistaril) (Pas-Depress [C]).	10-400 mg. daily. Oral. 25-100 mg. I.M. Available as a syrup, 10 mg./5 ml.	Used as an antiemetic, to overcome motion sickness, as a mild sedative and to reinforce the action of other drugs. It is a good antihistamine. Used in treatment of acute and chronic urticaria and allergic dematoses.	C.N.S. depressant, anticholinergic, antiemetic, antispasmodic, antihistaminic as well as local anesthetic effects. Well absorbed from G.I. tract. Biologic half-life and metabolic fate unknown.	Postural hypotension may occur, and decrease in granulocytes has been reported. Reduce dosage or stop drug as conditions indicate. Treat symptoms. If a vasopressor is needed, norepinephrine is preferred over epinephrine. Contraindicated in early pregnancy.	The injection should never be given subcutaneously. Use I.M. route only. Low incidence of side effects within recommended therapeutic dosage.
Hydroxyzine pamoate, N.F. (Vistaril).	25-100 mg. Dosage individually adjusted. Oral.				

Name, Source, Synonyms, Preparations	Dosage and Administration	Uses	Action and Fate	Side Effects and Contraindications	Nursing Implications and Remarks
VARIED. *Synthetic preparations.* (Continued)					
Lithium carbonate, U.S.P. (Eskalith, Lithane, Lithonate).	Dosage individually adjusted to maintain serum level of lithium between 0.5 and 1.5 mEq./L. Oral.	Used in control of the manic episodes of manic-depressive psychoses.	Lithium alters the transport in nerve and muscle cells and effects a shift toward intraneural metabolism of catecholamines, but the exact biochemical mechanism of lithium action is not known. Acetazolamide and chlorpromazine may cause increased excretion of lithium. Well absorbed. Appears to be well distributed, crossing the placenta. Lithium is excreted primarily in the urine and to some extent in feces, sperm, sweat and milk. It reaches levels in breast milk high enough to cause hypotonia, hypothermia and ECG changes in the nursing infant.	There are many adverse reactions to lithium therapy. The brochure should be studied in detail before administering the drug. Contraindicated in persons with significant cardiovascular or renal disease or evidence of brain damage. Lithium toxicity is closely related to its serum level and can occur at doses close to therapeutic levels.	The adequate intake of sodium and fluid must be maintained while lithium is being given, and the use of diuretics should be avoided. Facilities for prompt and accurate serum determinations should be available before initiating therapy. Lithium carbonate has been implicated in cases of neonatal goiter.
Mephenoxalone (Methoxydone, Tranpoise).	400 mg. given 100-200 mg. q.i.d. Oral.	Used like others of this group, especially when accompanied by muscle spasm associated with trauma or musculoskeletal disease.	Mild tranquilizer and skeletal muscle relaxant with action similar to that of meprobamate.	Skin rash, dizziness, nausea and drowsiness occur infrequently and may be controlled by reduction or discontinuance of dosage.	Blood picture should be watched with prolonged dosage.
Tybamate, N.F. (Solacen).	250-500 mg. t.i.d. or q.i.d. Dosage individually adjusted. Not more than 3 Gm. in any one day. Oral.	Used to treat a variety of psychoneurotic conditions, especially when anxiety and tension are the predominant symptoms.	Appears to exert its action on the hippocampal and limbic structures of the brain. Does not seem to affect cerebral cortical	Adverse symptoms are usually mild and require only dosage adjustment. However, many symptoms have been reported, including drowsiness,	

			activity to any appreciable extent. Fate in body similar to meprobamate.	dizziness, nausea, insomnia, euphoria, pruritus, skin rash, ataxia, confusion, headache, fatigue and gastrointestinal disturbances. Contraindicated, at present, during pregnancy and lactation, when the phenothiazine preparations are being used, and in children under 6 years of age.	
GENERAL ANESTHETICS	*See also local anesthetics and sedatives-hypnotics. These are synthetic preparations.*				
<u>Chloroform</u>, N.F. (Trichloromethane).	Dosage varies. Inhalation.	Used as a general anesthetic and also as an anodyne, carminative, sedative, antispasmodic, and as a counterirritant.	Descending, progressive central nervous system depressant. Produces surgical anesthesia in a very short time. Gives good muscle relaxation; tends to produce a steadily decreasing blood pressure. Induction fairly rapid. Rapidly passes lung barriers. Carried mainly by red blood corpuscles rather than plasma. Excreted largely unchanged by the lungs.	Local irritation, cardiac paralysis during anesthesia, acidosis during recovery. Treatment: symptomatic. Toxic symptoms: (delayed) hepatotoxia, progressive weakness, cyanosis, restlessness, vomiting, delirium, coma. Death may occur. Treatment: symptomatic. Contraindicated in cardiac disorders.	Use limited owing to toxicity. Not used for long anesthesia. Not flammable. Easy to administer, relatively pleasant to take. Chloroform can interact with sympathomimetics to produce cardiac arrhythmias.
<u>Chloroform liniment.</u> *External Chloroform Preparation.*	Dosage varies. Topical.	As a counterirritant.			

Name, Source, Synonyms, Preparations	Dosage and Administration	Uses	Action and Fate	Side Effects and Contraindications	Nursing Implications and Remarks
GENERAL ANESTHETICS (Continued)					
Cyclopropane, U.S.P. (Trimethylene).	Dosage varies. Inhalational. 10-20% with oxygen. 80-90% will maintain surgical anesthesia.	Used as a general anesthetic. Depth sufficient for major surgery and recovery rapid without adverse effects, except occasional nausea.	A potent central nervous system depressant, producing anesthesia with relatively low dosage. Sufficient oxygen can be given and still maintain adequate anesthesia. Muscle relaxation moderate. Induction about 5 minutes. Readily absorbed and excreted mostly unchanged by the lungs. A small amount is metabolized by the body into carbon dioxide and water.	Rarely sensitizes myocardium to epinephrine. Cardiac arrhythmia and failure may occur. Stop anesthesia and treat symptoms. Cyclopropane can interact with the sympathomimetics to produce cardiac arrhythmias. Also, in high dosage it can interact with the antibiotics—streptomycin, kanamycin, polymyxin-B, colistimethate, viomycin and paromomycin to give neuromuscular blockage and can cause respiratory arrest.	Is highly explosive; must be given in a closed circuit with pure oxygen, and where sparks cannot occur. Widely used in elderly and poor-risk patients. Cyclopropane can cross the placenta and cause neonatal respiratory depression.
Enflurane (Ethrane) *(a fluorinated ether).*	3.5-4.5% to induce surgical anesthesia. Maintenance, 1.5-3.0%.	Inhalation anesthesia. Induction in 7-10 minutes.	Induction and recovery fairly rapid. Levels of anesthesia change rapidly. Heart rate remains relatively constant, but there is an increase in amount of hypotension with increased level of anesthesia. Depth of ventilation is reduced as anesthesia is increased.	The nondepolarizing muscle relaxants are markedly potentiated and neostigmine does not reverse the direct effect of enflurane. Contraindicated in certain seizure disorders and in patients sensitive to the halogenated anesthesias. Motor activity shown by movement of various muscle groups and/or seizures may be encountered with deep levels of anesthesia. Hypotension and respiratory depression have occurred. Arrhythmias, shivering, nausea and vomiting have	Must be used only with equipment that can measure concentration. Safety for use in pregnancy has not been established.

				been reported and elevation of white blood cell count has been seen. This may be due to factors other than the anesthesia.	
<u>Ether</u>, U.S.P. (diethyl ether).	Dosage varies. Inhalational.	Used mainly for general anesthesia, especially when muscular relaxation is essential.	Progressive, descending central nervous system depressant. Gives good muscle relaxation. Somewhat slow induction and recovery. Absorbed through lung mucosa. About 90% excreted by the same route. It can be detected in expired air up to several hours later. A small amount is metabolized by the body. Some is excreted unchanged in urine, perspiration and other body fluids.	Local irritation, especially of mucous membranes; respiratory paralysis and circulatory involvement may occur. Stop drug and give artificial respiration. Epinephrine and caffeine may be used. Toxic symptoms: (delayed) symptoms of liver and kidney damage. Similar to vinyl ether. Treatment: symptomatic.	Ether is usually contraindicated in respiratory diseases. Ether vapor is explosive in some concentrations with oxygen. The fluid is not explosive. Ether can cross the placenta and cause apnea in the neonate. Nausea and vomiting are common after ether administration.
<u>Ethylene</u>, N.F. (Ethene).	Dosage varies. Inhalational.	Used as a general anesthetic.	Induction short, depth sufficient for major surgery and recovery rapid without adverse effects.	Rare in therapeutic dosage. Treatment: symptomatic, if needed.	Has an unpleasant odor. Is highly explosive; must be given in a closed circuit with pure oxygen and where sparks cannot occur.

Name, Source, Synonyms, Preparations	Dosage and Administration	Uses	Action and Fate	Side Effects and Contraindications	Nursing Implications and Remarks
GENERAL ANESTHETICS (Continued)					
Halothane, U.S.P. (Fluothane).	Dosage varies. Inhalational.	Liquid anesthetic agent that can be used in either open or closed method. Anesthetic of choice for patients with bronchial asthma.	Complete anesthesia causes continuous respiratory depression; is a bronchodilator and myocardial depressant; sensitizes myocardium to epinephrine, so that ventricular arrhythmias may occur. Absorbed through lung mucosa. About 60% excreted by lungs.	Cases of hepatic necrosis and dysfunction have been reported. Nausea and vomiting rare. Heavy dosage may cause cardiac arrest, severe hypotension or both.	It has not been shown that the use of this anesthetic will not have an adverse effect upon the fetus. Epinephrine, levarterenol and other sympathomimetics can cause cardiac arrhythmias. Halothane can interact with the antibiotics streptomycin, kanamycin, polymyxin-B, viomycin, colistimethate and paromomycin to give reduced neuromuscular blockage and can cause respiratory arrest.
Ketamine hydrochloride, N.F. (Ketaject, Ketalar).	1-4.5 mg./kg. I.V. anesthesia in 30 seconds, lasts 5-10 min. 6.5-13.0 mg./kg. I.M. anesthesia in 3-4 minutes, lasts 12-25 min.	Used for short anesthesia when muscle relaxation is not required, for induction and to supplement low potency agents such as nitrous oxide.	Rapid acting agent, produces good analgesia without muscle relaxation. Skeletal cardiac and respiratory muscles have slightly increased tone. Rapid administration may cause respiratory depression. Blood pressure is increased. Rapidly absorbed, widely distributed throughout the body, undergoes metabolic degradation. The degradation products are excreted in the urine, a small amount in feces.	Though toxicity is low, there are many warnings and precautions. Rapid administration may cause respiratory depression requiring resuscitative measures. Emergence reactions (anything from a dream-like state to hallucinations, confusion or excitement) are not uncommon. Contraindications: drug should not be used for the hypertensive patient. It is not used for an	Commercial brochure should be consulted before administering this drug. Ketamine should not be administered by the same equipment used for the barbiturates since a precipitate will be formed. Safe use during pregnancy or delivery has not been established. Emergence reactions occur in about 12% of patients and can be highly disturbing. Awakening is prolonged, lasting several

			Produces "dissociative anesthesia"; i.e., recipient feels dissociated from his environment.	acute or chronic alcoholic patient or for intracranial surgery.	hours with disagreeable dreams and hallucinations possible.
Methoxyflurane, N.F. (Penthrane) (Methofane [C]).	Dosage varies. Inhalational.	General inhalational anesthetic agent used chiefly for maintenance.	Complete anesthetic with moderate skeletal relaxation. Also lowers blood pressure. Slow onset of anesthesia and slow recovery may limit usefulness.	Respiratory and circulatory depression. Treatment: symptomatic. Epinephrine and levarterenol are contraindicated. See specific contraindications and interactions under halothane.	Used in either open or closed technique. Central nervous system depressant; dosage should be reduced. Usual eye signs do not apply.
Nitrous oxide, U.S.P. (nitrogen monoxide).	Dosage varies. Inhalational. Should always be given with at least 20% oxygen.	Useful in dentistry and 2nd stage of labor. Supplemented with other agents for surgical anesthesia.	Small amounts mixed with air act as an intoxicant; patient feels happy, laughs, is loquacious. Combination with other agents is required for deeper anesthesia.	Slow pulse; cyanosis; irregular rate, depth and rhythm of respiration. Stop drug and treat symptoms. See interactions under ether, page 169.	Unless ether is added there is little muscle relaxation. "Laughing gas" is the common name.
Trichloroethylene, U.S.P. (Trilene).	Inhalational.	Used as a general and specific anesthetic agent. Main use is in obstetrics for pain after cervix is dilated at least 3 cm. Is also used for minor surgery.	Produces a light plane of anesthesia. Does not produce muscle relaxation in usual dosage.	Cardiac arrhythmias, increasing muscular activity. Stop drug and treat symptoms. Trichloroethylene alone is not recommended for anesthesia or the induction of anesthesia. Epinephrine should not be used at the same time. Interactions same as for chloroform.	May be habit forming; apt to be dangerous. Should never be used in closed system with soda lime. Has been used in tic douloureux.

Name, Source, Synonyms, Preparations	Dosage and Administration	Uses	Action and Fate	Side Effects and Contraindications	Nursing Implications and Remarks
LOCAL ANESTHETICS AND ANODYNES. See also general anesthetics.					
BENZYL ALCOHOL (Phenylcarbinol). *Synthetic.* Benzyl alcohol, N.F.	Dosage varies. Topical and S.Q.	Used mainly for local and block anesthesia.	Produces insensitivity by blocking nerve impulses. If absorbed, it is converted to hippuric acid by the body.	Very rare. No treatment required.	Also used as a preservative.
COCAINE. Active principle of coca shrub. *Synthetic.* Cocaine hydrochloride, N.F.	1-10% solution. Topical.	Eye, ear, nose, throat, bronchoscopy.	It is a CNS stimulant but if used as it should be, local vasoconstriction limits absorption. That which is absorbed is detoxified by the liver and excreted unchanged by kidneys.	Excitement, anxiety, dizziness, severe headache, convulsions, fall in blood pressure. Death may occur from cardiovascular and respiratory failure. Treatment (prophylactic): barbiturates before surgery, slow administration of the local anesthetic agent, use of dilute solution, caution to prevent intravenous administration, use of epinephrine hydrochloride to delay absorption. Treatment (active): stop drug, give barbiturates, treat symptoms. If area of administration allows, use tourniquet. Idiosyncrasy is common even with small doses.	Cocaine comes under the jurisdiction of Drug Enforcement Agency. Surface anesthesia only. Action is prolonged.
Benoxinate hydrochloride, N.F. (Dorsacaine).	0.4% solution. Topical.	Used for surface, infiltration, conduction and regional, paravertebral, sacral and spinal anesthesia. All are used in dilute solutions. Ophthalmic.	In surface anesthesia, the nerve endings are rendered incapable of receiving and transmitting impulses. With other anesthetics of this type the conducting nerve fibers are rendered incapable of transmitting impulses. Some anesthetics have both types of action.		Epinephrine hydrochloride is often added to a local anesthetic to prolong its action.
Benzocaine, N.F. (Americaine).	5% ointment. Topical. 5% cream. Topical. 200-600 mg. suppositories. 20% aerosol.	For surface anesthesia of skin and mucous membranes.			

Bupivacaine hydrochloride (Marcaine hydrochloride).	0.25-0.75% solution.	Local anesthetic agent used for peripheral nerve block, infiltration, sympathetic block, caudal or epidural block.	Duration of action is significantly longer than with other commonly used local anesthetics.	Safe use in pregnancy or for children under 12 years of age has not been established.	Parenteral administration stabilizes the neuronal membrane and prevents initiation and transmission of nerve impulses. Warning: resuscitative equipment and drugs should be available when any local anesthetic is used parenterally.
Butacaine sulfate, N.F. (Amolyn, Optyn [C]).	2% solution. Topical.	Main use: eye, ear, nose and throat surgery.			
Butethamine hydrochloride, N.F. (Dentocaine) (Novocol [C]).	1-2% solution. Regional.	Similar to procaine but more toxic. Main use in dentistry.			
Butyl aminobenzoate, N.F. (Butesin, Butamben) (Planolorn [C]).	Dosage varies. Topical.				
Chloroprocaine hydrochloride, N.F. (Nesacaine) (Versacaine [C]).	1-3% solution. Injection.	Infiltration, nerve block, peridural and I.V. regional anesthesia.			
Cyclomethycaine sulfate, N.F. (Surfacaine).	0.5-1% solution, ointment and cream. Topical.				
Dibucaine hydrochloride, N.F. (Nupercainal, Nuperlone, Nupercaine) (cinchocaine [C]).	0.5-2% solution or ointment. Topical.	Used for local, infiltration, nerve block or spinal anesthesia.	Slow onset, up to 15 minutes, with duration of 3 to 4 hours.	Very toxic.	
Dimethisoquin hydrochloride, N.F. (Quotane).	0.5% lotion or ointment. Topical.			Too toxic for injection.	
Diperodon hydrochloride.	1% ointment or cream. Topical.				

Name, Source, Synonyms, Preparations	Dosage and Administration	Uses	Action and Fate	Side Effects and Contraindications	Nursing Implications and Remarks
LOCAL ANESTHETICS (Continued)					
Dyclonine hydrochloride, N.F. (Dyclone).	0.5% solution. Topical. 1% cream. Topical.	Eye, mouth, esophagus, oral endoscopy, bronchoscopy.			
Etidocaine hydrochloride (Duranest HCl).	0.5-1.5% solution (Maximum dose recommended not to exceed 400 mg.)	Infiltration anesthesia, peripheral nerve block, caudal and epidural blocks.	Amide type related to xylocaine. Metabolized in the liver and excreted via the kidney. Has duration of up to 8 to 10 hours in peripheral nerve block.	See lidocaine, page 198.	Safe use in pregnancy has not been established.
Hexylcaine hydrochloride, N.F. (Cyclaine).	2-5% solution or jelly. Topical.	Surface anesthesia of intact mucous membranes. Infiltration, nerve block, spinal, peridural, nose, throat, genito-urinary and rectal anesthesia.		Too toxic for injection.	
Lidocaine hydrochloride, U.S.P. (Xylocaine) (lignocaine, Octocaine, Topilidon [C]).	0.5-5.0% solution. Topical. Parenteral. 2.5-5% ointment. Topical.	Topical, infiltration, nerve block, epidural, spinal and I.V. regional anesthesia. This drug is used I.V. in the treatment of cardiac arrhythmias.		See page 198.	See page 198 for other information and interactions.
Mepivacaine hydrochloride, N.F., U.S.P. (Carbocaine).	1-2% solution. Parenteral	For infiltration, nerve block, epidural and I.V. regional anesthesia.			Mepivacaine can cross the placenta and cause fetal bradycardia and neonatal depression.
Oxethazine (Oxaine).	0.2% solution. Topical.	Mainly for gastric distress.			
Parethoxycaine hydrochloride (Diethoxin).	2-5% solution. Topical, and subcutaneous.				
Phenacaine hydrochloride, N.F. (Holocain, Holocaine).	1% solution. 1-2% ointment. Topical.	Main use as local anesthetic for eye.			

Piperocaine hydrochloride (Metycaine).	1-10% solution. Topical. 0.13-0.5% solution. S.Q.	Primarily for surface anesthesia, used only rarely for infiltration, nerve block and caudal anesthesia.			
Pramoxine hydrochloride, N.F. (Tronothane) pramocaine [C]).	1% cream, jelly, lotion or solution. Topical.	Topical.			Chemically different from amide and ester type compounds and may be useful in patients sensitive to these classes of compounds.
Prilocaine hydrochloride, N.F. (Citanest) (Xylonest [C]).	1%, 2%, 3% solution. Parenteral.	Therapeutic nerve block. Infiltration, nerve block, caudal, epidural and I.V. regional anesthesia.		Contraindications: patients hypersensitive to local anesthetic agents of the amide type. Also in congenital and idiopathic methemoglobinemia. Side effects: syncope, hypotension, headache, backache, apnea, nausea, vomiting and drowsiness.	Not recommended for spinal anesthesia.
Procaine hydrochloride, U.S.P. (Novocain, Syncaine) (Westocaine [C]).	0.2-2% solution. Parenteral.	Infiltration, nerve block and spinal anesthesia.	Readily absorbed from parenteral sites. Broken down in both liver and plasma and excreted in urine.		
Proparacaine hydrochloride, U.S.P. (Opthaine, Ophthetic) (proxymetacaine [C]).	0.5% solution. Topical.	In eyes.			
Propoxycaine hydrochloride, N.F. (Blockain, Ravocaine).	0.5% solution. Parenteral.	Used for infiltration and nerve block.			
Propylaminobenzoate (Propaesin).	Dosage varies. Topical as ointment.				
Tetracaine, N.F. Tetracaine hydrochloride, U.S.P. (Amethocaine, Pontocaine, Tetracel) (amethacaine, Anethaine [C]).	Dosage varies. Topical and parenteral. Maximum dose 50 mg. topically. Spinal dose rarely exceeds 15 mg.	Main use: eye, ear, nose, and throat surgery and spinal anesthesia.			

Name, Source, Synonyms, Preparations	Dosage and Administration	Uses	Action and Fate	Side Effects and Contraindications	Nursing Implications and Remarks
LOCAL ANESTHETICS (Continued)					
ETHYL CHLORIDE. *Synthetic.* Ethyl chloride, N.F.	Dosage varies. Topical and inhalational.	Used for short topical anesthesia. Used by inhalation for short general anesthesia and as an induction anesthetic agent.	Acts by freezing area.	Nausea, vomiting, cardiac failure, prostration. Stop drug and treat symptoms. Interactions as with chloroform when administered by inhalation.	Highly flammable.
QUININE AND UREA HYDROCHLORIDE. *Cinchona and synthetic.* Quinine and urea hydrochloride.	Dosage varies. Topical and S.Q.	Used for local and block anesthesia.	Painful, but then produces anesthesia lasting several days; also used as sclerosing agent.	Mainly local irritation, may cause sloughing. Treatment: symptomatic.	Solutions must be very dilute.

ANTIHISTAMINES

The antihistaminic drugs are used to relieve the symptoms of allergic reactions, especially nasal and conjunctival allergy. They are also used for treatment of allergic manifestations, such as dermatitis, urticaria, angioneurotic edema, occupational allergies; drug, food and cosmetic allergies and serum sickness. Some are used in Parkinson's disease; some are used as sedative or hypnotic agents, or both, and as antiemetics for active and prophylactic treatment of motion sickness.

These drugs block the action of histamine, which is present in excess in the blood of patients suffering from allergies and hypersensitivities. The basic ethylamine group is common to all antihistamines as well as to anticholinergic, ganglionic and adrenergic blocking agents, local anesthetics and antispasmodics, and therefore they may be expected to exhibit these other activities. Some demonstrate quinidine-like effects on myocardial conduction and may enhance the pressor effects of norepinephrine. The antiemetic and anti-motion sickness actions of some antihistamines appear to result from their central anticholinergic and C.N.S. depressant properties. Most are readily absorbed from the gastrointestinal sites. Most reach a peak level in 30–60 minutes, and effects last for 3–6 hours. Concentration in tissues is greatest in lungs, with progressively less in spleen, kidneys, brain, muscle and skin. Most metabolic transformation occurs in liver, but some also occurs in lungs and kidneys. Most of the metabolites are excreted by the kidneys.

Side effects and contraindications include drowsiness, dizziness, dryness of mouth and throat, disturbed coordination, lassitude, muscular weakness, gastrointestinal disturbances, nervousness, insomnia, xerostomia, nausea and vomiting. Should side effects occur, reduce the dosage or stop the drug and treat the symptoms.

These drugs can increase C.N.S. depression when given simultaneously with other C.N.S. depressants such as alcohol, narcotics, barbiturates, tranquilizers, anesthetics and reserpine. They give additive effects when used concurrently with anticholinergic drugs. They can reduce the effects of hormones by enzyme induction if given repeatedly. This property varies with the class of antihistamine. Persons whose occupations expose them to halogenated insecticides have a diminished effect from this class of drugs and need larger doses for therapeutic response. Antihistamines with phenothiazines or nylidin should probably not be used concurrently, since the action of both appears to be potentiated. Use of antihistamines in nursing mothers is contraindicated, and various ones are contraindicated in neonates and premies. Monoamine oxidase inhibitors prolong and intensify anticholinergic effects of antihistamines, and their concurrent use is also contraindicated.

Dosage of the antihistamines is individually adjusted, and patients should be cautioned about driving or operating machinery. Many of these drugs are available as both quick acting and delayed action tablets or capsules. The delayed action preparations are given once or twice daily; the others more often. Bioavailability of the delayed action forms can be unreliable and not uniform. Antihistamines should be used with caution, if at all, in patients with narrow angle glaucoma, stenosing peptic ulcer, prostatic hypertrophy, bladder neck obstruction and pyloric-duodenal obstruction. The ethylenediamine derivatives have relatively weak C.N.S. effects, but drowsiness does occur. G.I. effects are the most common.

These drugs have been grouped according to their chemical derivation into the ethylenediamine, ethanolamine, propylamine, phenothiazine, piperazine, and miscellaneous categories. All are of synthetic origin.

ETHYLENEDIAMINE DERIVATIVES. *Synthetic.*					The ethylenediamine derivatives have relatively weak C.N.S. effects, but drowsiness does occur. G.I. effects are the most common.
Antazoline hydrochloride (Antastan, Antistine [C]).	100 mg. Up to q.i.d. Oral.				
Antazoline phosphate, N.F. (Nasocon).	0.5% solution. Inhalational in nebulizer. 0.5% solution. Topical as eye drops.				
Pyrilamine maleate, N.F. (Histalon, Neopyramine, PYMA, Pyramaleate, Pyristan) (mepyramine maleate, pyranilamine, pyranisamin, Neo-Antergan [C]).	25-50 mg. Up to q.i.d. Oral.				
Tripelennamine citrate, U.S.P. (Pyribenzamine citrate).	25-100 q.i.d. Oral. Children 25-50 mg. q.i.d.				More palatable than the hydrochloride.
Tripelennamine hydrochloride, U.S.P. (Pyribenzamine hydrochloride)	50-100 q.i.d. Available for topical use and as an ingredient of cough mixtures. Oral.				Available in sustained release form.

Name, Source, Synonyms, Preparations	Dosage and Administration	Uses	Action and Fate	Side Effects and Contraindications	Nursing Implications and Remarks
ETHANOLAMINE DERIVATIVES. (Aminoalkyl Ethers) *Synthetic.*					The ethanolamine derivatives cause significant atropine-like activity; commonly cause C.N.S. depression, with drowsiness in 50% of patients. Usual G.I. side effects are low.
Bromodiphenhydramine hydrochloride, N.F. (Ambodryl) (bromazine [C]).	5-25 mg. Up to q.i.d. Oral or parenteral.				
Carbinoxamine maleate, NF. (Clistin) (paracarbinoxamine, [C]).	Children 0.5 mg./kg./day. 4 mg. q.i.d. Oral. 8-12 mg. b.i.d. Oral				
Clemastine fumarate (Tavist).	2.68 mg. q.d. or t.i.d. Oral.			Safety and efficacy in pregnancy and children under 12 years not established.	
Chlorphenoxamine HCl, N.F. (Phenoxene).	Children 0.35 mg./kg./day. 50-100 mg. q.i.d. Oral 10 mg. I.M. or I.V.	Main use in idopathic and postencephalitic Parkinson's disease.			
Diphenhydramine hydrochloride, U.S.P. (Benadryl) (Benhydramil [C]).	25-50 mg. q.i.d. Oral, parenteral, topical. Children 5 mg./kg./day in divided doses.	Uses same as those of others of this group. Also useful in asthma. Causes some muscular relaxation.		Causes more sedation than most antihistamines.	
Diphenylpyraline hydrochloride, N.F. (Diafen, Hispril) (Dorahist, Neo-Lergic [C]).	2 mg. t.i.d. Oral. 5 mg. sustained release capsule. Two or three times a day. Oral.				
Doxylamine succinate, N.F. (Decapryn).	12.5-25 mg. q. 4-6 h. Oral. Children 2 mg./kg./day in divided doses.			Effectiveness limited because of sedative action.	
Orphenadrine hydrochloride (Dispal).	50 mg. t.i.d. Oral.	Treatment of Parkinson's disease and drug-induced	Reduces skeletal muscle spasm primarily through	Typical anticholinergic effects of antihistamines.	

		extra pyramidal reactions.	an atropine-like central action on cerebral motor centers or on the medulla. Unlike diphenhydramine, produces slight C.N.S. stimulation.		
Phenyltoloxamine dihydrogen citrate (Bristimin, Floxamine).	25-50 mg. t.i.d. Oral	As antihistamines.			
Rotoxamine tartrate, N.F. (Twiston).	2 mg. three or four times a day, 4-6 mg. b.i.d. Oral.				
PROPYLAMINE DERIVATIVES (Alkylamines)					The propylamine derivatives cause less drowsiness and more C.N.S. stimulation, making them more suitable for daytime use.
Brompheniramine maleate, N.F. (Dimetane) (parabromdylamine [C]).	4 mg. q.i.d. Oral. Or 8-12 mg. b.i.d. Oral. 5-20 mg. b.i.d. Parenteral.				
Chlorpheniramine maleate, U.S.P. (Chlor-Trimeton, Histaspan, Teldrin) (chlorphenamine, chlorprophenpyridamine, Chlor-Tripolon, Chlortrone, Histalon, Novo-pheniram [C]).	4 mg. q.i.d. Oral. 8-12 mg. b.i.d. Oral. Children 0.35 mg./kg./ day.			Chlorpheniramine is contraindicated in severe cardiac conditions.	
Chlorpheniramine maleate injection, N.F. (Pheneton, Chlor-Trimeton).	5-40 mg. Parenteral.				
Dexbrompheniramine maleate, N.F. (Disomer).	8-12 mg. b.i.d. Oral.				
Dexchlorpheniramine maleate, N.F. (Polaramine) (*d*-chlorpheniramine [C]).	2 mg. q.i.d. Oral. Children 0.15 mg./kg./ day in divided doses. Oral.				
Dimethindene maleate, N.F. (Forhistal, Triten) (dimethpyrindine maleate [C]).	1 mg. q.i.d. Oral 2.5 mg. b.i.d. delayed release. Oral. Children over 6 years 0.1 mg./kg./day in divided doses. Oral.				

Name, Source, Synonyms, Preparations	Dosage and Administration	Uses	Action and Fate	Side Effects and Contraindications	Nursing Implications and Remarks
PROPYLAMINE DERIVATIVES (Alkylamines) (Continued)					
Pyrrobutamine phosphate, N.F.	15 mg. t.i.d. Oral.				
Triprolidine hydrochloride, N.F. (Actidil).	2.5 mg. t.i.d. or q.i.d. Oral.				
PHENOTHIAZINE DERIVATIVES					
Ethopropazine hydrochloride, U.S.P. (Parsidol) (profenamine, Parsitan [C]).	50-100 mg. q.i.d. Oral.	Treatment of Parkinsons's disease and drug-induced extrapyramidal reactions.	Strong parasympatholytic action plus antihistaminic, local anesthetic, ganglionic blocking and adrenolytic activity. Generally produces C.N.S. depression.	High incidence of side effects with therapeutic doses, with drowsiness, dizziness and lassitude occurring frequently, though they may be transient.	When an anti-Parkinsonian drug is to be discontinued and replaced by another drug, the first should be withdrawn slowly while the second is substituted. Administer with caution in cardiac disease, glaucoma, prostatic hypertrophy or pyloric obstruction.
Methdilazine hydrochloride, N.F. (Tacaryl) (Dilosyn [C]).	4-8 mg. two to four times daily. Children 0.3 mg./kg./day in two divided doses.	Used mainly in allergic pruritus.	Has antihistaminic and phenothiazine effects.	Although risk of phenothiazine adverse reactions has been minimal, the possibility of occurrence with prolonged therapy should be kept in mind. Methdilazine hydrochloride potentiates the action of hypnotics.	May suppress cough reflex and thus should be used with caution in patients with acute or chronic respiratory impairment. Use with caution in patients with history of G.I. ulceration.
Promethazine hydrochloride, U.S.P. (Phenergan) (Histanil [C]).	6-50 mg. p.r.n. Oral. Also available in cough medications. 25-50 mg. p.r.n. Rectal or parenteral. Children 0.13 mg./kg. in A.M. up to 0.5 mg./kg. at h.s.	Used for preoperative sedation, to control post-operative nausea and to potentiate action of analgesics. Also used for management of motion sickness.	C.N.S. depression with therapeutic doses. Slight antitussive activity, antihistaminic, antiemetic, anti-motion sickness and local anesthetic effects.	Anticholinergic side effects. Confusion and blood dyscrasias reported rarely. Photosensitivity, restlessness, akathisia and occasionally marked irregular respirations. Reverses vasopressor effect of epinephrine.	May cause false positive Gravidex and negative Prepurex and Dap tests. Sedative action limits usefulness as antihistamine.

Trimeprazine tartrate, U.S.P. (Temaril) (alimemazine, Panectyl [C]).	2.5-5 mg. q.i.d. Oral. Children under 2 yrs., 3.75 mg. q.d.; 3-12 yrs., 7.5 mg. q.d.	An oral dermatologic and systemic antipruritic.	A phenothiazine derivative with antipruritic action.	Mild drowsiness may occur. Stop drug. A few cases of jaundice and blood dyscrasias have been reported.	
PIPERAZINE DERIVATIVES					
Chlorcyclizine hydrochloride, N.F. (Perazil [C]).	50-mg. Up to q.i.d. Oral.	Slower acting, but longer duration than most antihistamines.			Doctor should weigh potential of use as an antiemetic during pregnancy against the possible teratogenic effect of the drug.
Cyclizine hydrochloride, U.S.P. (Marezine) (Marzine [C]).	50 mg. Up to q.i.d. Oral or rectal.	Used also as antiemetic and a tranquilizer.			
Cyclizine lactate, N.F. (Marezine).	50 mg. Up to q.i.d. Parenteral.				
MISCELLANEOUS					
Azatadine maleate (Optimine).	1-2 mg. b.i.d. Oral.	Systemic relief of seasonal rhinitis, nonseasonal allergic rhinitis and chronic urticaria.			
Chlorothen citrate (chlorothenylpyramine, Tagathen [C]).	25-50 mg. q.i.d. Oral.				
Clemizole hydrochloride (Reactrol).	20 mg. q.i.d. Oral.	Used especially for skin allergies; drug, food and cosmetic hypersensitivity; and serum sickness.			
Cyproheptadine hydrochloride, N.F. (Periactin).	4 mg. t.i.d. or q.i.d. Oral. Children 0.25 mg./kg./day in divided doses. Oral.	An antihistamine similar to atropine for treatment of allergy, cold urticaria and pruritus.	Also possesses anti-5-hydroxytryptamine and antikinin activity.		Has been said to increase appetite.
Isothipendyl hydrochloride.	4 mg. t.i.d. Oral.				
Thenyldiamine hydrochloride, N.F.	15-30 mg. t.i.d. Oral.				

Name, Source, Synonyms, Preparations	Dosage and Administration	Uses	Action and Fate	Side Effects and Contraindications	Nursing Implications and Remarks
Histamine azoprotein (Hapamine).	0.01-0.02 ml. S.Q.	Used to desensitize in cases of hypersensitivity.	Does not stimulate secretion of gastric juice.	May cause local and systemic reactions similar to those of hypersensitivity. Treatment: antihistaminic.	
Histamine phosphate, U.S.P. (Histapon).	0.3-1.0 mg. S.Q.	Used to desensitize in cases of hypersensitivity, as a diagnostic aid to stimulate secretion of the glands of the gastric mucosa, and in the treatment of peripheral vascular diseases.	Does stimulate secretion of gastric juice. Readily absorbed from parenteral sites but poorly absorbed from gastrointestinal tract. It diffuses rapidly into tissues and is metabolized. Metabolic products are excreted by the kidneys.	Rare in therapeutic dosage. Epinephrine is used if needed. Contraindicated in the elderly, bronchial asthma or cardiovascular disease.	For further information, see Diagnostic Drugs.

DRUGS ACTING ON THE CIRCULATORY SYSTEM

HEMATINICS
(hematopoietic agents)

Name, Source, Synonyms, Preparations	Dosage and Administration	Uses	Action and Fate	Side Effects and Contraindications	Nursing Implications and Remarks
COPPER, MANGANESE. *Mineral.*	These are added to other hematopoietic preparations. No specific preparation or dosage given for these.	Cobalt may be included in this group. These and possibly zinc and nickel are used with iron to treat iron deficiency anemia.	Believed to act as catalytic agents in the utilization of iron.	Rare in minute amounts used. Treatment: none usually required.	
IRON. *Mineral.*		Used to stimulate the hematopoietic system and to increase hemoglobin. There is a general tonic effect upon the entire body which is	Iron is contained in all hemoglobin as well as in other parts of the body. It is absorbed in the small intestines. Average daily	Disorders of the gastrointestinal system. Pasty, black stools are common. Fullness in the head, insomnia, tachycardia and skin eruptions	Give extra laxative foods during iron therapy. Give fluid preparations through a tube to protect teeth. Give with food (milk or

		probably due to better blood supply (better oxygen carrying ability). Used locally as a styptic. Especially valuable in treating iron deficiency anemia.	excretion is about 1 mg. If not replaced by the diet, the reserve is depleted. About 80% of iron from disintegrated red blood cells is retained and reused. Iron to be absorbed from the gastrointestinal tract must be in the soluble ferrous form. Many factors are involved in the absorption. But once absorbed it is transported in the blood to certain organs with a high concentration of iron. These are liver, spleen and marrow. The body excretes small amounts in the feces, urine and bile. The amount of iron is controlled through limited absorption and not by excretory processes.	may occur. The latter symptoms are most apt to occur after a single large dose. Treatment: (for severe symptoms) gastric lavage, emetics, tannic acid solutions orally and treat symptoms; (for mild symptoms) decrease or stop drug, give a laxative, and treat symptoms. Ingestion of liquid or tablets by children (overdose) can be *very toxic.* Mothers should be warned to keep drug out of child's reach. Administration of antacids with oral iron preparations may decrease absorption.	fruit juice) if diet allows. Iron is commonly given in combination with other drugs such as vitamins (especially B), liver and stomach extract. Products containing iron and an organic compound are available, but their effectiveness is open to question; hence they are not in common use. Iron preparations color the feces black. Large doses may give false positive guaiac tests for occult blood in stools. Benzidine tests are unaffected. Oral iron preparations are commercially available in combination with vitamins, minerals, antacids and stool softeners.
Ferric ammonium tartrate.	0.5-1 Gm. t.i.d. Oral.	For iron deficiency anemia.			
Ferric chloride.	Dosage varies. Topical.	Astringent for skin disorders.			
Ferric subsulfate solution (Monsel's solution).	Dosage varies. Topical.	Use undiluted as a styptic.			
Ferrocholinate (Chel-Iron, Ferrolip).	300-600 mg. Given as a solution or tablet, usually t.i.d. Oral.	For iron deficiency anemia.			
Ferroglycine sulfate complex (Ferronord).	40 mg. (40 mg. of ferrous iron in each dose) b.i.d. (between meals). Oral.	As above.			
Ferrous carbonate pills (Blaud's pills).	300 mg. t.i.d. Oral.	As above.			
Ferrous fumarate, U.S.P. (C-Ron, Fumasorb, Ircon, Prematinic, Toleron) (Feroton, Ferrofume, Fumiron, Irofume, Novofumar, Fersamal, Palafer, Tolifer [C]).	200 mg. t.i.d. Oral. Children 100-300 mg. q.d. in divided doses.	As above.			Also available in saccharated form.
Ferrous gluconate, N.F. (Fergon) (Novoferroglue [C]).	300 mg. t.i.d. Oral.	As above.			
Ferrous sulfate, U.S.P. (Feosol, Ferralyn) (Fer-in-Sol, Fesofor, Ferro-Gradumet, Ferrosulph, Novoferrosulf [C]).	300 mg. t.i.d. with meals or p.c. Available as tablets, solution, delayed action capsules. Oral. Children 125-375 mg. q.d. in divided doses.	As above.			

Name, Source, Synonyms, Preparations	Dosage and Administration	Uses	Action and Fate	Side Effects and Contraindications	Nursing Implications and Remarks
IRON (Continued)					
Iron-dextran injection, U.S.P. (Chromagen D, Imferon).	50-250 mg. Dosage and times individually adjusted. I.M. or I.V.	For treatment of iron deficiency anemia when oral administration is not advisable.	Absorbed from injection site primarily through lymphatics. Absorption is slow. Small amounts cross the placenta. Only traces of the unmetabolized drug are excreted in milk, urine, bile or feces.	Local irritation and staining may occur. Other side effects same as with any iron preparation. Sarcomata have been reported in experimental animals but not in man. Allergic or anaphylactoid reactions are not common, but have occurred, including 3 fatalities.	Use of "Z" technique will minimize skin staining. Avoid infiltration. Do not give subcutaneously. Many side effects and contraindications. Large doses color the serum brown and may give false elevated values of serum bilirubin and false decreased values of serum calcium.
Iron sorbitex, U.S.P. (Jectofer) (iron-sorbital citric acid complex [C]).	100 mg. of iron (1 ampule) 10 to 20 injections as indicated by condition. I.M.	As above.	Absorbed directly into blood stream as well as from lymphatic system. Absorption more rapid than with iron-dextran.	As above.	As above. During therapy, urine may turn dark on standing.
Polyferose (iron carbohydrate complex) (Jefron [C]).	4-8 ml. t.i.d. Oral. 5 ml.=100 mg. iron.)	See ferrous sulfate.			
LIVER AND STOMACH PREPARATIONS. *Animal.*		Used to stimulate the production of red blood cells. Owing to increased oxygen carrying power of the blood, these preparations also cause an increase in the activity of all the body organs.	Increase the activity of the hematopoietic organs.	Probably none in therapeutic dosage. May cause local irritation. Change site of injections regularly.	Liver extract is often added to other tonic and antianemic drugs. Liver injection is obsolete and should not be used.
Liver injection.	1-20 mcg. of B_{12} q. 1-3 weeks. I.M.				
Liver injection, crude (Campolon, Pernaemon).	1-2 mcg. of B_{12} q. 1-3 weeks. I.M.				
Liver extract with stomach extract (Extralin).	1 U. o.d. Oral.				

VASODILATORS—ANTI-HYPERTENSIVES

See also Drugs Affecting the Central and Autonomic Nervous Systems, Intoxicants, Histamines and Diuretics.

GANGLIONIC BLOCKING AGENTS

These are synthetic quaternary ammonium compounds unless otherwise stated.

Pentolinium tartrate, N.F. (Ansolysen) (pentolonium [C]).	20-200 mg. Usually started q. 8 h. Individually adjusted. Oral, S.Q. or I.M. Not given I.V.	A potent ganglionic blocking agent whose main use is for hypertension. It is also useful in some peripheral vascular disorders.	These drugs all block passage of impulses of both the sympathetic and parasympathetic ganglia and produce symptoms similar to those of the sympatholytic and parasympatholytic drugs. Drugs are mainly confined to the extracellular fluids. Penetration of the blood-brain barrier is limited. Most are excreted unchanged by the kidneys.		

Name, Source, Synonyms, Preparations	Dosage and Administration	Uses	Action and Fate	Side Effects and Contraindications	Nursing Implications and Remarks
GANGLIONIC BLOCKING AGENTS (Continued)					
Mecamylamine hydrochloride, N.F. (Inversine) (dimecamine [C]).	2.5-10 mg. Dosage individually adjusted. Oral.	Exerts a strong hypotensive action. Usually used only in severe cases of hypertension.	Completely absorbed from the gastrointestinal tract. Widely distributed. Found in high concentration in liver and kidneys. It penetrates the blood-brain barrier. Slowly excreted unchanged by the kidneys.	Orthostatic hypotension occurs commonly. G.I. side effects include anorexia, dry mouth, nausea, vomiting, diarrhea, constipation and paralytic ileus. Glossitis, dysphagia and nasal congestion have occurred. Causes dilated pupils, blurred vision, decreased libido, impotence, dysuria, and urinary retention. C.N.S. side effects have occurred rarely. May cause weakness, fatigue, malaise, headache, sedation and paresthesias. Contraindicated in patients with coronary insufficiency, recent myocardial infarction, uremia, glaucoma or organic pyloric stenosis. Also contraindicated in patients with chronic pyelonephritis receiving antibiotics and sulfonamides.	Not a quaternary. Patients should be told of postural hypotension, especially upon arising in morning and should be advised of measures to take if it develops. Mecamylamine therapy is withdrawn gradually and other anti-hypertensive therapy is substituted at that time. Hypotensive effects potentiated by diuretics, other anti-hypertensives, alcohol, bethanechol. Avoid use during pregnancy.
Trimethaphan camsylate, U.S.P. (Arfonad) (trimetaphan [C]).	1-4 mg./minute. Usually given in 1 mg./ml. concentration in 5% dextrose or normal saline as continuous drip until blood pressure has reached desired level. I.V.	Main use for controlled hypotension during neurosurgery. Also used in hypertensive crisis and in treatment of pulmonary edema in patients with pulmonary hypertension associated with systemic hypertension.	Ganglionic blocking agent with direct vasodilating action. Lowers both diastolic and systolic pressure in normotensive and hypertensive patients.	Toxicity low. Use with caution in patients with arteriosclerosis, cardiac disease, hepatic or renal disease, degenerative disease of the CNS, Addison's disease, diabetes and in patients on steroids.	Not a quaternary ammonium compound. Side effects include urinary retention, orthostatic hypotension, tachycardia, angina pectoris, anorexia, nausea, vomiting, dry mouth, weakness, restlessness,

			Crosses the placenta. Metabolites excreted by kidneys.	Contraindicated in uncorrected anemia, hypovolemia, shock and uncorrected respiratory insufficiency.	cycloplegia, urticaria and itching. Avoid use during pregnancy.
VASODILATORS. *Synthetic preparations unless otherwise noted.*					
Nicotinyl alcohol (Roniacol).	25-50 mg. t.i.d. Oral.	Used for vasodilation: peripheral vascular disease, migraine headache, neuralgia, and other conditions in which vasodilation of the superficial blood vessels is desired.	Vasodilation of superficial blood vessels.	Transient flushing gastric disturbances, minor skin rashes and allergies in some patients. Contraindicated in patients with active peptic ulcer or gastritis.	Also prepared in a delayed release tablet (150 mg. o.d.).
Cyclandelate (Cyclospasmol).	100-200 m.g. q.i.d. Oral.	Use for adjunctive therapy in intermittent claudication, arteriosclerosis obliterans, thrombophlebitis (to control associated vasospasm and muscular ischemia), nocturnal leg cramps, Raynaud's phenomenon and for selected cases of ischemic cerebral vascular disease.	Musculotropic agent acting directly on vascular smooth muscle. Has no significant adrenergic stimulating or blocking action. Absorbed rapidly and completely. Metabolic fate unknown, probably excreted in urine.	Toxicity low, but flushing, tachycardia and nausea may occur. Adjust dosage.	Safe use during pregnancy and lactation has not been established.

Name, Source, Synonyms, Preparations	Dosage and Administration	Uses	Action and Fate	Side Effects and Contraindications	Nursing Implications and Remarks
VASODILATORS (Continued)					
Diazoxide (Hyperstat, Proglycem).	300 mg. in 20 ml. given undiluted, rapidly, intravenously. Do not give I.M., S.Q. or into body cavity. Use a superficial vein. May be repeated in 30 minutes, if required. Can be repeated in 4 to 24 hours to maintain reduction.	For the reduction of malignant hypertension in hospitalized patients, when rapid reduction of diastolic pressure is essential. Used as a temporary expedient. Orally effective drugs should be started as soon as possible.	Pressure usually reduced to lowest level in 5 minutes. Increases fairly rapidly for next 10 to 30 minutes, slowly for next 2 to 12 hours. Rarely reaches pretreatment level. Acts by relaxing smooth muscle tissue in peripheral arterioles. Cardiac output is increased as pressure is reduced. Renal blood flow is increased.	Side effects are frequent and serious: sodium and water retention after repeated injections, especially in patients with impaired cardiac reserve. Hyperglycemia is frequent, but usually requires treatment only in patients with diabetes mellitus. Infrequent but serious: hypotension to shock levels, myocardial and/or cerebral ischemia, atrial or ventricular arrhythmias, marked changes in ECG, unconsciousness, convulsions, paralysis, confusion, persistent retention of nitrogenous wastes in the blood stream after repeated injections, many other adverse reactions. Most are transient in nature.	Proglycem is the oral form. Should be administered only to hospitalized patients where close monitoring of electrolytes, glycemic levels, cardiac and renal functions is possible. This drug is not effective against hypertension caused by pheochromocytoma. Has been shown to have teratogenic effects in animal studies. Concurrent administration of thiazides or other potent diuretics may potentiate the hyperglycemic and hyperuricemic effects. Safe use in pregnancy not established.
	3-8 mg./kg./day in divided doses q. 8-12 h. Oral.	Treatment of hypoglycemia *due to hyperinsulinism.*	When given orally, diazoxide acts to raise blood glucose levels primarily by inhibiting the release of insulin from the pancreas, but also by an extrapancreatic effect. The hypotensive effects of the orally administered drug are usually not marked.		
Dioxyline phosphate (Paveril phosphate) (dimoxyline, Paverone [C]).	100-400 mg. 3 or 4 times daily. Oral.	Used for angina and in conditions in which there are reflex spasms of blood vessels in arms, legs or lungs.	Action similar to that of papaverine. Metabolized primarily in liver and excreted in urine.	Rare in therapeutic dosage but include nausea, dizziness, sweating, flushing and abdominal cramping.	Safe use in pregnancy not established.
Dipyridamole (Persantine).	25-50 mg. Before meals t.i.d. Oral.	Long-term therapy of chronic angina pectoris. Not of value in acute angina attack.	A spasmolytic agent with special action on the myocardium. It is metabolized in the liver and excreted in	Headache, dizziness, nausea, flushing, mild gastrointestinal disturbances, syncope and weakness. Reduce	2-3 months of continuous therapy may be required before a clinical response is achieved.

			the feces, either unchanged or as the glucuronide.	dosage or stop drug. Used with caution in hypotensive states. Not advised for acute phase of myocardial infarction.	
Hydralazine hydrochloride, U.S.P. (Apresoline) (hydralazine [C]).	40-300 mg. daily in divided doses. Oral. 20 mg. I.M. or I.V. Dosage individually adjusted.	Used to treat hypertension.	Lowers blood pressure through direct action on arteriolar smooth muscle. Has little effect on capacitance of vessels and causes reflex stimulation of the heart. Sustains or can increase renal blood flow. Well absorbed from gastrointestinal tract or parenteral sites. After oral dose maximum blood levels reached in 3 to 4 hours. Fate and excretion not well understood.	Headache, tachycardia, palpitation aggravates angina, fluid retention, nasal congestion and gastrointestinal disturbances. There have been reports of cases resembling acute systemic lupus erythematosus and rheumatoid arthritis, which usually disappear when drug is withdrawn. Contraindications: coronary artery disease and mitral valvular rheumatic heart disease.	With high dosage, arrhythmias are seen. Use with caution in patients taking MAO inhibitors. Teratogenicity has been demonstrated in mice and rabbits, so use in pregnancy only if benefits justify risk.

Name, Source, Synonyms, Preparations	Dosage and Administration	Uses	Action and Fate	Side Effects and Contraindications	Nursing Implications and Remarks
VASODILATORS (Continued)					
NITRITES. *Salts and esters of nitrous acid and organic nitrates.*		Used for vasodilation; will lower blood pressure. Used also in angina pectoris.	The nitrite ion relaxes smooth, muscle tissue, especially of the coronary vessels. Anti-hypertensive action is less potent than that of some other drugs, but action on coronary vessels is stronger. These drugs also increase pulse rate, increase the rate and depth of respirations, and are antispasmodic in action. Amyl nitrite is absorbed through the lungs. Nitroglycerin and others such as isosorbide dinitrate and erythrityl tetranitrate are best absorbed sublingually. Other nitrates such as pentaerythritol tetranitrate, trolnitrate, sodium nitrite and mannitol hexanitrate are readily absorbed from the gastrointestinal tract. Some nitrate preparations can be absorbed through the skin. Both nitrite ions and organic nitrates disappear rapidly from the blood stream. The blood concentration from a single dose does not appear to be directly correlated with the	Irregular pulse, headache, dizziness, rise in intraocular pressure, blurred vision, flushed face, palpitation, vomiting, diarrhea, mental confusion, muscular weakness, cyanosis, slowing of heart rate and respiratory rate. Any or all symptoms may occur. Deaths are rare. Stop drug and give evacuants. Cold applications to the head, artifical respiration and shock therapy as indicated. Digitalis, strychnine and sodium sulfate should be available.	All these substances become nitrites in the body. Tolerance may occur, requiring change in form or dosage.
Amyl nitrite, N.F. (isoamylnitrate).	0.2 ml. inhalation. Comes prepared in perles, ready for crushing and inhaling.				
Erythrityl tetranitrate, N.F. (Cardilate) (erythrol tetranitrate [C]).	5-30 mg. p.r.n. Oral. 5-15 mg. p.r.n. Sublingual.				
Isosorbide dinitrate (Isordil, Sorbitrate) (Coronex [C]).	2.5-20 mg. q. 4 h. or p.r.n. Oral or sublingual.				Both nitroglycerin and pentaerythritol are available in sustained release form.
Mannitol hexanitrate (Maxitate).	15-60 mg. q. 4-6 h. Oral.				Mannitol hexanitrate is used cautiously in anemia, as it tends to produce methemoglobin.
Nitroglycerin, U.S.P. (glyceryl trinitrate).	0.1-0.6 mg. p.r.n. Oral. 2.5-6.5 mg. b.i.d. sublingual. 2% ointment. Topical.				
Pentaerythritol tetranitrate, N.F. (Glynite, Niglycon, Nitroglyn, Nitrol, Nitrostabilin, Trinitrine [C]).	5-20 mg. One or 2 tablets as needed for anginal attacks. t.i.d. or q.i.d. for prophylaxis. Oral.				There are any number of proprietary names for nitroglycerin and pentaerythritol in the United States and Canada. Space does not permit their inclusion.
Sodium nitrite, U.S.P. (Anti-Rust, Filmerine).	Found in cyanide antidote package with sodium thiosulfate and amyl nitrate. I.V.				Main use now is in instrument sterilizing solutions as an antirust agent.

			therapeutic effects. About 2/3 of the nitrite ions disappear in the body and the exact fate and excretion are not well known.		
Sodium nitroprusside (Nipride).	3 mcg./kg./min. (range 0.5-8.0 mcg./kg./min.) (3 mcg./kg./min. is usually sufficient to maintain B/P at 30-40% lower than pretreatment diastolic levels.) Patients receiving other antihypertensive drugs should have lower dosage. Used only in infusion with 5% dextrose in water I.V. Not as a direct injection. Maximum recommended dose 8 mcg./min.	Used to treat hypertensive crisis with change to oral drugs as soon as possible. May be used concomitantly during transfer.	Action is believed to be due to nitroso group. It is rapidly converted to thiocyanate, hence effective action is short. The hypotensive effect is caused by peripheral vasodilation by direct action on blood vessels. Rapidly metabolized. Metabolites excreted primarily in urine, exhaled air and probably in feces.	Nausea, retching, diaphoresis, apprehension, headache, restlessness, palpitation, dizziness, abdominal pain. If given for a prolonged period, signs of hypothyroidism may appear. The thiocyanate blood level should be monitored. Safe use during pregnancy or for children has not been established.	Drug is photosensitive. Solution should be wrapped in foil to protect from light. Drug is stable for only 4 hours. Adequate facilities (equipment and personnel) should be available for monitoring of B/P because hypotensive effects occur rapidly. I.V. administration should allow precise measurement of flow rate as determined by blood pressures. Recommend use of infusion pump, micro-drip regulator or similar devices.
Trolnitrate phosphate (Metamine, Nitretamin).	2-4 mg. t.i.d. p.c. and h.s. Oral.				
PAPAVERINE. *Active principle of the opium poppy.* Papaverine hydrochloride, N.F.	30-100 mg. three to four times daily. Oral or parenteral. Long acting, 150 mg. b.i.d. Oral.	Used for vasodilation and as an antispasmodic to relieve gastric, intestinal, bronchial, biliary and urethral colic. Also used in peripheral vascular disease and pulmonary embolism. It produces some sedation (mild), some coronary dilation and some hypotension.	Smooth muscle tissue relaxant. Acts more on muscles in spasm than on those with normal tonus. Well absorbed from all routes. Some is localized in the fat tissue of the liver. A considerable amount is bound to plasma proteins. The exact extent of therapeutic effectiveness is not known, but every 6 hour dosage appears adequate. It is excreted in an inactivated form by the kidneys.	Side effects include general discomfort, intense flushing of the face, perspiration, increase in depth of respiration and heart rate, rise in blood pressure and some sedation. Hepatic hypersensitivity has been reported. Contraindicated: I.V. injection in the presence of complete AV heart block.	No tolerance or habituation has been demonstrated. The sedative effect of papaverine is very limited and probably due to its antispasmodic action.

Name, Source, Synonyms, Preparations	Dosage and Administration	Uses	Action and Fate	Side Effects and Contraindications	Nursing Implications and Remarks
VASODILATORS (Continued)					
PARGYLINE HYDROCHLORIDE. *Synthetic.* Pargyline hydrochloride, N.F. (Eutonyl).	10-50 mg. daily. Oral.	Antidepressant and anti-hypertensive agent used to treat most types of hypertension, but not recommended for labile hypertension or patients amenable to treatment with sedatives and the thiazide diuretics.	Monoamine oxidase inhibitor mainly used in the treatment of hypertension. Exact mechanism is not known, but effect is greatest when patient is in standing position.	Postural hypotension, gastro-intestinal disturbances, insomnia, urinary frequency, dry mouth, nightmares, impotence and edema have been reported. Congestive failure may occur in patients with reduced cardiac reserve. Used with caution, if at all, in labile or malignant hypertension, pregnancy, pheochromocytoma, renal failure, paranoid schizophrenia and hyperthyroidism. Pargyline is a monoamine oxidase inhibitor. For interactions, see under Monoamine Oxidase Inhibitors, Page 109. Meperidine is contraindicated in patients taking pargyline. This drug should be discontinued 2 weeks before elective surgery.	Blood and liver tests should be done frequently. Patients should be warned against taking any of the following: over-the-counter cold preparations or anti-histamines, alcoholic beverages, certain types of cheese and foods with high amine content. (See interactions of MAO inhibitors. Page 109).
VERATRUM. *Veratrum viride (green hellebore).* Alkavervir (Veriloid).	3-5 mg. t.i.d. q. 6-8 h. Oral.	Used as a vasodilator in the treatment of hypertension, angina pectoris, some cases of asthma. It is also used to treat emergency conditions such as toxemia of pregnancy, acute glomerulonephritis and hypertensive encephalopathy.	The hypotensive action is due chiefly to direct central nervous system action resulting in vasodilation. It reduces both the systolic and the diastolic pressure. It produces some bradycardia through reflexes in heart and lungs. It tends	Substernal or epigastric burning sensation, anorexia, nausea, vomiting. Reduce dosage or stop drug and treat symptoms. In acute poisoning there may be cardiovascular collapse. Epinephrine or similar drug is used in treatment.	Varied preparations of *Veratrum* differ in their hypotensive effect. Dosage is individually adjusted. With continued use there is a tendency to gain weight. All preparations listed are a mixture of alkaloids.

			to reduce urinary output. Only 5-20% of these alkaloids is absorbed from the gastro-intestinal tract. The absorption is not only limited but also variable. Little is known of the fate of these drugs in the body. Only a very small percentage is excreted unchanged by the kidneys.	Thiazide diuretics may potentiate hypotensive effects.	Narrow range between therapeutic and toxic doses.
Cryptenamine acetate (Unitensin acetate).	1-2 mg. Used in emergencies. Repeated at 1-2 h. intervals until desired pressure is secured. I.M. or I.V.				
Cryptenamine tannate (Unitensin tannate) (Unitensyl [C]).	1-2 mg. two or three times a day. Oral.				
Protoveratrine A & B (Veralba).	0.1-0.5 mg. two or three times a day. Oral.				
Protoveratrine A & B maleates (Provell maleate).	0.5-2.5 mg. two or three times a day. Oral.				

Name, Source, Synonyms, Preparations	Dosage and Administration	Uses	Action and Fate	Side Effects and Contraindications	Nursing Implications and Remarks
CARDIOTONICS (indirect heart stimulants)					
DIGITALIS *(glycosides, digitoxin). Digitalis purpurea and lanata.*	Dosages listed are maintenance doses. usually o.d.	Main use is to treat cardiac decompensation and to control the ventricular rate with atrial fibrillation. Used as an emergency drug and also for maintenance of the chronic patient. Preparations from *Digitalis purpurea* (primarily digitoxin) have slower and more prolonged action than those from *Digitalis lanata* (primarily digoxin).	Stimulates the vagus nerve, thus increasing the strength of the heart beat while decreasing its rate. The pulse is slower and stronger. Improvement in heart action relieves cyanosis, dyspnea and cardiac edema. It also benefits all body processes by improving blood supply. Reduces high blood pressure and increases low blood pressure caused by circulatory disorder. Urinary output is increased in individuals with edema of cardiac origin. Most glycosides are absorbed from the intestinal tract, a little from the stomach. Absorption from parenteral sites, subcutaneous or intramuscular, is irregular and uncertain. Lanatoside C is absorbed only about 10%, digitalis, digilanid and digifolin about 20%, digoxin 50% and digitoxin 100%. Much of these drugs is bound to plasma protein, but this does not appear to greatly decrease their effectiveness. Ouabain is unbound and lanatoside C only slightly bound. Digoxin, more active than	Cumulative: slow pulse (below 60), anorexia, vomiting, irregular and intermittent pulse. Rapid change in pulse rate, diarrhea, abdominal pain, weakness, headache, vertigo and visual disturbances may occur. Cardiac arrhythmias may occur with or without other signs of toxicity. These often precede other toxic side effects. Treatment: withhold further digitalis until the physician is notified. Keep patient quiet. Apply ice bag to precordium. Atropine and caffeine should be available. Other drugs that may be required include epinephrine, sodium phenobarbital, bromide or the opiates. Electrolyte imbalances, especially hypokalemia and to a lesser extent hypomagnesemia and hypercalcemia may predispose patients to cardiotoxic effects of cardiac glycosides. Administer with caution to patients with severe pulmonary disease, hypoxia, myxedema, acute myocardial infarction, severe	Digitalis and similar products are given in a number of circumstances. Emergency: usually one large dose given intravenously to cover immediate needs. Rapid digitalization. One large dose or several doses given close together to produce desired effect in a few hours. Gradual digitalization: give in lesser doses and over a longer time so that digitalization takes several days. Safe use during pregnancy and lactation not established. Narrow range between therapeutic and toxic doses. Before administering the dose during digitalization or when dosage is being altered, be sure to: (1) check serum electrolyte and digitalis lab. reports, (2) take apical pulse for 1 full minute; note rate, rhythm and quality, (3) if the patient is on ECG monitor, note for changes in rhythm, (4) check for signs of toxicity. Digitalis products are irritating to the tissues and are never given subcutaneously and rarely intramuscularly.
Deslonoside, N.F. (Cedilanid-D).	0.4-0.8 mg. I.M. or I.V.				
Digitoxin, U.S.P. (Crystodigin, Myodigin, Purodigin, Unidigin) (digitoxoside [C]).	0.1-0.2 mg. Acetyl salt also available. Oral.				
Digitoxin injection, N.F.	0.2 mg. I.V.				
Digoxin, U.S.P. (Lanoxin) (Natigoxin-Nativelle, Reugoxin, Winoxin [C]).	0.125-0.5 mg. Oral.				
Digoxin injection, U.S.P.	0.1-0.5 mg. I.V.				
Gitalin amorphous (Gitaligin).	0.3-0.8 mg. Oral.				
Lanatoside C, (Cedilanid).	0.5 mg. Oral.				
Lanatoside C injection.	0.5 mg. I.V.				

			digitoxin, is excreted much more rapidly. Digoxin and lanatoside C are excreted by the kidneys largely unchanged. Digitoxin is broken down by the liver, and the degradation products are excreted by the kidneys.	congestive heart failure, acute myocarditis, since the likelihood of arrhythmias is increased. Aluminum hydroxide, magnesia hydroxide, magnesium trisilicate, kaolin-pectin, aminosalicylic acid and sulfasalazine may reduce G.I. absorption of digoxin.	Since drug is apt to cause cumulative poisoning, patients on long-term use should skip an occasional dose as directed by the physician. Many plants contain glycosides that act similarly to digitalis. However, digitalis, digitoxin, digoxin or ouabain are the drugs most commonly used. If one of these preparations is not effective, usually another will be. The other glyosides are not considered reliable.
STROPHANTHUS (*Strophanthin, Ouabain*). *Strophanthus bispidus* and *kombe.* <u>Ouabain</u>, U.S.P. (injection).	0.5 mg. I.V. or I.M.	Used mostly for patients who need digitalis but do not respond to that drug. It is sometimes used to sustain a patient who has cumulative toxic symptoms from digitalis and cannot use that drug for a time.	Similar to digitalis but less reliable. The active principals act quickly.	Similar to digitalis but not so severe. Stop drug and treat symptoms.	Ouabain acts faster than digitalis and is used intravenously in emergencies.

Name, Source, Synonyms, Preparations	Dosage and Administration	Uses	Action and Fate	Side Effects and Contraindications	Nursing Implications and Remarks
			CARDIAC DEPRESSANTS		
Bretylium tosylate (Bretylol).	5-10 mg./kg. over 8 min. I.V., repeated in 1-2 h. p.r.n. or constant infusion of 1-2 mg./min. 5-10 mg./kg. I.M. q. 6-8 h.	Short term management of life threatening ventricular arrhythmias.	Inhibits norepinephrine release by depressing adrenergic nerve terminal excitability. Suppresses ventricular fibrillation and arrhythmias. Mechanism of action not established. Suppression of ventricular fibrillation is rapid, usually within minutes after I.V. administration. Suppression of ventricular tachycardia and other arrhythmias develops more slowly, usually 20 min. 2 h. after parenteral dose. Eliminated unchanged by kidneys. About 70-80% excreted in first 24 h. with additional 10% excreted over the next 3 days.	Some degree of hypotension present in about 50% of patients while they are supine. Transient hypertension and increased frequency of arrhythmias may occur in some. Nausea and vomiting occur, primarily when administered I.V. at fast rate. Vertigo, dizziness, light-headedness and syncope, which sometimes accompanies hypotension. Bradycardia, increased frequency of premature ventricular contractions, precipitation of anginal attacks and sensation of substernal pressure have also been reported.	Patients should be kept in supine position until tolerance to hypotensive effect develops. Tolerance occurs unpredictably but may be present after several days. Dosage of bretylium should be under ECG monitoring and should be reduced and discontinued after 3-5 days.
Disopyramide phosphate (Norpace).	150 mg. q. 6 h. Oral. Individually adjusted.	Suppression and prevention of recurrence of cardiac arrhythmias occurring singly or in combination in digitalized and nondigitalized patients.	Shown to shorten the sinus node recovery time, to lengthen effective refractory period of the atria and to have minimal effect on the effective refractory period of the AV node. Electrophysiology studies have shown prolonged conduction in accessory pathways. At recommended doses, produces significant blood pressure alterations.	Most common side effects are anticholinergic and may be transient or require dose reduction: dry mouth, nose and eyes, blurred vision, constipation and urinary hesitancy. Cardiovascular side effects include edema, weight gain, chest pain, dyspnea, syncope, hypotension. Less frequent were dizziness, fatigue, muscle weakness,	Safe use in pregnancy, lactation and children has not been established. Additive effects when given with other antiarrhythmic or anticholinergic drugs.

			Has anticholinergic properties, which may affect G.I. and/or G.U. systems; these effects may be transitory or may disappear with dose reduction. Rapidly absorbed from G.I. tract with 60-83% reaching systemic circulation unchanged. Crosses the placenta. With therapeutic levels, 50% is protein bound. Metabolized by liver. Unchanged drug and its metabolites excreted in urine.	headache, malaise, anorexia, diarrhea, vomiting, cardiac conduction disturbances, generalized rash and dermatoses. Use with caution in patients with prostatic hypertrophy, narrow angle glaucoma, myasthenia gravis. In patients with marginally compensated heart failure the drug has precipitated heart failure. Conduction disorders have occurred in patients with preexisting conduction disorders. Administer with caution to patients with renal and hepatic insufficiency. Contraindicated in patients with preexisting 2nd. and 3rd. degree AV block (if no artificial pacemaker has been inserted), cardiogenic shock, or previous hypersensitivity to the drug.	

Name, Source, Synonyms, Preparations	Dosage and Administration	Uses	Action and Fate	Side Effects and Contraindications	Nursing Implications and Remarks
Lidocaine hydrochloride 2% solution, U.S.P. (Xylocaine 2%). (lignocaine [C]).	50-100 mg. I.V. under electrocardiographic monitoring at a rate of approximately 25-30 mg./min. If initial dose does not give desired response, dose may be repeated in 5 minutes. No more than 200-300 mg. should be given in a one-hour period. For a continuous infusion the rate is from 1-4 mg./min. under electrocardiographic monitoring. 100 mg. I.M. but only by physician when ECG equipment is not available or by paramedical persons when transmitted ECG is being viewed by a physician.	Used in the management of acute ventricular arrhythmias.	Has been reported to exert antiarrhythmic effect by increasing the electrical stimulation threshold of the ventricles during diastole. Ninety per cent of dose is metabolized by the liver and 10 per cent is excreted unchanged by the kidneys. A C.N.S. depressant producing sedative, analgesic and anticonvulsant effects. Also suppresses cough and gag reflexes.	Side effects generally involve the CNS and are dose related. These include drowsiness, dizziness, disorientation, apprehension, euphoria, tinnitus or decreased hearing, swallowing or breathing. Stupor, convulsions and respiratory depression may occur. Anaphylactoid reactions may occur.	Constant monitoring with the electrocardiograph is essential for the proper administration of this drug. Contraindicated in patients with a history of sensitivity to local anesthetics of the amide type, in patients with Adams-Stokes syndrome or with a severe degree of sinoatrial, atrioventricular or intraventricular block. Use with caution in the following: repeated use for patients with severe renal or liver disease, as it can induce toxic phenomena as a result of accumulation of the drug; patients with sinus bradycardia in whom this drug is used to eliminate ventricular ectopic beats if patient has had prior accelerated heart rate since it may provoke more frequent and serious ventricular arrhythmias.
PROCAINAMIDE HYDROCHLORIDE *Synthetic* from procaine.					
Procainamide hydrochloride, U.S.P. (Procamide, Procapan, Pronestyl).	250-500 mg. q. 4-6 h. Oral. 200 mg.-1 Gm. (100 mg./ml.) I.V. Dosage regulated to suit patient and condition.	Used in the treatment of ventricular tachycardia, premature ventricular contractions, atrial fibrillation and paroxysmal atrial tachycardia.	Decreases the irritability of the ventricular muscles, thus slowing pulse. Rapid and almost complete absorption after oral dose.	With oral therapy, G.I. side effects include anorexia, bitter taste, nausea, vomiting, diarrhea. With long term therapy, anti-	Continuous ECG and vital sign monitoring is important during I.V. therapy. Patients on prolonged

		Maximum blood level is reached in about 1 hour, after I.M. dose about 15 minutes. Widely distributed and except for brain, tissue concentrations are higher than plasma concentrations. Most is excreted unchanged by the kidneys.	nuclear antibodies may be found in 50% of patients. These patients may develop a syndrome resembling systemic lupus erythematosus. Other hypersensitivity reactions may occur. May cause agranulocytosis in susceptible individuals. Hypotension may occur. Stop drug and treat symptoms. Contraindicated in kidney or liver disorders. When used shortly after surgery or in the immediate postsurgical period in which a polarizing or non-polarizing muscle relaxant has been given, procainamide can cause a recurarization to occur.	therapy should be monitored closely for hypersensitivity reactions. Complete blood count, LE cell preparation and ANA determinations should be done before and during therapy.

Name, Source, Synonyms, Preparations	Dosage and Administration	Uses	Action and Fate	Side Effects and Contraindications	Nursing Implications and Remarks
QUINIDINE. *Active principle of cinchona.*		Used to decrease pulse rate in many cardiac and cardiovascular disorders.	Slows rate of impulses of the sinoauricular node. Depresses all activity of the heart muscle. There is reduced force, reduced tonus and a prolonged refractory period. Produces a lessened heart rate. Also posseses anticholinergic properties. Rapidly and completely absorbed from the gastrointestinal tract. Maximum effects occur in 1-3 hours and last 6-8 hours. After I.M. dose, maximum effect in 1-1½ hours. An appreciable amount is bound to plasma protein. About half of the quinidine is excreted unchanged by the kidneys within 24 hours. The remainder is excreted as metabolic degradation products.	Same as quinine: ringing in ears, nausea, vomiting, dizziness, headache. Reduce or stop drug and treat symptoms. Antiarrhythmic effects of quinidine are enhanced in the presence of reserpine. When given together, the dose should be reduced. Quinidine, like procainamide, can cause recurarization in the immediate postoperative period. See page 149. Quinidine exerts a mild hypoprothrombinemic effect which can potentiate the action of warfarin-like compounds. Aluminum hydroxide and related antacids can cause a delay in the absorption of quinidine.	In usual doses, quinidine may cause syncope, probably due to ventricular tachycardia or fibrillation. Continual ECG and vital sign monitoring is important with parenteral and initial oral therapy. Severe hypotension may occur with vascular collapse, respiratory distress and respiratory arrest. Symptomatic measures may be required and should be available during therapy. Should not be used in pregnancy unless the possibility of the benefits outweigh potential risks.
Quinidine gluconate, U.S.P. (Quinaglute) (Quinate [C]).	300-500 mg. I.M. or I.V. 200-400 mg. q. 12 h. Oral.				
Quinidine hydrochloride, U.S.P.	200-400 mg. p.r.n. Oral, I.M. or I.V.				
Quinidine polygalacturonate (Cardioquin).	275 mg. two to three times daily. Oral.				
Quinidine sulfate, U.S.P. (Quinidate, Quinidex, Quinora) (Kinidine, Novoquinidin, Quincardine [C]).	200-300 mg. three or four times a day. 400 mg. (long-acting) two or three times a day. Oral. 300-500 mg. I.M. or I.V.				

BLOOD SUBSTITUTES
(blood replacement)

Name, Source, Synonyms, Preparations	Dosage and Administration	Uses	Action and Fate	Side Effects and Contraindications	Nursing Implications and Remarks
See also Biologicals. COLLOIDAL SOLUTIONS. *Animal* and *vegetable.*	These are all given p.r.n.	Used as substitutes for blood plasma; especially valuable in the control of shock resulting from hemorrhage. They are called plasma expanders.	These preparations maintain blood volume until nature can replenish it or whole blood or plasma can be secured.	Varied: drug may stay in the organs and act as a foreign body, but this is relatively rare. Treatment: symptomatic.	Patients should be observed closely during the first minute of infusion for hypersensitivity reactions.

Dextran (Expandex, Gentran, Plavolex) (Dextraven, Macrodex).	6-12% solution. 250-500 ml. I.V.	A glucose polymer used to expand plasma and to maintain blood pressure in emergencies.	They remain in the body for 12-24 hours, are partly metabolized and usually excreted by the kidneys.	Contraindications: thrombocytopenia, hypofibrinogenemia, renal disease with anuria or severe oliguria.	Dosage should not exceed 20 ml./kg. during the first 24 hours and 10 mg./kg. each day after the first day. With dosage over recommended limits prolongation of bleeding time may occur.
Dextran-40 (LMD 10 per cent, Rheomacrodex).	10-20 ml./kg. as sole primer or additive varying with volume of perfusion circuit. 10% solution added to normal saline or 5% dextrose I.V.	Used as a priming fluid, either as sole primer or an additive in pump oxygenator during extracorporeal circulation. Flow improver for cardiopulmonary bypass.	See uses.	Use with caution in poorly hydrated patients.	
PLASMA AND SERUM. *Human blood.*		General use same as for whole blood.	These contain all blood factors except cells, thus they do not produce any additional oxygen-carrying ability. Serum does not contain the clotting elements.	Rare: allergic reaction if any. Treatment: if needed, is anti-allergic.	
Albumin, normal human serum, U.S.P. (Albumisol, serum albumin).	2.2 ml./kg. body weight. Given slowly, usually 250-500 ml. I.V.			Since this is made from pooled human blood, it could contain the causative agent of serum hepatitis. This should be considered when it is administered.	Expiration date should be carefully checked.
Antihemophilic human plasma, U.S.P.	50 ml. in 250 ml. diluent I.V.	Contains clotting factors. Used in hemorrhagic conditions.			Pulse rate should be taken before administration and if there is a significant increase during therapy, the rate of administration should be decreased or discontinued.
Antihemophilic factor (Factor VIII, AHF, AHG).	Varies with circumstances and with different patients. Parenteral.	Used in the treatment of hemophilia.	A stable dried preparation of human antihemophilic factor in concentrated form with minimal quantities of other protein. Action is substitutive.	Side effects are generally related to rate of infusion and can include headache, flushing, tachycardia, paresthesias, nausea, vomiting, hypotension.	
Citrated normal human plasma.	250-1000 ml. I.V. Occasionally given in small doses I.M.				
Fibrinogen, U.S.P.	1-2 Gm. with 50-200 ml. of diluent. I.V.	Used in hemorrhagic conditions due to fibrinogenemia.			
Plasma, normal human, U.S.P.	250-1000 ml. I.V. occasionally given in small doses I.M.				

Name, Source, Synonyms, Preparations	Dosage and Administration	Uses	Action and Fate	Side Effects and Contraindications	Nursing Implications and Remarks
PLASMA AND SERUM *(Continued)*					
Plasma protein fraction, U.S.P. (Plasmanate).	5% solution, 250 ml. I.V.	Used to combat hypoproteinemia and in same conditions as albumin.			
Salt poor serum albumin 25%.	50-100 ml. Usually given every 24 hours until symptoms subside. I.V.	Used in nephrosis and other conditions in which there is hypoproteinemia.			
SALINE SOLUTIONS. *Water and various salts.*		Used to restore blood volume in hemorrhage and blood pressure in shock, and to compensate for fluid loss from burns, dehydration and many similar conditions. Also as a means of giving needed I.V. medications.	Electrolyte solutions given to maintain balance. The type used depends upon the needs of the patient. Isotonic sodium chloride is used if sodium is depleted, potassium preparations in potassium depletion. Other solutions contain several electrolytes and are used as general replacement.	Rare in therapeutic use.	
Sodium chloride solution (0.9%) isotonic, U.S.P. (normal saline solution).	100-1000 ml. I.V. or S.Q.				
Sodium chloride solution (0.45 per cent) (one-half isotonic).	100-1000 ml. I.V.				
Sodium chloride solution (0.2 per cent).	100-1000 ml. I.V.				
Lactated Ringer's solution, U.S.P., (Hartmann's solution).	100-1000 ml. I.V. or S.Q.				
Multiple (balanced) electrolytes (Butler's solution, Ionosol MB, Talbot's solution, Travert's solution).	100-1000 ml. I.V. or S.Q.				
Potassium acetate, bicarbonate and citrate solution.	100-1000 ml. I.V. or S.Q.				
Potassium chloride injection, U.S.P.	0.3% solution 1000 ml. I.V. (over 4 hour period).				
Potassium chloride in dextrose (Kadalex).	100-1000 ml. I.V. or S.Q.				
Potassium lactate solution (Darrow's solution, Potassic saline, Ionosol P.S.L.).	40-100 ml./kg. of body weight. I.V. or S.Q.				
Ringer's solution, N.F. (3 Chlorides, Triple Chloride).	100-1000 ml. I.V. or S.Q.				
Sodium lactate, injection, U.S.P.	1000 ml. 1/6 molar solution I.V.				

SUGAR SOLUTIONS. *Water and various monosaccharides and disaccharides.*					
Dextrose solution, U.S.P.	100-1000 ml. Dextrose is used in strengths varying from 2 to 50% I.V.	Used for the same purposes as the saline solutions, with added nutrients. Strong solutions are diuretic in action and reduce edema, especially meningeal.	Dextrose is prepared in isotonic sodium chloride and also in distilled water for use as patient's condition indicates. These solutions provide an easily metabolized source of calories.	Rare in therapeutic use.	
Fructose injection, N.F. (Levugen).	10% solution. 100-1000 ml. I.V.				
WHOLE BLOOD. *Human blood.*					
Citrated whole human blood, U.S.P.	200-1000 ml. I.V.	Used to replace blood. Also used in the treatment of shock, burns, debility and certain diseases (especially diseases of the blood).	If blood is compatible, action is same as that of patient's blood.	If blood is compatible there is usually no toxic reaction. Otherwise, chills, anxiety, back pain, flushing of the face, tachycardia, dyspnea, and allergic symptoms may occur. Treatment: anti-allergic and symptomatic.	Blood may be obtained from public or private donors or from blood banks. The possibility of the transfer of viral diseases such as serum hepatitis or of protozoal infections such as malaria should not be overlooked. Typing and cross matching are required.
Packed human blood cells, U.S.P.	Equivalent of 1 unit (500 ml.) of whole blood I.V.	As above.			

SCLEROSING AGENTS

SODIUM MORRHUATE. *Cod liver oil.*					
Sodium morrhuate injection	0.5-5 ml. of a 5% solution into varicosities. Used with vein ligation in large veins and without ligation in small veins.	Used to produce sclerosing, thrombosis, and obliteration of varicose veins and hemorrhoids.	Action of these solutions varies slightly, but most destroy the endothelium and set up a fibrosing (scarring) process, which eventually obliterates the vein.	Rare in therapeutic usage. Treatment: none usually required.	
SODIUM TETRADECYL. *Synthetic.*		See above.	See above.	As above. This drug is contraindicated during pregnancy.	
Sodium tetradecyl sulfate (Sotradecol, Trombovar [C]).	1-5% solution. Injection into varicosities.				

Name, Source, Synonyms, Preparations	Dosage and Administration	Uses	Action and Fate	Side Effects and Contraindications	Nursing Implications and Remarks
		ANTICOAGULANTS			
		(*Prothrombin time should be checked regularly when giving any of these drugs.*)			
IN VITRO					
SODIUM CITRATE AND SIMILAR PREPARATIONS. *Chemical, Food, Synthetic.*		Used to prevent blood clotting outside the blood vessels, as in indirect transfusions.	Prevents clotting in vitro but does not prevent clotting in vivo.		
Sodium citrate solution, anticoagulant, N.F.	For whole blood. 50 ml. will prevent coagulation of 450 ml. of whole blood.		Binds calcium ion, preventing thrombin formation.		
IN VIVO					
BISHYDROXYCOUMARIN. *Spoiled sweet clover hay. Synthetic.*	Dosages are adjusted daily as indicated by the prothrombin time.	Used to prolong the clotting time of blood and to treat thrombophlebitis; pulmonary embolism, certain cardiac conditions, or any disorder in which there is excessive or undesirable clotting. It is especially valuable in thrombosis and embolism, except in cases of bacterial endocarditis.	Prolongs the clotting time of blood by preventing the production of prothrombin in the liver. The action of these drugs is slower but more prolonged than that of heparin. They are often given with heparin to secure both immediate and delayed action. Coumarin products are used for maintenance. Oral absorption is slow and erratic and varies widely with the individual. Most is bound to plasma proteins, widely distributed throughout the body, but little reaches the brain. Slowly metabolized by the body, but a small percentage is excreted by the	Not common, but hemorrhage may occur, either as one large local hemorrhage or as a number of smaller bleeding points. Stop drug, give whole blood or coagulants. Phytonadione (vitamin K_1) may be ordered. Cumulative action may occur. Also seen are alopecia, urticaria, dermatitis, fever, nausea, diarrhea and hypersensitivity reactions. Oral anticoagulants cross the placental barrier and danger of fatal hemorrhage in the fetus in utero may exist even within the accepted therapeutic range of maternal prothrombin level. The doctor must determine if	Many factors can influence the prothrombin time of people on anticoagulant therapy. Among these are: diet, environment, physical state and other medications. The patient should understand that other drugs should be added or stopped only under the physician's direct observation so that additional prothrombin times can be taken to determine the effect. See brochures for the endogenous and exogenous factors which may influence the prothrombin time response. Oral anticoagulants appear in only insignificant quantities in breast milk.
Acenocoumarol (Sintrom) (acenocoumarin, nicoumaline [C]).	2-10 mg. Oral.				
Bishydroxycoumarin, U.S.P. (Dicumarol) (dicoumarin, Dufalone [C]).	50-200 mg. q.d. Oral.				
Phenprocoumon, N.F. (Liquamar) (Marcumar [C]).	1-4 mg. Oral.				

			kidneys. Plasma levels may be maintained for up to 5 days.	potential benefits outweigh possible risks.	
WARFARIN *Synthetic.* Warfarin sodium, U.S.P. (Athrombin, Coumadin, Panwarfin) (Warfilone, Warnerin [C]).	2-25 mg. Dosage is adjusted as indicated by prothrombin time. Oral, I.V. or I.M.	As above.	Action: similar to that of bishydroxycoumarin. Fate: after oral dose, absorption is practically complete. Maximal plasma concentration reached in 2-12 hours. It is largely bound to plasma protein. Maximal effects in 36-72 hours. Blood levels effective 4-5 days.	Aspirin, phenylbutazone, large doses of vitamin E, or C-17 alkylated androgens can increase the hypoprothrombinemic effect of coumarins and warfarin. Their action is antagonized by the barbiturates, glutethimide and griseofulvin. Quinidine exerts a mild direct hypoprothrombinemic effect and can potentiate the action of the anticoagulants. Their concurrent use with tolbutamide can cause a hypoglycemic effect.	As above.
Warfarin potassium (Athrombin-K).	2.5-10 mg. Dosage adjusted as indicated by prothrombin time. Oral.				

Name, Source, Synonyms, Preparations	Dosage and Administration	Uses	Action and Fate	Side Effects and Contraindications	Nursing Implications and Remarks
HEPARIN SODIUM. *Intestinal mucosa or lungs of animals.* Depo-heparin sodium, U.S.P. (contains heparin, gelatin, dextrose, and water) (Depo-Heparin).	20,000-40,000 U. I.M.	Used to prolong the clotting time of blood and to treat thrombophlebitis, pulmonary embolism, certain cardiac conditions or any disorder in which there is excessive or undersirable clotting.	Action not fully understood but believed to inhibit conversion of prothrombin to thrombin and also fibrinogen to fibrin. It does not dissolve clots but it does prevent extension of old clots and formation of new ones. After injection it slowly disappears from the blood. The larger the dose, the longer levels can be seen in the plasma. Most is metabolized by the liver and excreted by the kidneys. With large doses as much as 50% may be excreted unchanged. Does not cross the placenta or appear in mothers' milk.	Not common, but hemorrhage may occur, either as one large hemorrhage or as a number of smaller bleeding points. Stop drug. Vitamin K_1 may be ordered. Toluidine blue is sometimes used, as is protamine. I.M. administration may cause local irritation and ecchymosis.	During heparin therapy, clotting time should be checked frequently. Watch closely for any signs of hemorrhage, external or internal.
Heparin Sodium, U.S.P., (Hepathrom, Lipo-Hepin, Liquaemin, Panheprin) (Hepalean [C]).	5000-30,000 U. May be intermittent, or in continuous drip with saline or dextrose solution. I.V. or S.Q.				I.M. or S.Q. injection of heparin may produce local irritation, hematoma and tissue sloughing. To minimize these effects, drug should be administered by deep S.Q. injection.
PHENINDIONE AND SIMILAR DRUGS. *Synthetic.*	All doses individually adjusted.	As above.	Action same as coumarin.	Side effects similar to those of coumarin, but considered less toxic.	
Anisindione (Miradon).	25-250 mg. daily. Oral.		Well absorbed from the gastrointestinal tract. Therapeutic effectiveness reached in 24-48 hours and lasts 1-4 days.		Anisindione is chemically related to phenindione; claimed to give greater control because of speed and uniformity of response and absence of accumulation.
Phenindione N.F. (Danilone, Hedulin) (phenylendanedione [C]).	200-300 mg. daily in divided doses in acute conditions. Oral. 50-100 mg. daily in divided doses for maintenance. Oral.		Exact fate in the body is not known, but a metabolic product produces a red-orange color in alkaline urine.		

COAGULANTS

See also Vitamins

TOPICAL

ABSORBABLE GELATIN. *Gelatin.* Absorbable gelatin sponge, U.S.P. (Gelfoam).	Size and amount used varies.	Used as a local hemostatic agent.	Gives a good surface for and aids in clot formation.	None.	
CELLULOSE, OXIDIZED. *Vegetable.* Cellulose, oxidized, U.S.P. (Hemo-Pak, Oxycel).	Size and amount used varies.	Used as a local hemostatic agent.	As above.	None	An absorbable oxidized cellulose in sterile gauze or cotton-like form.
Microfibrillar collagen hemostat (Avitene).	Topical.	Adjunct to hemostasis when control of bleeding by ligature or conventional procedures is ineffective or impractical.	It is an absorbable topical hemostatic agent of purified bovine corium collagen. It must be applied directly to the source of bleeding in its dry state.	Because of its adhesiveness it may seal over the exit site of deeper hemorrhage and conceal an underlying hematoma as in penetrating liver wounds. It is inactivated by autoclaving. Cannot be used for injection and should not be wetted with saline or thrombin.	

Many other preparations are used to stop bleeding locally. They are mainly from animal sources, although some are mineral or synthetic. Some of these preparations from animal sources (in addition to those given above) are brain lipoid (impure, cephalin), brain and lung extract, thromboplastin, thrombin, blood fractions and fibrinogen. Ferropyrin (antipyrine and ferric chloride), ferric chloride, alum, burnt alum, chromium trioxide, silver nitrate and cotarnine biphthalate (Styptol) are made from chemical sources. The following are synthetic preparations unless otherwise noted.

SYSTEMIC

Aminocaproic acid, N.F. (Amicar).	4-5 Gm. first hour followed by 1 Gm./h. for up to 8 hours or until bleeding is controlled. Oral or I.V.	Used in hemorrhage resulting from overactivity of the fibrinolytic system.	Inhibits both plasminogen activator substances and to a lesser degree plasmin activity. Good absorption orally. Peak	Nausea, cramps, diarrhea, dizziness, tinnitus, malaise, conjunctival suffusion, nasal stuffiness, headache and skin rash have been reported.	Use with caution in patients with cardiac, hepatic or renal disease. Administration of more than

Name, Source, Synonyms, Preparations	Dosage and Administration	Uses	Action and Fate	Side Effects and Contraindications	Nursing Implications and Remarks
SYSTEMIC (Continued)					
			plasma levels in about 2 hours. Excreted rapidly in urine, mostly unchanged.	Contraindicated when there is evidence of an active intravascular clotting process during the first and second trimesters of pregnancy, unless the need outweighs possible hazards.	30 Gm. in 24 hours is not recommended.
Calcium chloride, U.S.P. (Calcivitam [C]). Calcium lactate, N.F. (Novocalcilac [C]).	1 Gm. p.r.n. Oral. 1 Gm. Oral or S.Q.	Used to control bleeding in such conditions as purpura, intestinal bleeding and any multiple small hemorrhages.	Calcium salts are essential for clot formation and if blood level is low, bleeding is apt to occur.	Rare in therapeutic dosage.	The chloride is more irritating than the lactate when given parenterally.
Carbazochrome salicylate (Andrenosem) (Adrestat, Statimo [C]).	Surgical use: 10 mg. preoperatively. Oral or I.M. 10 mg. q. 2 h. p.r.n. postoperatively. Oral or I.M. Nonsurgical use: 2.5 mg. t.i.d. Oral or I.M.	For control of capillary oozing and bleeding and to prevent capillary permeability.	Action not completely understood.	Low.	
Protamine sulfate, U.S.P.	5-8 mg./kg. of body weight. Dosage should not exceed 50 mg. at any one time or 300 mg. in any one day. I.V. or I.M.	Used as a heparin antagonist.	Protamine by itself is an anticoagulant and will cause an increase in clotting time. When given with heparin the drugs are attracted to each other and form a stable salt. Rapid onset of action after I.V. administration, with neutralization of heparin occurring within 5 min.	I.V. injections may cause sudden fall in BP, bradycardia, dyspnea, transitory flushing and a feeling of warmth.	Protamine solution should be stored under refigeration. Each mg. of protamine neutralizes about 90 units of heparin derived from lung tissue and 115 units of heparin derived from intestinal mucosa.

THROMBOLYTIC AGENTS

FIBRINOLYSIN. *Naturally derived fraction of human plasma.*					
Fibrinolysin (Thrombolysin).	50,000 to 100,000 U. q./h. for 1 to 6 hours per day. Given as I.V. infusion.	For I.V. dissolution of thrombi, thrombophlebitis and pulmonary embolism.	Normal blood plasma fraction which causes lysis of blood clots.	Precautions as for any anticoagulant. Contraindicated in hemorrhagic disorders, fibrinogen deficiency or major liver dysfunction.	Effectiveness of this drug is questionable.
Streptokinase (Streptase).	250,000 U loading dose and maintenance dose of 100,000 U/h. Thrombin time must be monitored during therapy and should be 2-5 times normal control value. If it does not fall in this range, streptokinase resistance levels should be checked. If levels are over 1,000,000 U, Streptase should not be administered.	Lysis of pulmonary emboli (massive) and lysis of acute extensive thrombi of the deep veins in adults; also for arteriovenous cannula occlusion.	Streptokinase is an enzyme that acts on the endogenous fibrinolytic system to produce sufficient amounts of plasmin for lysis of intravascular fibrin.	Contraindicated in patients with predisposition to bleeding, such as recent surgery, liver or renal biopsy, cerebral hemorrhage, recent trauma, G.I. bleeding, severe hypertension, etc. Severe bleeding is the major risk. Mild allergic reactions have been reported, so contraindicated in patients with history of allergies. Concurrent use of drugs that alter platelet function (aspirin, indomethacin and phenylbutazone) should be avoided.	All invasive procedures (I.M. injections, etc.) must be avoided. Venipunctures should be performed as carefully and infrequently as possible. Pressure should be applied for at least 15 min., a pressure dressing applied and site checked frequently for evidence of bleeding. Patient should be monitored carefully to detect internal bleeding. Safe use in pregnancy or children has not been established.
Urokinase (Abbokinase).	For priming: 4,400 IU/kg. I.V. over 10 min., then 4,400 IU/kg./h. I.V. for 12 h.	Lysis of pulmonary emboli if treatment initiated within 5 days after onset.	See streptokinase. I.V. infusion is followed by prompt increase in fibrinolytic activity, with effect persisting up to 12 h. after dose discontinued.	See streptokinase. Rethrombosis has been observed following termination of urokinase therapy. To minimize this risk, the use of I.V. heparin followed by oral anticoagulant therapy is considered necessary.	See streptokinase.

Name, Source, Synonyms, Preparations	Dosage and Administration	Uses	Action and Fate	Side Effects and Contraindications	Nursing Implications and Remarks
	Antineoplastic drugs are highly toxic with low therapeutic indices. A therapeutic response may not occur without some evidence of toxicity. Because of their effect on rapidly proliferating tissues, the drugs frequently cause varying degrees of myelosuppression, with the risks of infection and bleeding. They also frequently cause gastrointestinal disturbances and alopecia. Toxicity is often the limiting factor in the usefulness of antineoplastic drugs. The patient's hematologic status must be carefully monitored during and after therapy. Observations of fever, sore throat, bruising or unusual bleeding need to be reported immediately. Resistance, both natural and acquired, is another limitation of therapy. Combination therapy is widely used in an effort to delay the emergence of resistance and to attain an additive or synergistic therapeutic effect with minimum toxicity. Therefore these drugs should be used only under the supervision of a qualified physician who is experienced in the use of cancer chemotherapeutic agents.				
CHEMOTHERAPY OF NEOPLASTIC DISEASES. See also Hematinics and Radioactive Drugs.					
L-Asparaginase (Elspar).	I.V. combination regimen: 1000 I.U./kg./day for 10 days beginning day 22 of chemotherapy. I.M. combination regimen: 9 doses of 6000 I.U./m^2 beginning day 4 and q. 3 days thereafter. 100 I.U./kg./day I.V. for 28 days when given alone.	Induction of remission of acute lymphocytic leukemia. Maintenance therapy not recommended.	Reduces concentration of circulating asparagine, on which growth of malignant cells depend. Normal cells synthesize asparagine, hence are less affected.	Asparaginase therapy carries the risk of serious toxicity. Adverse reactions include allergic reactions, including anaphylaxis, hemorrhagic pancreatitis, hyperglycemia, depressed clotting factors, abnormal hepatic function, C.N.S. reactions, azotemia, hyperthermia, leukopenia and rarely transient bone marrow depression. Contraindicated in patients with history of pancreatitis.	Intradermal skin test for allergy is recommended before starting therapy. Be prepared and observant for allergic reactions, since anaphylaxis has been known to occur in absence of an initial positive skin test. Limit I.M. dose to 2 ml. at any one injection site. Because of toxicity, patients receiving therapy should be hospitalized for close observation.
Bleomycin sulfate (Blenoxane). From *Streptomyces verticillus.*	0.25 U./kg. weekly or twice weekly I.V., I.M., intra-arterial or subcutaneously. Doses over 400 U. given with great caution. Toxicity appears dose-related.	Used for palliative treatment or adjunct to surgery or radiation therapy in squamous cell carcinoma, lymphomas (Hodgkin's disease, reticulum cell sarcoma, lymphosarcoma),	Bleomycin is a mixture of basic cytotoxic glycopeptide antibiotics. Exact mode of action is not known, but the main mode appears to be the inhibition of DNA synthesis and, to a lesser	Most serious is interstitial pneumonitis, 10% which occurs mainly with higher doses in elderly patients and may progress to pulmonary fibrosis and even death, 1%. Skin changes are relatively	When used in combination with other agents, pulmonary toxicity can occur at lower dosage levels. Observe for early signs of bleomycin pneumonitis, which include dyspnea,

	1st dose should be 2 units or less.	testicular carcinoma and some renal carcinomas.	extent, inhibition of RNA and protein synthesis. Has minimal immunosuppressive activity in mice. Absorbed systemically from parenteral sites. Metabolic fate unknown Exreted in urine.	common, but rarely severe enough to require discontinuing drug. Fever, chills, idiosyncratic reactions, pain at tumor site, phlebitis, anorexia and weight loss (these last two may remain after the drug has been discontinued).	fine rales, nonproductive cough, sore throat.
SYNTHETIC PREPARATIONS. (Except as noted) Busulfan, U.S.P. (Myleran) (busulphan [C]).	4-8 mg. q. d. until maximum hematologic response and clinical improvement obtained, then reduce to maintenance of 1-3 mg./day. Oral.	Used in the treatment of chronic myelocytic leukemia. Also useful in polycythemia vera.	It is an alkylating agent that depresses bone marrow but not lymphoid tissue. Produces remissions of a few weeks to several months. May depress thrombocytes. Well absorbed orally. Found mainly in the nuclei of the myelocytic cells. It is slowly excreted almost entirely as methanesulfonic acid in the urine.	After small or average doses, nausea and vomiting may occur. After heavy doses, bone marrow depression has been reported. Reduce dosage or stop drug and treat symptoms.	The doctor should weigh potential benefits of the use of these drugs during pregnancy or in women of child-bearing age against the possible teratogenic effects. Frequent blood counts, including platelets (at least weekly), should be done during therapy.
Carmustine (BiCNU).	Initial dose in previously untreated patients is 200 mg./n^2 every 6 weeks. I.V. If used in combination, the dose is based on the blood picture and adjusted for the individual patient.	As palliative therapy or combination therapy in treatment of brain tumors, multiple myeloma, Hodgkin's disease and non-Hodgkin's lymphomas.	Carmustine alkylates DNA and RNA and has also been shown to inhibit several enzymes by carbamoylation of amino acids in proteins. When given I.V., it is rapidly degraded and no intact drug is detectable after 15 minutes. Based on radioactive-labeled carmustine, high levels are found in the CSF. 60-70% of a dose is excreted in the urine in 96 hours, 10% as respiratory CO_2 and the remainder undetermined.	Most severe adverse effects are related to the hematopoietic system, among them delayed myelosuppression. Thrombocytopenia is usually more severe than leukopenia. Anemia also occurs but is usually less severe. Nausea and vomiting follow doses by 2 to 4 hours. A reversible hepatic toxicity is seen with high doses. There can be burning at site of I.V. injection and with rapid infusion, flushing will occur.	Carmustine is embryotoxic, teratogenic and carcinogenic in rats. It should not be given to individuals with decreased circulating platelets, leukocytes or erythrocytes. Complete blood counts and liver function should be monitored during therapy. Safe use in pregnancy has not been established. The manufacturer reports that cross-resistance between carmustine and lomustine has occurred.

Name, Source, Synonyms, Preparations	Dosage and Administration	Uses	Action and Fate	Side Effects and Contraindications	Nursing Implications and Remarks
SYNTHETIC PREPARATIONS. (Continued)					
Chlorambucil, U.S.P. (Leukeran).	0.1-0.2 mg./kg. of body weight, usually 4-10 mg./day reduced to maintenance dose of 2-4 mg./day. Oral.	Used for the treatment of chronic lymphatic leukemia and malignant lymphomas, including Hodgkin's disease, giant follicular lymphoma and lymphosarcoma.	A derivative of nitrogen mustard drugs that is cytotoxic. Gives symptomatic relief and general remissions of varying lengths. Produces a rapid reduction in total white blood cell count. Good oral absorption, but fate in body is not known.	As above (Busulfan).	See above (Busulfan).
Cyclophosphamide, U.S.P. (Cytoxan) (Procytox [C]).	1.5-2 mg./kg daily. Oral. 100-500 mg. into tumor. 10-15 mg./kg. every 7-10 days I.V. Dosage individually adjusted. I.V., I.M., I.P.	Used for palliative treatment of Hodgkin's disease, lymphomas, acute and chronic leukemias, multiple myeloma, mycosis fungoides, neuroblastoma, adenocarcinoma of ovary, retinoblastoma.	A nitrogen mustard derivative with similar but more prolonged action. Readily absorbed after oral dose or from parenteral site. Cyclophosphamide and its metabolites are excreted by the kidneys, but the amount excreted by other routes is not known. It is distributed throughout the body, including the brain.	Immunosuppression and hematologic toxicity occur. In addition, sterile hemorrhagic cystitis, alopecia, gonadal suppression, as well as C.N.S. and cardiotoxic effects have been reported. Dosage must be reduced in adenocarcinoma of ovary.	See package insert for details of administration, toxicity, etc. Cytoxan should not be stored at temperatures above 90°F. Cyclophosphamide is teratogenic in animals and is excreted in breast milk. Adequate fluid intake and frequent voiding will help prevent development of cystitis.
Cytarabine, U.S.P. (Cytosar) (cytosine arabinoside [C]).	Dosage individually adjusted. For induction of therapy, the I.V. route is usually best, with subcutaneous for maintenance. 1 mg./kg. weekly or semiweekly S.Q. has been found	Used for the induction of remission of acute myeloblastic leukemia and secondarily for other acute leukemias in adults and children.	This drug is cytotoxic to a variety of mammalian cells in tissue culture. It is believed to exert its primary effect by inhibition of deoxycytidine synthesis. After I.V. administration, only 5-8% is excreted unaltered in	Leukopenia, thrombocytopenia, bone marrow suppression, megaloblastosis, anemia, nausea, vomiting, diarrhea, oral inflammation or ulceration, thrombophlebitis, hepatic dysfunction and fever occur most often. For	When this drug is used, the patient should be under close medical supervision, and during induction therapy should have daily leukocyte and platelet counts. In patients with poor liver function, dosage should be reduced.

	satisfactory for maintenance in the majority of patients.		the urine after 24 hours. It is deaminated to arabinofuranosyl uracil (an inactive metabolite) by the liver and possibly by the kidneys. 15 minutes after a single high I.V. dose, the blood level falls to unmeasurable amounts in most patients. The drug is excreted by the kidneys as the above mentioned metabolite.	other side effects and the drug's use for children, see package insert. Contraindications: patients with pre-existing drug-induced bone marrow suppression, unless the physician feels that such management offers the most helpful alternative.	In use of this drug during pregnancy or in women of child-bearing age, the potential hazards must be weighed against possible benefits. Safe use in infants has not been established.
Dacarbazine (DTIC).	2-4.5 mg./kg. body wt. daily for 10 days. I.V.	Used for treatment of metastatic malignant melanoma, Hodgkin's disease, soft tissue sarcoma and neuroblastoma.	Mechanism of action unknown, thought to exert its cytotoxic effects as an alkylating agent. Poorly absorbed from the G.I. tract. Probably localized in some body tissues, possibly the liver. Metabolized in the liver and excreted in the urine.	Over 90% of the patients experience G.I. discomfort; however, tolerance develops to this within 1-2 days of therapy. Bone marrow depression, predominantly leukopenia and thrombocytopenia, generally appear 2-4 weeks after the last dose. Fever, myalgia and malaise may occur during or after treatment. Alopecia, hypersensitivity and CNS symptoms have also been reported.	Administered to hospitalized patients under the supervision of experienced physicians. The drug should be well diluted and administered by intravenous infusion. Avoid extravasation into tissues.

Name, Source, Synonyms, Preparations	Dosage and Administration	Uses	Action and Fate	Side Effects and Contraindications	Nursing Implications and Remarks
DACTINOMYCIN. *Streptomyces parvelbus.* Dactinomycin, U.S.P. (Cosmegen) (Actinomycin D [C]).	0.5 mg. daily for a maximum of 5 days. I.V. Children: 15 micrograms/kg. daily for a maximum of 5 days. I.V.	Used only in palliative treatment of hospitalized patients with Wilms' tumor, rhabdomyosarcoma and carcinoma of the testis and uterus.	Exact mechanism is not known. It is believed that this drug concentrates in the submaxillary glands, liver and kidneys. About half is excreted unchanged in the bile, about 10% in the urine.	Toxic reactions are frequent and may be severe. This is not dose dependent. These include bone marrow depression. G.I. effects include: stomatitis, proctitis and ulceration of oral mucosa. Skin eruptions, alopecia, malaise, fatigue, lethargy, myalgia and epistaxis also occur.	As above. Commercial brochure should be consulted before administering this drug.
Doxorubicin hydrochloride (Adriamycin, Hydroxyduanomycin hydrochloride), from *Streptomyces peucetius* var. *caesius.*	Dosage individualized. Usual adult dose is 60-75 mg./sq. meter of body surface as a single dose at 21-day intervals. I.V.	Treatment of solid tumors, soft tissue and osteogenic sarcomas, neuroblastomas and Wilms' tumor; malignant lymphomas and acute lymphoblastic and acute myeloblastic leukemias.	Action similar to daunorubicin and dactinomycin. Precise mechanism of action not fully understood. Not absorbed from G.I. tract. Rapidly metabolized, probably by the liver. Rapidly and widely distributed with some tissue binding. Does not cross blood-brain barrier. Excreted primarily in the bile.	A toxic drug with a low therapeutic index having effects on the G.I. tract, bone marrow and hair. Leukopenia is the most predominant manifestation, severity is dose related. Cardiotoxicity may occur. The drug has reactivated latent effects of previous irradiation in some patients, producing erythema and desquamation. Extravasation produces severe local necrosis and should be avoided. Contraindicated in patients with pre-existing myelosuppression or in patients with impaired cardiac function.	Doxorubicin imparts a red color to the urine for 1-2 days after administration and patients should be so advised. Administered to hospitalized patients under the supervision of experienced physicians. Complete alopecia almost always accompanies doxorubicin therapy, and patients should be advised of this effect.

Floxuridine, N.F. (FUDR).	0.1-0.6 mg./kg. daily. Intra-arterial infusion only. (Higher doses usually used in hepatic artery infusion, since liver metabolizes drug. Less risk of toxicity.)	Palliative management of carcinoma by regional, intra-arterial infusion in patients considered incurable by surgery or other means. Best results are achieved by use of pump to overcome pressure in large arteries.	It is rapidly metabolized to 5-fluorouracil. Its action is to interfere with the synthesis of DNA and, to a lesser extent, of RNA.	Has all the toxic manifestations of 5-fluorouracil. Side effects: nausea, vomiting, diarrhea, enteritis, stomatitis and localized erythema. Laboratory abnormalities include anemia, leukopenia, elevations of alkaline phosphatase, serum transaminase, serum bilirubin and lactic dehydrogenase. See brochure for others.	Therapy is continued until adverse symptoms occur. May be restarted as they subside. Floxuridine is a highly toxic drug with a narrow margin of safety. For this reason, close supervision is required, since therapeutic response is unlikely to occur without some evidence of toxicity. Caution: therapy should be discontinued at first signs of stomatitis, pharyngitis, leukopenia (WBC below 3500) or a rapidly falling WBC, vomiting, intractable diarrhea, gastrointestinal ulceration, thrombocytopenia, platelet count below 100,000 or hemorrhage.
Fluorouracil, U.S.P. (Fluorouracil, Efudex).	Dosage individually adjusted. I.V. but no more than 800 mg. daily.	Used in the palliative treatment of carcinoma of breast, colon, rectum, stomach and pancreas.	It is believed to block the methylation reaction of deoxyuridilic acid to thymidylic acid. It then interferes with the synthesis of DNA.	Bone marrow depression, alopecia, stomatitis, diarrhea, gastrointestinal ulcerations and bleeding, and hemorrhage may occur. Relatively toxic drug.	Not an antileukemic drug.
	Solution 2-5% or cream 1-5% b.i.d. Topical.	Used to treat solar keratoses.	The drug is usually administered I.V. since the oral route attenuates its effectiveness. It is reduced in the body to urea, CO_2 and fluoroalanine. 60-80% of the carbon dioxide (CO_2) is excreted through the lungs.	Given with caution in patients considered poor risks. Local adverse reactions include: dermatitis, scarring, soreness and tenderness.	With topical use, if an occlusive dressing is applied, there may be an increase in the incidence of inflammatory reactions. During therapy, prolonged exposure to ultraviolet light should be avoided.

Name, Source, Synonyms, Preparations	Dosage and Administration	Uses	Action and Fate	Side Effects and Contraindications	Nursing Implications and Remarks
Hydroxyurea, U.S.P. (Hydrea).	80 mg./kg. every third day, orally, or 20-30 mg./kg. daily, orally (each based on actual or ideal weight, whichever is less). 20-30 mg./kg. daily (single dose), orally.	Indicated for use in melanoma, recurrent metastatic or inoperable carcinoma of the ovary and with irradiation in treatment of primary squamous cell carcinoma of the head and neck. Myelocytic leukemia (resistant chronic).	Mechanism of action is not known. It is believed to act by inhibition of the synthesis of DNA without affecting RNA or protein synthesis. About 80% of an oral dose is recovered from the urine in 12 hours.	Side effects: bone marrow depression (leukopenia, thrombocytopenia, anemia), gastrointestinal symptoms (stomatitis, nausea, vomiting, diarrhea), some dermatological reactions (maculopapular rash), alopecia and some neurological symptoms have been reported. Contraindications: marked bone marrow depression (below 2500 WBC), thrombocytopenia (below 100,000) or severe anemia and in women of childbearing age.	Precautions: complete blood picture including bone marrow examination and liver function tests should be done prior to – and repeatedly during – treatment with this drug. Hemoglobin, leukocyte and platelet counts should be done weekly.
Lomustine (CeeNU).	130 mg./M^2 as a single dose every 6 weeks. If bone marrow function is compromised, dose should be reduced to 100 mg./M^2. Dose is adjusted to hematologic response.	Palliative therapy with other agents in treatment of brain tumors and Hodgkin's disease.	Lomustine acts as an alkylating agent and may also inhibit other enzymatic processes. It penetrates the blood-brain barrier because of its high lipid solubility at physiological pH. Measured radioactively it is well absorbed orally and about ½ of radioactivity given was excreted in 24 hours.	Nausea and vomiting occur 3-6 hours after oral dose. Thrombocytopenia occurs in about 4 weeks and persists 1-2 weeks. Leukopenia occurs at about 6 weeks and lasts 1-2 weeks. Other effects include alopecia, stomatitis, anemia, hepatic toxicity, disorientation, lethargy, ataxia and dysarthria.	Major toxic effect is delayed bone marrow suppression so blood counts should be done weekly for at least 6 weeks after a dose. It is teratogenic in animals; safe use in pregnancy has not been established. The manufacturer reports that cross-resistance between carmustine and lomustine has occurred.
Mechlorethamine hydrochloride, U.S.P. (Mustargen) (Methyl bis beta chloroethylamine hydrochloride) (chlomethine, mustine [C]).	Dosages individually adjusted. 10 mg. in 20 ml. I.V. 0.1 mg./kg. of body	Used to reduce the white blood cell count, especially in leukemia. Also used in lymphosarcoma, Hodgkin's	A polyfunctional alkylating agent cytotoxic to cell tissue; affects the mitotic cells first, thereby destroy-	Nausea, vomiting, moderate lymphopenia, neutropenia, anemia and thrombocytopenia may occur. Occasion-	The doctor should weigh potential benefits of use of these drugs during pregnancy or in women of

	weight given in isotonic saline solution. Do not give into tissues, as severe damage may occur. I.V.	disease, lymphoblastoma of the skin and mycosis fungoides.	ing malignant tissue before normal tissue. Readily absorbed, but usually given I.V. Rapidly metabolized. Little or none is excreted unchanged by the kidneys.	ally bleeding occurs. Stop drug and treat symptoms. Toxic to tissue, vesicant to skin; avoid infiltration; margin of safety narrow.	childbearing age against the teratogenic effects. Frequent blood counts, including platelets, should be done during therapy. Use only freshly prepared solutions.
Megestrol acetate (Megace).	40 mg. daily in divided doses. Oral. Given as long as beneficial results are seen. Adequate trial period is 2 months of continuous therapy.	Used as adjunct or palliative treatment of recurrent or metastatic endometrial carcinoma and inoperable carcinoma of the breast or endometrium.	Mechanism of action is not known but it is thought to act by an antiluteinizing effect mediated through the pituitary gland. The compound possesses biological properties similar to progesterone.	No serious side effects in doses up to 800 mg./day. Caution: used with caution in patients with a history of thrombophlebitis.	Has been shown to be teratogenic in dogs.
Melphalan, U.S.P. (Alkeran).	6 mg. daily for 2-3 weeks; discontinue for up to 4 weeks; then start maintenance dose of 2 mg. daily.	Used in the treatment of multiple myeloma.	Alkylating agent consisting of phenylalanine nitrogen mustard, which has been found useful in multiple myeloma. Good oral absorption. Exact fate in body is not known, but it is believed the metabolic products are excreted through the kidneys.	Nausea and vomiting, depression of the bone marrow. Should not be given concurrently with radiation treatment.	
Mercaptopurine, U.S.P. (Purinethol).	2.5-5 mg./kg. daily. Oral.	Used to reduce white blood cell count, especially in children with acute lymphoblastic or stem cell leukemia.	A purine antagonist. Depresses bone marrow. Reduces white cell count. Causes temporary remission. Readily absorbed from the intestinal tract. Plasma half-life about 1½ hours. Rapidly metabolized. Metabolites excreted by the kidneys.	Nausea, vomiting, moderate lymphopenia, neutropenia, anemia and thrombocytopenia may occur. Occasionally bleeding occurs. Stop drug and treat symptoms. When mercaptopurine and allopurinol are given concurrently, the dose of mercaptopurine must be reduced to as little as $1/3$ to ¼ of the usual dose. Reported to both potentiate and diminish effects of warfarin.	Also available as the methyl derivative. Frequent blood counts should be done. If a sudden large reduction in white blood cells occurs, stop drug. Complete cross-resistance between mercaptopurine and thioguanine exists.

Name, Source, Synonyms, Preparations	Dosage and Administration	Uses	Action and Fate	Side Effects and Contraindications	Nursing Implications and Remarks
Methotrexate, U.S.P. (amethopterin).	Dosage individually adjusted. Oral or parenteral.	Effective in trophoblastic tumors. Useful in carcinoma of the testes and stages III and IV of lymphosarcoma. Also used in carcinoma of the breasts, lungs, and ovaries and in acute lymphoblastic leukemia in children. Chemotherapy of psoriasis.	A folic acid antagonist that acts by the competitive inhibition of the enzyme folic acid reductase. Well absorbed from the gastrointestinal tract. Part is rather rapidly excreted in the urine. Significant amounts of the drug are retained in the body, particularly in the liver and kidneys, for long periods (sometimes for months).	As with all such drugs, hemopoietic system depression may occur. Leucovorin is an effective antidote if given soon enough after dose of methotrexate. When given concurrently with sulfisoxazole, methotrexate is replaced from plasma binding sites, and this can raise the levels of methotrexate to possible toxic amounts..	Blood counts twice weekly recommended. Citrovorum factor. I.M. aids in avoiding damage to such structures as intestinal mucosa and bone marrow. The patient should be fully informed of the risks involved and should be under the constant supervision of the physician.
Mithramycin, U.S.P. (Mithracin). From *Streptomyces plicatus.*	25-30 mcg./kg. daily for 8-10 days. Dose not to exceed 30 mcg./kg. Drug should be diluted in 5% glucose in water and given slowly. I.V. over a 4-6 hour period. 25 mcg./kg. for 3-4 days. If desired reduction is not secured, course may be repeated in one week or more to achieve normal calcium levels in serum and urine. A single weekly dose may maintain normal levels once they are obtained.	Used for certain inoperable testicular malignancies. In patients with hypercalcemia and hypercalciuria associated with a variety of advanced neoplasms not responsive to conventional treatment.	The exact mechanism of action is not known, but it has been shown to form a complex deoxyribonucleic acid (DNA) and to inhibit cellular ribonucleic acid (RNA) and enzymic synthesis. The binding of the DNA (in presence of divalent cation) is responsible for inhibition of DNA-dependent or DNA-directed RNA synthesis.	The most important side effect is a bleeding syndrome. For others refer to package insert. Contraindications: thrombocytopenia, thrombocytopathy, any coagulation disorder or an increased susceptibility to bleeding due to other causes, in patients with bone marrow impairment or in patients who are not hospitalized.	

Mitomycin (Mutamycin) From *Streptomyces caespitosus.*	0.05 mg./kg./day for 5 days. I.V. After 2 day interval can be repeated. After 2-3 weeks regimen may be repeated if no toxicity has occurred. See last column.	Used as adjunct therapy in adenocarcinoma of stomach and pancreas.	Inhibits synthesis of deoxyribonucleic acid (DNA). Metabolized mainly by the liver but about 10% is excreted unchanged in the urine.	Fever, anorexia, nausea, vomiting. Severe toxicity: bone marrow depression (mostly thrombocytopenia and leukopenia). Mouth ulcers, alopecia, induration, pruritus, bleeding, paresthesia, necrosis or slough at injection site (especially if extravasation has occurred); hemoptysis, dyspnea, coughing, pneumonia; rise in BUN.	If white cell count falls below 4,000 or platelet count below 75,000, or there is a significant prolongation of prothrombin time or bleeding, termination of therapy should be considered.
Mitotane (Lysodren).	9-10 Gm. daily either t.i.d. or q.i.d. Oral.	In palliative treatment of inoperable functional and nonfunctional adrenocortical carcinoma.	Precise mechanism of action not determined. Appears to suppress adrenal cortex and adrenocortical neoplastic tissue. It also alters the peripheral metabolism of steroids. About 35-40% is absorbed from the G.I. tract. Detectable blood levels may persist for 6-9 wks. after the drug has been discontinued. Distributed to all tissues with fat being the primary storage site. Metabolized in part by the liver and kidneys, excreted in the bile and urine.	High incidence of side effects, the most frequent being anorexia, nausea, vomiting and diarrhea. CNS symptoms of mental depression, lethargy, dizziness or vertigo and skin reactions also occur frequently. Patients may develop adrenal insufficiency, which can be treated with higher than normal doses of corticosteroids. Other CNS symptoms, hypotension and hemorrhage occur less frequently. Hypersensitivity has been reported.	Safe use during pregnancy or lactation has not been established. Patients performing hazardous tasks involving mental alertness or physical coordination should be advised of the CNS side effects of this drug. Responses to mitotane are usually obtained within 3 months of therapy at maximum tolerable dosage.

Name, Source, Synonyms, Preparations	Dosage and Administration	Uses	Action and Fate	Side Effects and Contraindications	Nursing Implications and Remarks
Pipobroman, N.F. (Vercyte).	Initial dose 1 mg./kg./day. Larger doses up to 1.5-3.0 mg./kg./day may be used. Not to exceed 30 days. When hematocrit is 50-55%, maintenance dose is 0.1-0.2 mg./kg./day. Oral.	To treat polycythemia vera.	This is classified as an alkylating agent. Exact mechanism of action is not known. Readily absorbed after oral administration. Metabolic fate and route of excretion unknown.	Principal toxic effect is bone marrow suppression with resulting leukopenia, thrombocytopenia, and anemia. Skin rashes and G.I. effects may occur and are usually transient. Should not be given to patients with bone marrow depression following x-ray or cytotoxic chemotherapy.	Not recommended for children or during pregnancy.
	1.5-2.5 mg./kg./day initial dose. Oral. Maintenance dosage individually adjusted.	To treat chronic myelocytic leukemia.			
Platinol (Cisplatin).	20 mg./M^2 I.V. daily for 5 days every 3 or 4 weeks for 3 or 4 courses.	For testicular tumors.	Activity of this drug is not well understood, but alkylation and enhancement of tumor immunogenicity have been suggested as possible mechanisms.	Renal damage, which can occur after a single dose, is dose related and cumulative. Ototoxicity, tinnitus and loss of high frequency hearing can occur. Leukopenia and thrombocytopenia may occur with higher doses. Marked nausea and vomiting occur in almost all patients. Peripheral neuropathy, anaphylactic-like reactions, facial edema, wheezing, tachycardia, and hypotension can occur.	To minimize nephrotoxicity, adequate pretreatment hydration is essential.
	50 mg./M^2 I.V. once q. 3 weeks as part of combination therapy or 100 mg./M^2 I.V. once q. 4 weeks as a single agent.	For ovarian tumors.			

Procarbazine, U.S.P. (Matulane) (Natulan [C]).	100-200 mg. daily for 1st week, then 200 mg. daily until white count falls below 4000 per cu. mm. or the platelet count is below 100,000 per cu. mm. or until maximum response is obtained. For children the dose is highly individualized and very close monitoring is essential because of possible adverse side effects. Dosage is usually started with 50 mg. daily for one week, then maintained at 100 mg./sq. m. of body surface (to the closest 50 mg.) until leukopenia, thrombocytopenia or maximum response is reached. Oral.	Indicated for the palliative treatment of generalized Hodgkin's disease and for those patients who have become resistant to other forms of therapy.	The exact mode of action has not been clearly defined, but it is believed the drug may act by inhibition of protein, DNA and RNA synthesis. No cross resistance with other chemotherapeutic agents, radiotherapy or steroids has been demonstrated.	Occurring frequently: leukopenia, anemia, thrombocytopenia, nausea and vomiting. There are many other less common side effects; refer to package insert. Contraindications: in patients known to be hypersensitive or those with inadequate bone marrow reserve. This should be considered in patients who have leukopenia, thrombocytopenia and/or anemia. Use during pregnancy or for women of child-bearing age requires first carefully weighing potential benefits against possible hazards. Meperidine should not be used in patients taking procarbazine.	Alcoholic intake should be stopped when this drug is given, as it can possibly give a disulfiram-like reaction. Procarbazine has some monoamine oxidase inhibitor activity. Foods high in tyramine content should be avoided, as should sympathomimetic drugs and the tricyclic antidepressants. One month interval should be allowed following termination of therapy with radiation or with drugs with bone marrow depressant action before starting this drug.

Name, Source, Synonyms, Preparations	Dosage and Administration	Uses	Action and Fate	Side Effects and Contraindications	Nursing Implications and Remarks
Tamoxifen citrate (Nolvadex).	10-20 mg. q. 12 h.	Palliation of advanced breast cancer in postmenopausal women with positive assays for estrogen receptors.	Competes with estrogen for binding sites in target tissues; thus inhibits stimulation of tumor growth by endogenous estrogen and causes regression of established tumor of this origin. Most of drug is excreted in feces with small amounts in urine. Blood levels after oral doses show peak values at 4-7 h. after dosing. Initial half-life is 7-14 h., with secondary peaks 4 or more days later.	Most frequent side effects are hot flashes, nausea and vomiting, but these are generally not severe enough to interrupt therapy. Less frequently reported effects include: vaginal bleeding or discharge, menstrual irregularities, and skin rash. Increased bone and tumor pain and also local disease flare-up have occurred but appear to be associated with good tumor response. Other effects include: hypercalcemia, peripheral edema, distaste for food, pruritus vulvae, depression, dizziness, light headedness and headache. Use with caution in patients with existing leukopenia and thrombocytopenia. It is uncertain whether tamoxifen causes these changes in the blood picture.	Periodic complete blood count and platelet counts should be done before and during therapy.
Testolactone, N.F. (Teslac).	100 mg. three times a week I.M. 250 mg. q.i.d. Oral. However, up to 2000 mg./day have been given.	Used as adjunctive therapy in the palliative treatment of advanced disseminated breast cancer in postmenopausal women when hormone therapy is indicated. It may be used	The precise mechanism of action is not known. The chemical configuration is similar to that of the androgens, but it is devoid of androgenic activity in the commonly	Maculopapular erythema, increased blood pressure, paresthesia, aching and edema of extremities, nausea, vomiting and hot flashes; however, some of the adverse symptoms	Treatment should be continued for at least 3 months in order to evaluate the response unless there is active progression of the disease. The drug has been found to be effective in

		for premenopausal women in whom ovarian function has been terminated.	employed dosage. Well absorbed from G.I. tract. Metabolized primarily in liver and excreted in urine.	could be due to the disease and cannot always be attributed to the drug. Pain and local inflammation at site of injection are seen. Contraindicated in the treatment of breast cancer in men.	about 15% of the patients treated. Warning: Calcium levels should be monitored routinely, especially during times of active remission of bony metastases. If hypercalcemia occurs, steps should be taken to lower this level.
Thioguanine, N.F.	Dosages individually adjusted. Usually, initial dose is 2 mg./kg./day. If not effective after 14-21 days, 3 mg./kg./day may be tried. Effective maintenance dose is usually 2 mg./kg./day. Oral.	Used to treat acute leukemia and chronic granulocytic leukemia.	Purine antagonist interfering with nucleic acid synthesis and interconversion of purines. Partially absorbed from G.I. tract. Assumed to be partially detoxified in the liver. Excreted in both urine and feces.	Nausea, vomiting, anorexia and stomatitis may occur. Toxic hepatitis may be related to this drug. If jaundice appears, drug should be stopped. Dosage should be reduced if used concurrently with allopurinol. Principal toxic effect is bone marrow depression with resulting thrombocytopenia, leukopenia, and anemia.	Not used in chronic lymphocytic leukemia. Not advised during the first trimester of pregnancy. Weekly blood counts are recommended. Drug should be discontinued at first signs of abnormal bone marrow depression.
Triethylene-thio-phosphoramide (Thio-Tepa).	0.2 mg./kg. daily for no more than 5 days. I.M. 40-50 mg. intracarotid q. 6-8 weeks. 10-60 mg. intratumor. 10-50 mg. intraserosal.	Used in the palliative treatment of adenocarcinoma of the breast and ovaries, malignant lymphomas, bronchogenic carcinoma and for controlling intracavitary effusions.	Usually given by injection because of erratic oral absorption. It rapidly acts with cellular elements. Most of the drug appears to be excreted unchanged in the urine.	Nausea, vomiting, anorexia and headache may occur. Hemopoietic depression (all formed elements) mild to severe has been reported. This drug is actively teratogenic.	As with others of this group.

Name, Source, Synonyms, Preparations	Dosage and Administration	Uses	Action and Fate	Side Effects and Contraindications	Nursing Implications and Remarks
VINBLASTINE. *Alkaloid of Vinca rosea linn.* Vinblastine sulfate, U.S.P. (Velban) (Velbe [C]).	0.1-0.5 mg./kg. of body weight weekly. I.V.	Used to treat Hodgkin's disease and choriocarcinomas that are resistant to other therapy, histiocytosis, lymphosarcoma and reticulum cell sarcoma. Indicated in the palliative treatment of lymphoma, Hodgkin's disease, lymphosarcoma, reticulum-cell sarcoma, mycosis fungoides, neuroblastoma, histiocytosis X, choriocarcinoma resistant to other agents, embryonal carcinoma of the testes and carcinoma of the breast unresponsive to other therapy.	It is believed to interfere with metabolic pathways of amino acids, leading from glutamic acid to the citric acid cycle and to urea. Also, vinblastine has an effect on cell energy production required for mitosis and interferes with nucleic acid synthesis. Following I.V. administration, is rapidly localized in body tissues. Penetrates blood-brain barrier poorly. Extensively metabolized by the liver. Excreted slowly in urine, feces and bile.	Degree of toxicity appears dose related as well as dependent on functional capacity of the patient's bone marrow. Toxic side effects include G.I. symptoms and bone marrow depression. Other side effects include alopecia, mental depression, neuritis, paresthesias, psychoses and convulsions. Contraindicated if WBC is under 4000/cu. mm. and in bacterial infections.	These drugs may possibly have teratogenic effects. Consult commercial brochure for more complete details. Vinblastine is a tissue irritant and may cause phlebitis and necrosis. Extravasation can cause pain and cellulitis and should be avoided. Care must be taken to avoid contact of vinblastine with the eyes, as severe irritation and possible corneal ulceration may result.
Vincristine sulfate, U.S.P. (Oncovin).	Dose in children 2 mg./M^2. Weekly, I.V. Adults: 1.4 mg./M^2. Weekly, I.V.	Acute leukemia in children. It is indicated in acute leukemia and is useful in combination with other oncolytic agents in Hodgkin's disease, lymphosarcoma, reticulum-cell sarcoma, rhabdomyosarcoma, neuroblastoma, and Wilms' tumor.	Mechanism of action is not known, but it may cause arrest of mitotic division at the stage of metaphase. Drug leaves blood stream rapidly after infusion. Most is excreted through the bile and feces, only a small amount by way of the kidneys.	Neurological and neuromuscular manifestations are the most frequent and severe signs of toxicity. These include paresthesias, loss of deep tendon reflexes, muscle weakness, ptosis, ocular changes, dysphagia, paresis, ataxia, convulsions and coma. Abdominal pain and constipation occur frequently. G.I. distress and alopecia may also occur. Vincristine is less toxic to the bone marrow than vinblastine.	If extravasation occurs, it may cause considerable irritation.

DIAGNOSTIC DRUGS

These are all synthetic preparations, except as noted.

Drug	Dosage	Use	Action	Side effects	Remarks
ETHYL ALCOHOL. *Grain.*					
Alcohol, ethyl, U.S.P. (Ethanol).	7% solution. Amount individually determined. Oral.	Used for the same purpose as histamine, when measuring gastric secretion.	A gastric stimulant that indicates the ability of the mucosa to secrete hydrochloric acid. 90-98% of ingested alcohol is metabolized by the body. Only 2-10% is excreted unchanged chiefly in the urine and to a lesser extent in expired air.	May cause symptoms of intoxication. Treat symptoms. Has a large number of drug interactions. See pages 110–111.	
FLUORESCEIN PREPARATIONS.					
Fluorescein (Fluorescite) (Fluor-I-Strip [C]).	5-25% solution. See circular for various doses depending on use.	Determine circulation time, determine if tissue is viable. String test.	It is a strongly fluorescent dye that can readily be seen under ultraviolet light.	Nausea.	
Sodium fluorescein ophthalmic solution, U.S.P.	0.1 ml. of a 2% solution. Topical in conjunctival sac.	Used to reveal ulcers and foreign bodies in the eyes.	Outlines the foreign body or lesion, making it easier to locate.	Rare in therapeutic dosage.	
HISTAMINE PREPARATIONS *Animal, synthetic.*		Used to test secretion of gastric juice and the amount of acid secreted by the gastric mucosa.	Similar to ethyl alcohol, but is a stronger stimulant.	Urticaria, severe dyspnea, bronchial spasms, severe vasomotor reactions. Treatment: epinephrine (1 mg. will neutralize 10 mg. of histamine). Ephedrine and aminophylline will help to relieve symptoms. Use with care, especially in cases of allergy. Have epinephrine ready.	
Histamine phosphate injection, U.S.P. (Histapon).	0.3 mg. S.Q.				
Betazole hydrochloride, U.S.P. (Histalog).	50 mg. I.M. or S.Q.				Betazole produces fewer side effects than histamine.
Indocyanine green, U.S.P. (Cardio-Green).	1.25 to 5 mg. I.V.	Test cardiac function.	A dye that is easily measured to derive the dilution curve to determine cardiac output.	May color the feces green. Low incidence of side effects.	Use the day it is reconstituted.

Name, Source, Synonyms, Preparations	Dosage and Administration	Uses	Action and Fate	Side Effects and Contraindications	Nursing Implications and Remarks
MANNITOL. *Vegetable.* Mannitol, N.F. (d-Mannitol, Mannite, Manna Sugar) (Osmitrol [C]).	25% solution. Amount determined individually. I.V.	Used to measure glomerular filtration.	A hexahydric alcohol that is neither absorbed nor secreted by the kidney tubule. Thus the amount excreted gives an accurate estimation of glomerular filtration.	Relatively nontoxic when administered in small doses.	Also see under Diuretics (page 306).
Metyrapone, U.S.P. (Metopirone) (methapyrapone [C]). Metyrapone tartrate, N.F. (Metopirone).	Usual dosage is 750 mg. q. 4 h. for six doses. Oral. 100 mg. I.V.	Used to test for residual pituitary function. A drug used as diagnostic test for hypothalamico-pituitary function.	Selectively inhibits 11-β-hydroxylation in the biosynthesis of the three main corticosteroids—cortisol, corticosterone and aldosterone.	Transient vertigo, dizziness, headache, sedation and allergic rash. Treat symptoms. Adrenal insufficiency may develop in patients with minimal adrenal function.	Refer to package for complete dosage schedule and interpretation of results.
Pentagastrin (Peptavlon).	Adults: 6 mcg./kg. S.Q.	Diagnostic aid to evaluate gastric acid secretory function.	Acts as a physiologic gastric acid secretagogue. It stimulates gastric acid secretion about 10 minutes after S.Q. injection, peak effect in 20-30 minutes and duration of activity is usually 60-80 minutes. It has other physiological actions that include stimulation of pepsin secretion, pancreatic enzyme and bicarbonate secretion, gastric motility stimulation and intrinsic factor secretion.	Majority are related to G.I. tract, including abdominal pain, desire to defecate, nausea, vomiting, borborygmi and blood-tinged mucus. Others: flushing, tachycardia, dizziness, faintness, drowsiness, transient blurring of vision, headache and allergic and hypersensitivity reactions.	Safe use in pregnancy and children has not been established.
Phenolsulfonphthalein injection, U.S.P.	6 mg. Exact dosage and directions vary. I.M. or I.V.	Used to test kidney function.	A dye that is excreted by the kidneys after I.V. administration. 25-45%	Rare in therapeutic dosage.	Safe use during pregnancy has not been established.

			should be eliminated in 15 minutes. After I.M. administration 40-50% should be eliminated the first hour.		
Phentolamine hydrochloride, N.F. (Regitine) (Rogitine [C]).	5 mg. I.M. or I.V.	Test for pheochromocytoma. Also administer small amounts with norepinephrine I.V. to combat tissue damage if extravasation is found to occur.	Adrenalytic and sympatholytic. In patients with pheochromocytoma that is secreting epinephrine or norepinephrine, the response to phentolamine is an immediate marked decrease in both systolic and diastolic blood pressure, with maximum effect within 2 min. Blood pressure returns to pretest levels within 15-30 min.	Tachycardia, weakness, dizziness, orthostatic hypotension, nasal stuffiness and gastrointestinal disturbances.	Before administration, the patient should rest in a supine position in a quiet room for at least 30 min. until a basal blood pressure is established. Careful monitoring of blood pressure during and after the test is important.
Sincalide (Kinevac).	0.02 mcg./kg. I.V. over a 30-60 second interval; may repeat in 15 minutes with dose of 0.04 mcg./kg. I.V. if satisfactory contracture of gall bladder does not occur.	To provide a sample of gall bladder bile that must be aspirated from the duodenum for analysis of its composition. Also used in conjunction with secretin to stimulate pancreatic secretion for analysis of composition and cytology.	Causes a prompt contraction of the gall bladder. It is a synthetic C-terminal octapeptide of cholecystokinin.	Nausea, dizziness and flushing occur occasionally. G.I. symptoms such as abdominal discomfort or pain and urge to defecate frequently seen after injection.	Safe use in pregnancy and children has not been established.

Name, Source, Synonyms, Preparations	Dosage and Administration	Uses	Action and Fate	Side Effects and Contraindications	Nursing Implications and Remarks
SODIUM RADIOIODINE (^{131}I). *Mineral, synthetic.*		Used to diagnose and to treat certain malignant tumors, especially those of the thyroid gland.	Since the thyroid cells have a definite affinity for iodine, the radioactive form affects these cells (normal or malignant) first; thus, by using a scanner, the area of the gland, metastatic tumor, or both, may be determined and treated. The iodine is converted to iodide in the gastrointestinal tract and absorbed as such. Widely distributed in the extracellular fluid, but mainly concentrated in the thyroid tissue with lesser amounts in saliva and gastric secretions. Most iodine is excreted in the urine.	As for both iodine and radiation. Treat symptoms as they occur.	
Sodium iodide (^{131}I), U.S.P. (Iodotrope, Oriodide, Radiocaps, Theriodide, Tracervial).	1-100 microcuries. Oral or I.V. 1-100 millicuries. Oral or I.V.	As a diagnostic aid. For treatment of malignant lesions.			
BROMSULPHTHALEIN Sodium sulfobromophthalein. U.S.P. (Bromsulphthalein).	See circular (2-5 mg./kg.) I.V.	To determine hepatic function.	Bromsulphthalein (BSP) when injected is removed by the liver and excreted in the bile. The amount removed from the blood gives a measure of hepatic function.	Anaphylactic reactions have occurred. Use with caution in patients with allergic history or bronchial asthma.	Check brochure for drugs that interfere with test.

DRUGS ACTING ON THE GASTROINTESTINAL SYSTEM

STOMACHICS, BITTERS, APPETIZERS

The therapeutic value of these drugs has never been proved, and they are not now used to any great extent. Sometimes they are added to other drugs, or used alone for the psychologic effect only. Unless otherwise ordered, all these drugs are given ½ hour before meals, diluted only slightly.

CINCHONA. *Bark of any species of Cinchona.* Compound tincture of cinchona.	4 ml. t.i.d. a.c. Oral.	Used to increase appetite and to stimulate the secretion of the digestive juices.	The bitter taste is thought to stimulate the flow of the digestive juices.	Rare in therapeutic dosage. In excessive amounts will cause the same symptoms as quinine (page 56). Treatment: see quinine.	Contains cinchona, serpentaria, bitter orange peel.
GENTIAN. *Gentiana Intea.* Compound tincture of gentian.	4 ml. t.i.d. a.c. Oral.	Used to increase appetite and to stimulate the secretion of the digestive juices.	See above.	None.	Contains gentian, cardamom, bitter orange peel.
IRON, QUININE, AND STRYCHNINE. *Mineral, vegetable.* Elixir of iron, quinine, and strychnine.	4 ml. t.i.d. a.c. well diluted and through a straw or tube. Oral.	Used to increase appetite and to stimulate the secretion of the digestive juices. Also used as a general alternative.	As above.	Rare in therapeutic dosage. In excessive amounts same as for drugs, mainly strychnine. Pasty, dark stools may result.	

Name, Source, Synonyms, Preparations	Dosage and Administration	Uses	Action and Fate	Side Effects and Contraindications	Nursing Implications and Remarks
			ALKALINE DRUGS (antacids, carminative drugs)		
These are all mineral preparations unless otherwise noted. There are many combinations of these drugs. They are all used for the treatment of peptic ulcers and other gastric disorders.					
ALUMINUM PREPARATIONS.					
Aluminum hydroxide gel, suspension, U.S.P. (A1-U-Creme, Co-Lu-Gel, Creamalin, Gelumina, Hartgel, Hydroxal) (algeldrate [C]).	5-30 ml. Given between or before meals with generous amount of water. All q.i.d. or p.r.n. Oral.	Used as an antacid in the treatment of gastric ulcers and any gastric hyperacidity. Also used as a carminative, protective and astringent.	Aluminum hydroxide acts as an antacid by combination with hydrochloride of the stomach acid to give $AlCl_3$ (aluminum chloride) and H_2O. Acts more slowly than soluble alkalies, but there is much less incidence of acid rebound. Dried aluminum hydroxide gel is less antacid than the fluid. Aluminum phosphate gel is less antacid than the hydroxide but more demulcent and adsorptive. Little if any absorption occurs.	Rare in therapeutic dosage, but may cause constipation. It is not absorbed to any appreciable extent. These compounds have been shown to reduce the absorption of tetracycline, and concurrent use should be avoided or the tetracycline given one hour before or two hours after the aluminum-containing preparation.	Patients on dialysis take these preparations to decrease the possibility of phosphatic stone formation.
Aluminum hydroxide gel (concentrate) 600 mg./5 ml. (Alernagel)	5-15 ml. Oral.				
Aluminum hydroxide gel, dried, N.F. (Adsogil, AluCaps, AluTabs, Co-Lu-Gel, Creamalin, Dialume). (A-H-Gel, Alocol, Alugel, Amphojel, Chem-Gel [C]).	300-600 mg. Oral. 5-6 times daily and h.s.				Tablets should be chewed before swallowed and taken with milk or water.
Aluminum phosphate gel, N.F. (Phosphajel) (Uigel [C]).	15 ml. Oral				
Basic aluminum carbonate (Basaljel).	30 ml. Oral.				
Dihydroxy aluminum aminoacetate, N.F. (Alglyn, Alkam, Robalate).	500 mg. Oral.				Dihydroxy aluminum aminoacetate is a combination of aluminum hydroxide and glycine. Less apt to cause constipation than the hydroxide.
Magaldrate, U.S.P. (Riopan) (magaldrate [C]).	400-800 mg. Oral.				

ALKALINE BISMUTH SALTS					
Bismuth, milk of, N.F. (Cremo-Bismuth, Lac-Bismo).	4 ml. q.i.d. Oral.	Used to decrease gastric acidity and as a demulcent in gastric ulcers. Also used as a carminative, antiemetic and antacid.	They are demulcent, astringent and mildly antiseptic. They tend to coat irritated or denuded surfaces, as in peptic ulcers. Being basic, they also help neutralize excess gastric acidity. Not absorbed to any degree because of insolubility.	Rare except in presence of a large raw surface, in which case the bismuth may be absorbed, causing such toxic symptoms as black gums, swelling of the tongue, dysphagia, salivation, gastrointestinal disorders. Stop drug and treat symptoms.	
Bismuth subcarbonate, (Cremo-Carbonate).	1 Gm. q.i.d. Oral.				
Bismuth subgallate.	1 Gm. q.i.d. Oral.				
ALKALINE CALCIUM SALTS.					
Precipitated calcium carbonate (precipitated chalk) (Calcibarb [C]).	1-2 Gm. q.i.d. Oral.	Used mainly as an antacid and protective for raw surfaces.	Good long acting antacid with less chance of alkalosis or rebound because it is relatively insoluble.	Rare in therapeutic dosage but may cause constipation. Stop drug and treat symptoms.	Releases carbon dioxide in the stomach; is not absorbed.
Calcium carbonate tablets.					
MAGNESIUM PREPARATIONS					
Magnesia, milk of, U.S.P. (magnesia magma, magnesium hydroxide).	4 ml. q.i.d. as antacid. Oral.	Used mainly as an antacid and as a laxative.	Acts as antacid, and in sufficient dose following interaction with stomach acid acts as saline laxative. Little if any absorption occurs.	Rare in therapeutic dosage. Interaction with the tetracyclines same as aluminum compounds.	Magnesia magma also comes in tablet form.
Magnesium carbonate.	600 mg. } q.i.d. as antacid. Oral.				
Magnesium oxide, U.S.P.	250 mg. } q.i.d. as antacid. Oral.				
Magnesium trisilicate, U.S.P. (Trisomin) (Neutrasil [C]).	1 Gm. p.r.n. Oral.				Magnesium trisilicate is a rapid powerful adsorbent used in toxic conditions; gives slow long-continued action but is not systemic.
PHOSPHATE PREPARATIONS.					
Calcium phosphate dibasic, N.F.	1 Gm. q.i.d. or p.r.n. Oral.	Used mainly as an antacid and as a laxative.	Similar to others of this group. Tribasic calcium phosphate tends to cause systemic action. Raises blood calcium. Tribasic magnesium phosphate is similar to magnesium trisilicate.	Same as the constituent drugs. May cause mild constipation and acid rebound.	
Magnesium phosphate.	1 Gm. q.i.d. or p.r.n. Oral.				

DRUGS ACTING ON THE GASTROINTESTINAL SYSTEM (Continued)

ALKALINE DRUGS *(Continued)*

Name, Source, Synonyms, Preparations	Dosage and Administration	Uses	Action and Fate	Side Effects and Contraindications	Nursing Implications and Remarks
ALKALINE SODIUM SALTS. Sodium acetate. Sodium bicarbonate, U.S.P. (baking soda) Sodium citrate, U.S.P.	1.5 Gm. p.r.n. Oral. 1-2 Gm. p.r.n. Oral. 44.6 mEq. ampul. I.V. 1 Gm. p.r.n. Oral.	Used for many purposes, such as to decrease gastric acidity, to reduce acidity systemically and locally as an antipruritic. The citrate also is used to prevent blood clotting in blood to be used for transfusions.	Alkaline salts that act as antacid because of their basic nature. These salts are soluble and are widely distributed. They are excreted by the kidneys and will cause the urine to be alkaline.	Rare in therapeutic dosage. Excessive amounts may cause alkalosis. Stop drug and give mild acids. Sodium salts, especially the bicarbonates, are more apt to cause alkalosis. Sodium bicarbonate may cause acid rebound and increase in CO_2 in the stomach.	Sodium bicarbonate is used intravenously to combat metabolic acidosis, especially in cardiac arrest. When sodium citrate is given to alkalinize the urine, the patient should be on a low-calcium diet (no milk or milk products), since calcium will precipitate in an alkaline urine.
MISCELLANEOUS Cimetidine (Tagamet). Cimetidine hydrochloride.	300 mg. q.i.d. with meals and h.s. Oral. 300 mg. q. 6 h. I.V. injected over 1-2 min. or infused 15-20 min. for hospitalized patients. Total dose not to exceed 2.5 G. daily.	Treatment of duodenal ulcers and pathological hypersecretory conditions.	Competitively inhibits action of histamine on receptors of parietal cells, reducing gastric acid output and concentration. Indirectly reduces pepsin secretion. Rapidly and well absorbed from G.I. tract. Food may slightly decrease absorption. Widely distributed with 15-20% protein bound. Crosses placenta and secreted in milk. Metabolized in liver. 80-90% excreted in urine within 24 h.	Mild and transient diarrhea, dizziness, transient maculopapular or acne-like rashes, urticaria and muscle pains reported in a few patients. Mental confusion, agitation, restlessness, lightheadedness, diaphoresis and flushing noted in patients receiving 1-2 G./day. Rarely adynamic ileus, gynecomastia, perforation of chronic peptic ulcer, neutropenia.	Safe use in pregnancy, lactation and children under 16 years not established.

EMETICS

Name, Source, Synonyms, Preparations	Dosage and Administration	Uses	Action and Fate	Side Effects and Contraindications	Nursing Implications and Remarks
ALUM. *Mineral.* Alum, N.F.	1-2 Gm. Oral.	Used as an emetic and locally as an astringent.	Powerful astringent and styptic with irritant qualities; if taken in sufficient quantities is an emetic and purgative.	Rare in therapeutic dosage. If taken in large quantities can cause gastrointestinal irritation.	Do not use in cases of corrosive poisoning.

ANTIMONY AND POTASSIUM TARTRATE *(tartar emetic). Mineral and vegetable.* Antimony potassium tartrate, U.S.P.	30-120 mg. Oral.	Used as an emetic and expectorant. It is also used as an anti-infective. Used more frequently as an expectorant than as an emetic.	It acts as an emetic because of its irritating effect.	Rare in therapeutic dosage. Treatment: see antimony poisoning. Page 49.	
APOMORPHINE HYDROCHLORIDE. *Synthetic derivative of opium (morphine).* Apomorphine hydrochloride, N.F.	5 mg. S.Q. Range: 2-10 mg. Do not repeat.	Used as a centrally acting emetic.	Acts as a direct stimulant on the vomiting center in the medulla. It is metabolized mainly by the liver, and degradation products are excreted in the urine.	Salivation, lacrimation, weakness, dizziness, convulsions. Stop drug, treat symptoms, maintain respiration. Contraindicated in impending shock, corrosive ingestions, narcosis due to CNS depressants or if patient is too inebriated to stand.	Prepared solutions should be sterilized prior to use.
COPPER SULFATE. *Mineral.* Copper sulfate.	300 mg.-1 Gm. Either one dose or 300 mg. q. 15 minutes for three doses. Oral.	Used as an emetic and as a catalyst with iron given for anemia. Also acts as an antidote in phosphorus poisoning.	Acts as an irritant to mucous membranes.	Rare in therapeutic dosage.	Do not use in cases of corrosive poisoning.
IPECAC (emetine, cephaeline). *Cephaelis ipecacuanha.* Ipecac, U.S.P. Ipecac syrup, U.S.P.	500 mg. Oral. 10-30 ml. Oral.	Used as an emetic and expectorant.	Produces emesis by stimulation of medullary chemoreceptor trigger zone and by irritation of gastric mucosa. Vomiting is slower than with apomorphine, but ipecac produces less depression.	Rare in therapeutic dosage. Sweating and depression may occur. Can exert a cardiotoxic effect if drug is not vomited and is absorbed.	Action of these preparations as emetics is uncertain, especially if ingested substance is an anti-emetic.

Name, Source, Synonyms, Preparations	Dosage and Administration	Uses	Action and Fate	Side Effects and Contraindications	Nursing Implications and Remarks
MUSTARD. *Sinapis nigra.* Ground mustard.	4-10 Gm. Dissolve in warm water. Oral.	Used as an emetic and locally as a counterirritant.	Action uncertain but often effective; frequently used in emergencies, especially in the home.	Rare in therapeutic dosage.	Safe, but not very effective.
ZINC SULFATE. *Mineral.* Zinc sulfate, U.S.P. (Orazinc).	600 mg.-1 Gm. Give well diluted. Oral. 220 mg. t.i.d. Oral.	Used as an emetic and also general treatment with trace elements. Treatment of zinc deficiencies and leg ulcer in diabetic patients.	Same as copper sulfate. As an emetic it is an irritant to mucous membranes. Zinc also functions as an integral part of a number of enzymes important to protein and carbohydrate metabolism and is essential for normal growth and tissue repair.	Rare in therapeutic dosage. Some gastric distress may occur.	Do not use in cases of corrosive poisoning. Said to help increase the ability to taste in patients shown to have lower than normal serum levels of zinc.

ANTIEMETICS–ANTINAUSEANTS

See also Antacids, Antihistamines, Tranquilizers and Vitamins. Patients should be warned about operating machinery and driving cars when taking these drugs (especially for the first time) or upon initiation of treatment. These are all synthetic preparations.

Name, Source, Synonyms, Preparations	Dosage and Administration	Uses	Action and Fate	Side Effects and Contraindications	Nursing Implications and Remarks
Benzquinamide hydrochloride (Emete-con).	50 mg. Repeat in 1 hour if needed, then q. 3-4 h. p.r.n. I.M. 25 mg. I.V. given over period of ½ to 1 minute (if this route is used).	Prevention and treatment of nausea and vomiting associated with anesthesia and surgery in patients in whom emesis would endanger results of surgery or result in harm to the patient.	Onset of action within 15 minutes is usual. Method of action is not known. Has antiemetic, antihistaminic, mild anticholinergic and sedative action. Rapidly absorbed and distributed. Metabolized in the liver, excreted in bile and urine.	Side effects: dry mouth, drowsiness, hyper- or hypotension, dizziness, mild cardiac arrhythmias, anorexia, twitching, tremors, shaking, urticaria, rash, fatigue, chills, increased temperature. Sudden increase in BP and transient arrhythmias have been reported following I.V. administration. Safe use during pregnancy or for children has not been established.	Reconstituted drug maintains potency for 14 days at room temperature. This drug can mask signs of overdosing of toxic drugs or may obscure diagnosis of such conditions as intestinal obstruction. Safe use in pregnancy has not been established.

Dimenhydrinate, U.S.P. (Dramamine, Dramocen, Reioamine) (Dramavol, Dymenol, Gravol, Neo-Matic, Novodimenate, Travamine, Traveller's Friend [C]).	50-100 mg. q. 4 h. p.r.n. Oral, parenteral or rectal.	Used as an antiemetic, to overcome vertigo and dizziness of motion sickness.	Has C.N.S. depressant, anticholinergic, antiemetic, antihistaminic and local anesthetic effects. Has a depressant action on hyperstimulated labyrinthine function. The fate of this drug is the same as that of the antihistamines. They are readily absorbed and widely distributed. They are of short duration of action since they are rapidly metabolized. The degradation products are usually eliminated in the urine.	Rare in therapeutic dosage, but drowsiness can occur. Patients should be cautioned about operating autos or dangerous machinery. Tolerance to C.N.S. effects occurs within a few days of therapy. May enhance effects of other C.N.S. depressants and anticholinergic drugs.	Use with caution when given in conjunction with ototoxic drugs, as ototoxic effect may be masked.
Diphenidol (Vontrol).	25-50 mg. q. 4 h. p.r.n. Oral. 50 mg. q. 4 h. p.r.n. Rectal. 20-40 mg. q. 4 h. p.r.n. I.V. or I.M. Children's dosage: 0.4 mg./lb. Oral or rectal. 0.2 mg./lb. by injection.	Limited to hospitalized patients or those under professional supervision because of side effects. Used for vertigo due to labyrinthitis and Meniere's disease and for control of nausea and vomiting postoperatively and that seen with malignant neoplasms.	Apparently acts on vestibular apparatus to control vertigo and on the chemoreceptor trigger zone to control nausea and vomiting. Very weak C.N.S. depressant, anticholinergic and antihistaminic activity. Metabolic fate in man unknown. Animal studies indicate excretion within 3-5 days.	Contraindications: Anuria. Safety for nausea of pregnancy has not been established. Side effects: dry mouth, drowsiness, gastrointestinal irritation, blurred vision, dizziness, skin rashes, malaise, headache, slight transient lowering of blood pressure. May cause hallucinations, disorientation or confusion.	Cautions: do not inject subcutaneously. Drug may mask overdose of drugs and may obscure the diagnosis of other conditions (such as intestinal obstruction or brain tumor).

Name, Source, Synonyms, Preparations	Dosage and Administration	Uses	Action and Fate	Side Effects and Contraindications	Nursing Implications and Remarks
Meclizine hydrochloride, U.S.P. (Antivert, Antivert-25, Bonine) (histamethizine, meclozine, Bonamine, Mecazine, Nauzine [C]).	12.5-25 mg. t.i.d. p.r.n. Oral.	Used as an antiemetic, to overcome vertigo, dizziness, motion sickness, labyrinthitis and nausea.	Exhibits CNS-depressant, anticholinergic, antiemetic, antispasmodic and antihistaminic properties. Action is similar to dimenhydrinate. Prolonged duration of action, with effects lasting 8-24 hours. Metabolic fate unknown. It is probably metabolized in the liver. The metabolites are well distributed, crossing the placenta. Excreted in feces and urine.	Drowsiness, dry mouth, fatigue and rarely blurred vision have occurred. May enhance effects of other CNS depressants and antihistamines.	Not for use in women who are pregnant or may become pregnant. Drug has possible teratogenic effects.
Thiethylperazine maleate, N.F. (Torecan).	10-30 mg. Daily. Oral. 10-20 mg. Daily. I.M.	Antiemetic and antinauseant for the treatment of all forms of nausea, vomiting and vertigo.	Same fate as that of the phenothiazines.	Drowsiness, dry mouth, orthostatic hypotension. Contraindicated in pregnancy, severely depressed or comatose patients and patients sensitive to phenothiazine.	
Trimethobenzamide hydrochloride, N.F. (Tigan).	100-250 mg. q.i.d. p.r.n. Oral, parenteral, I.M., rectal.	Used like thiethylperazine and also for motion sickness.	Controls nausea and vomiting by depressing the chemoreceptor trigger zone in the medulla. Has weak antihistaminic activity. Antiemetic action apparent in 10-40 min. and lasts 3-4 h. Metabolized in liver, excreted in feces and urine.	Incidence of drowsiness claimed to be rare. Pain, stinging, burning, redness and swelling may occur at I.M. injection site. To minimize, inject into deep muscle and avoid escape of medication along needle track.	There is some suspicion that in children this drug may lead to development of Reye's syndrome or unfavorably alter the course of this syndrome.

SUBSTITUTIVE AGENTS (Digestants)
(See also Acidifiers.)

BILE AND BILE SALTS. *Animal.*					
Cholic acid and ketocholanic acid (Chodile).	100 mg. t.i.d. Oral.	Used to aid digestion of fats. Also increases peristalsis and aids absorption of fat-soluble vitamins. Treatment of biliary stasis. Replacement therapy.	These preparations act in the body like the natural bile salts.	Rare in therapeutic dosage but may cause mild diarrhea if taken in excessive amounts. Stop drug and treat symptoms.	
Dehydrocholic acid, N.F. (Cholan-D H, Decholin, Ketacholanic acid, Neocholan (Biocholin, Dehydrocholin, Dycholium, Idrocrine, Novodecholin, Transibyl [C]).	250-500 mg. t.i.d. Oral.	Stimulant laxative as well as hydrocholeretic.	Readily absorbed from G.I. tract. Concentrated presumably in liver and excreted in bile.	Dehydrocholic acid is contraindicated in patients with cholelithiasis, partial or complete obstruction of common or hepatic ducts or in jaundice or hepatic insufficiency.	
Desiccated whole bile (Desicol).	325 mg. t.i.d. Oral.				
Ox bile extract.	300 mg. t.i.d. Oral.				
Sodium dehydrocholate injection, N.F. (Decholin sodium, Dilabil sodium).	5-10 ml. of a 20% solution. Usually given daily for 3 days. I.V.	Used to test circulation time in cholecystography and cholangiography.			
DILUTE HYDROCHLORIC ACID. *Chemical.*					
Hydrochloric acid, diluted, N.F.	0.6-1 ml. t.i.d. a.c. Should be given well diluted through a straw to protect teeth. Oral.	To aid in gastric digestion when there is insufficient hydrochloric acid.	Aids in protein digestion in cases of achlorhydria.	Rare in therapeutic dosage.	
DRIED DUODENUM. *Animal.*					
Dried duodenum (Viodenum) Desiccated and defatted.	500 mg.-1 Gm. t.i.d. a.c. Oral.	Used in the treatment of gastric and duodenal ulcers.	Hormone-like substance, whose exact mechanism of action is not known.	None.	Similar to urogastrone.
GLUTAMIC ACID AND HYDROCHLORIDE. *Chemical.*					
Glutamic acid hydrochloride, N.F. (Acidulin) (Acidogen, Antalka [C]).	1-2 capsules before meals. Oral.	To aid in gastric digestion when there is insufficient hydrochloric acid.	Action same as that of hydrochloric acid.	Rare in therapeutic dosage. Contraindicated if hyperacidity or peptic ulcers are present.	Not unpleasant to take, and does not injure teeth.

DRUGS ACTING ON THE GASTROINTESTINAL SYSTEM (Continued)

SUBSTITUTIVE AGENTS *(Continued)*

Name, Source, Synonyms, Preparations	Dosage and Administration	Uses	Action and Fate	Side Effects and Contraindications	Nursing Implications and Remarks
MALT. *Vegetable.*					
Malt extract.	15 Gm. With meals. Oral.	Used to aid digestion of carbohydrates and as a nutrient.	Is able to convert at least five times its weight of starch into sugar.	None.	
PANCREATIN. *Animal.*					
Pancreatin, N.F. (Panopsin, Panteric, Viokase).	325 mg. With meals. Oral.	Used to assist digestion of protein and carbohydrate foods and to aid digestion of fats, especially in pancreatic insufficiency. Used also to peptonize milk.	Action is the same as that of the enzymes of the pancreatic juice.	Use with caution in patients allergic to pork protein.	Each Viokase tablet digests: 23 Gm. fat; 32 Gm. protein; 48 Gm. starch.
PANCRELIPASE. *Animal; concentrated pancreatic enzyme.*					
Pancrelipase, N.F. (Cotazym) (lipanereatin [C]).	Up to 18 tablets or capsules daily with meals. Oral.	Used to treat pancreatic insufficiency.	As above.	As above. Rare, but sensitivity may occur.	Each Cotazym capsule contains digestive enzymes, sufficient to digest, as follows: lipase, 17 Gm. fat; trypsin, 34 Gm. protein; amylase, 40 Gm. starch.
SACCHARIN. *Synthetic.*					
Saccharin, U.S.P. (Benzosulfimide, Gluside, Saxin).	15-60 mg. With food. Oral.	Used as a sugar substitute in diabetes, reducing diets, and other conditions in which sugar is not allowed.	A sweetening agent with no caloric value.	None. Thought to be rare but possibly implicated in cancer of the bladder in rats and humans.	
Sodium saccharin, N.F. (sodium benzosulfimide, Sweeta) (Crystallose, (Crystallose, Hermesetas [C]).	15-60 mg. With food. Oral.				
TAKA-DIASTASE. *Proprietary from enzyme of Aspergillus oryzae.*					
Taka-Diastase, Elixir. Taka-Diastase (*Aspergillus oryzae* enzyme [C]).	4 ml. With meals. Oral. 1 Gm. With meals.	Used to aid digestion of carbohydrates and to relieve indigestion.	A mixture containing the active enzymes of malt.	Rare in therapeutic dosage.	

ANTISEPTIC

(See also Anti-infectives and Urinary Antiseptics.)

FURAZOLIDONE. *Synthetic.* Furazolidone, N.F. (Furoxone).	50-100 mg. q.i.d. Oral.	Used as an anti-infective for the intestinal tract.	Action and use are similar to those of the poorly absorbed sulfonamides.	Nausea and vomiting most common side effects. Toxicity usually low, but sensitivity reactions may occur. Hypertensive crisis can occur. Safe use during pregnancy has not been established.	Has effects similar to disulfiram (Antabuse), so alcohol must not be used. Also acts as a monoamine oxidase inhibitor. The usual precautions and interactions prevail. See page 109.

ADSORBENTS (ABSORBENTS), PROTECTIVES, ANTIDIARRHEICS

(See also Antacids and Astringents.)

ACTIVATED CHARCOAL *(purified organic charcoal).* Activated charcoal (Charcocaps, Charcotabs).	1-8 Gm. p.r.n. Oral.	Mainly used to treat flatulence and in accidental ingestion of various substances.	An effective adsorbent of a wide variety of drugs and chemicals; it prevents absorption of these agents. Not absorbed or metabolized; excreted with feces. Colors feces black.	Drugs of this type, when given concurrently with other medication, can significantly reduce absorption of the drug. Remember that it adsorbs enzymes, vitamins, amino acids, minerals and other nutrients from the G.I. tract. This can produce adverse nutritional effects when this drug is used indiscriminately.	An ingredient of many proprietary preparations. The powder should be mixed with sufficient water to form consistency of thick soup. Palatability can be improved by adding a small amount of concentrated fruit juice or chocolate powder. Adsorptive properties are decreased when added to ice cream or sherbet.
BENTONITE *(hydrous aluminum silicate). Earth (clay).* Bentonite magma, U.S.P.	Dosage varies p.r.n. Oral.	Used to treat flatulence and nonspecific diarrhea.	Acts as an adsorbent and protective.	As above.	Often used in combination with other drugs.
DIATOMACEOUS EARTH *(purified siliceous earth). Earth (clay).* Purified siliceous earth.	Dosage varies. Oral or topical.	Also used to treat flatulence and nonspecific diarrhea.	Acts as an adsorbent and protective.	As above.	

Name, Source, Synonyms, Preparations	Dosage and Administration	Uses	Action and Fate	Side Effects and Contraindications	Nursing Implications and Remarks
DIPHENOXYLATE. *Synthetic.* Diphenoxylate hydrochloride, N.F. (Clonil, Lomotil).	2.5-5 mg. three or four times daily. p.r.n. Tablets or liquid.	Used in diarrhea or in any condition in which there is gastrointestinal hypermotility.	Chemically related to narcotic drugs so addiction is theoretically possible at high doses. Not analgesic. Only important action appears to be decreased intestinal peristalsis. Onset of action in 45 min.-1 h. Effects last 3-4 h. Metabolized in liver and excreted in bile and feces.	Toxicity includes those symptoms associated with atropine: respiratory depression, drowsiness, toxic megacolon, paralytic ileus, nausea and vomiting, headache, depression, urticaria and pruritus. Use with caution in patients with glaucoma or advanced liver disease. Contraindicated in children less than 2 years of age and in patients with pseudomembranous enterocolitis.	Clonil and Lomotil contain a subtherapeutic amount of atropine sulfate. Concurrent use with MAO inhibitors may precipitate hypertensive crises. Careful attention should be given to fluid and electrolyte replacement especially with children. Safe use in pregnancy and lactation should be weighed against possible hazards to mother and child.
Loperamide hydrochloride (Imodium).	4 mg. now, then 2 mg. after each unformed stool, to a maximum of 16 mg. daily.	Acute nonspecific diarrhea and chronic diarrhea associated with inflammatory bowel disease. Also to reduce the volume of discharge from ileostomies.	Acts by slowing intestinal motility. Inhibits peristaltic activity by a direct effect on the circular and longitudinal muscles of the intestinal wall. Plasma ½ life is about 40 hours. Studies in monkeys at high doses produced physical dependence of the morphine type.	Side effects include abdominal pain, distention, constipation, drowsiness, dizziness, dry mouth, nausea, vomiting, skin rash, and tiredness. Contraindicated in acute diarrhea associated with organisms that penetrate the intestinal mucosa, such as salmonella, shigella, *E. coli* and in pseudomembranous colitis seen with certain broad-spectrum antibiotics.	Loperamide is a Schedule V drug under the Federal Controlled Substances Act. Safe use in pregnancy, lactating women and children under 12 has not been established.
KAOLIN *(aluminum silicate). Earth (clay, china clay).*					
Kaolin, N.F. (Collo-Kaolin [C]).	50-100 Gm. p.r.n. Oral.	Used to treat dysentery, food poisoning, nonspecific diarrhea.	Acts as a protective and adsorbent.	Kaolin should not be given concurrently with lincomycin, since the absorption of lincomycin can be	
Kaolin mixture with pectin, N.F. (Kao-con, Kaopectate, Kalpec,	5-30 ml. p.r.n. Oral				

Ka-Pek, Paocin, Pargel, Pektamalt).				reduced by as much as 90 per cent.	
Kaomagma (kaolin and magnesia).	5-15 ml. p.r.n. Oral.				
MISCELLANEOUS					
Lactobacillus acidophilus (Bacid). Lactobacillus bulgaricus (Lactinex).	2 capsules b.i.d. or q.i.d. Oral. 3-4 tabs. or 1 packet of granules t.i.d. or q.i.d. Oral.	Treatment of uncomplicated diarrhea, particularly that due to modification of the intestinal flora.	*Lactobacillus acidophilus*, a natural inhabitant of the G.I. tract, creates an environment unfavorable to the overgrowth of potentially pathogenic fungi and bacteria. Both preparations establish an aciduric flora through the production of lactic acid.	Initially may produce an increase in flatus, but this subsides with continued therapy. No known contraindications.	*Lactobacillus acidophilus* should be administered with at least 120 ml. milk or tomato juice. Granules may be sprinkled on food or cereal.
Lactulose (Cephulac).	20-30 Gm. t. or q.i.d. Adjust dose for 2 or 3 soft stools daily.	Prevention and treatment of portal-systemic encephalopathy including the stages of hepatic pre-coma and coma. It does not alter the serious underlying liver disease with its complications.	Lactulose reaches the colon essentially unchanged; there it is metabolized by bacteria with the formation of low molecular weight acids that acidify the colonic contents. This changes the ammonia present to ammonium ion, and it is not absorbed but is eliminated with the feces. Therapy can reduce the blood ammonia levels by 25-50%.	Reactions include gaseous distention with flatulence or belching, abdominal discomfort and cramping in about 20% of patients. Excessive doses lead to diarrhea. Nausea and vomiting also seen. Contraindicated in patients who require low galactose diet. Concurrent therapy with neomycin is counterproductive.	Other laxatives should not be given when drug is being administered, as this drug is titrated by the resulting loose stools. The sweet taste of the syrup can be minimized by administration with water, fruit juice or food.
SIMETHICONE. *Synthetic.*					
Simethicone, N.F. (Antiform, Mylicon, Silain).	40-80 mg. p.c. and h.s. Oral.	Used to relieve flatulence due to functional or organic disease.	Physiologically inert. Changes surface tension, causing collapse of foam bubbles.	None.	Tablet should be chewed thoroughly.

CATHARTICS

The use of cathartic drugs should be confined to such conditions as relief of temporary constipation, presurgery or prediagnostic procedures, relief of edema, to lessen the work of the kidneys and in treatment of disorders and diseases of the gastrointestinal tract. Other measures should be used for the treatment of chronic or persistent constipation. Cathartics may be classified in a variety of ways. The more common classifications are as follows: According to degree of action–laxative, mild; purgative, more severe; drastic purgative, very severe. According to method of action–increase bulk of intestinal content; lubrication; chemical irritation of the mucosa; selective action. Varying the amount of the drug or the type of drug will produce different degrees of action. Cathartics are contraindicated when abdominal pain, nausea, vomiting or other signs or symptoms of appendicitis are present.

SALINE CATHARTICS AND ANTACID MINERAL SALTS

Name, Source, Synonyms, Preparations	Dosage and Administration	Uses	Action and Fate	Side Effects and Contraindications	Nursing Implications and Remarks
MAGNESIUM, SODIUM, POTASSIUM SALTS. *Mineral.*		Used to increase the intestinal content by "salt action," producing fluid or semi-fluid stools. Used also to reduce edema, obesity, milk secretion and intracranial pressure. Most of the cathartics are given at bedtime. Liquid saline preparations are given early in the morning, usually before breakfast and, except in edema, with ample fluid.	The carbonate or hydroxide derivatives of these salts have an antacid action. These preparations withdraw fluid from the blood and the tissues. They produce a semi-fluid or watery stool within 3-6 h. after oral dose.	Nausea, colic and polyuria may occur. Force fluids, if indicated; otherwise no treatment is needed. These compounds have been shown to reduce the absorption of tetracycline, and concurrent use should be avoided or the tetracycline given one hour before or two hours after the aluminum-containing preparation.	Compound effervescent powders contain potassium and sodium tartrate 7.5 Gm. and sodium bicarbonate 2.5 Gm. in the blue paper. Tartaric acid 2.2 Gm. in the white paper. Dissolve separately in about one-fourth glass of water, mix at bedside and administer as soon as possible.
Compound effervescent powders (Seidlitz powders).	See last column. Oral.				
Magnesium carbonate.	8 Gm. Oral.				
Magnesium citrate solution, N.F.	200-300 ml. Oral.				
Magnesia, milk of, U.S.P. (magnesia magma).	15-20 ml. Also comes in tablet form, often given h.s. Oral.				
Magnesium oxide, U.S.P. (calcined magnesia).	4 Gm. Oral.				
Magnesium sulfate, U.S.P. (Epsom salts).	15 Gm. Oral.				Bitter taste of magnesium sulfate can be masked by mixing with lemon juice.
Potassium sodium tartrate, N.F. (Rochelle salts).	10 Gm. Oral.				
Sodium phosphate, U.S.P.	4 Gm. Oral.				
Sodium phosphate, dried, N.F.	2 Gm. Oral.				
Sodium phosphate, effervescent, N.F.	10 Gm. See last column. Oral.				Effervescent sodium phosphate contains sodium phosphate, citric and tartaric acid and sodium bicarbonate.
Sodium sulfate (Glauber's salt).	15 gm. Oral.				

BULK LAXATIVES

AGAR *(agar-agar). Dried seaweed.*					
Agar, U.S.P. (Agar-agar, Benzal gelatin).	These drugs are often added to food. Dosage varies. Oral.	Used in both temporary and chronic constipation. Especially valuable in spastic conditions.	Produce colloidal bulk in the intestines, thus promoting peristalsis and formation of soft stools. Slow acting.		Laxative effects from bulk laxatives are usually apparent within 12-24 h., but full effect may not be apparent for 2-3 days. A minimum of 240 ml. of water must be given with the colloidal bulk laxatives to prevent the formation of hard dry stools. Obstruction may occur if sufficient fluid is not administered.
BASSORAN. *Proprietary compound from Sterculia gum, bassorin and magnesium sulfate.*					
Bassoran.	Dosage varies. Oral.	As above.	As above.	None.	Sterculia gum granules coated with magnesium trisilicate.
BRAN. *Outer covering of cereal grain.*					
Bran.	Dosage varies. Oral.	As above.	As above.	None.	Usually added to food, as are many of the bulk laxatives. Bran is not a lubricant, as are most of the bulk laxatives.
FLAXSEED *(linseed)* Flax.					
Oxyphenisatin acetate (Acetphenolisatin, Bisatin, Endophenolphthalein, Isocrin, Phenylisatin) (acetphenolisan, Lavema, Normalax [C]).	5 mg. Oral.	As above.	As above.	None	A constituent of many bulk laxatives.
Linseed.	Dosage varies. Oral.				
METHYLCELLULOSE. *Cellulose.*					
Methylcellulose, U.S.P. (Cellothyl, Cologel, Hydrolose, Melozets, Methocel, Nicel) (conjunctival lubricant; Gonioscopic fluid, Lacril, Syncelose, Tearisol, Visculose) (Gonicosol, IpsO-tears [C]).	1.5 Gm. p.r.n. Oral. 0.5% Ophthalmic solution.	Used as a bulk laxative, as is agar; also as an anorexic agent and for conjunctival lubrication.	As above.	Binds orally administered digitalis, nitrofurantoin and salicylates.	There are several proprietary preparations that contain either methylcellulose or vegetable gums, such as Imbicoll, Saraka, Serutan, Effergel.

DRUGS ACTING ON THE GASTROINTESTINAL SYSTEM (Continued)

CATHARTICS *(Continued)*

Name, Source, Synonyms, Preparations	Dosage and Administration	Uses	Action and Fate	Side Effects and Contraindications	Nursing Implications and Remarks
METHYLCELLULOSE. (Continued)					
Hydroxypropyl Methylcellulose, U.S.P. (Isoto-Tears, Ultra-tears, Goniosol).	0.5-2.5% Ophthalmic solution.	Conjunctival lubrication. 2.5% used with gonioscopic prisms.	Provides moisture in eyes that are deficient in tear production and prolongs contact time.	None.	
PSYLLIUM SEED. *Plantago psyllium.*					
Plantago ovata coating (Betajel; Metamucil, L.A. formula).	5-10 Gm. p.r.n. Oral.	See agar.	As above. See agar.	Binds orally administered coumarin derivatives in the G.I. tract.	Metamucil contains psyllium and other ingredients.
Plantago seed, N.F. (Konsyl, Psyllium, Plantain seed).	7.5 Gm. p.r.n. Oral.				
TRAGACANTH. *Astragalus gummifer.* See agar.					
Tragacanth.	Dosage varies. p.r.n.	See agar.	As above	None.	
LUBRICANTS					
LIQUID PETROLATUM *(Mineral oil.)*		Used to lubricate the intestinal tract and to produce soft stools. Useful in certain types of chronic constipation.	Action similar to that of olive oil, but it is less demulcent and is not usually absorbed. Has been thought to prevent the absorption of some of the fat-soluble vitamins.	None. Can give rise to chronic inflammatory reaction in tissue if absorbed. Can produce lipid pneumonia if any gets into the trachea.	Liquid petrolatum in large doses tends to "seep" through the rectum and soil the clothes.
Mineral oil, emulsion (Milkinol).	15-30 ml. Oral.				
Mineral oil, light, U.S.P. (Nujol, Albolene).	15 ml. Oral. 60-150 ml. rectally as enema.				
Petrogalar, plain (Agoral, Kondremul).	15-30 ml. Oral.				
OLIVE OIL. *Vegetable. Olive fruit.*					
Olive oil.	30 ml. Usually given in divided doses during the day and at bedtime. Oral.	As above.	Acts as a demulcent. Tends to empty the gall bladder. Some of the oil is absorbed and acts as any fat.	None.	
IRRITANT CATHARTICS (Antracene, Emodin or Anthraquinone). This group of cathartics includes rhubarb, senna, aloe, cascara and related substances.			These drugs act, after partial hydrolysis, as irritants of the large bowel.		Orally administered anthraquinone drugs produce their effects with 6-12 h. but may be delayed until 24 h. Rectally administered preparations produce their effects in 30-120 min.

ALOE *(aloin). Aloe vera and similar plants.*		Used as a purgative–mild to moderate–according to dosage. Used to relieve temporary constipation, atonic chronic constipation or both.	Aloe yields anthraquinones in the alkaline portion of the small intestine; some are absorbed and later secreted in the large intestine where they produce irritant effect.	Rare in therapeutic dosage. Causes congestion of pelvic organs and is therefore contraindicated in pregnancy, during menstruation or when hemorrhoids are present.	
Aloe, U.S.P.	250 mg. Oral.				
Aloin.	15 mg. Oral.				
Aloin, belladonna, cascara, podophyllin pills (Hinkle pills).	1 pill. Oral. These should be given at bedtime because of their action on the colon.				
CASCARA SAGRADA. *Rhamnus purshiana.*					
Casanthranol (Peristim).	30 mg. Oral. Should be given at bedtime because of its action on the colon.	Used as a purgative–mild to moderate–according to dosage. Most useful in chronic constipation to improve tone of intestinal muscles. Does not cause increased constipation.	Action is mainly on large bowel. Acts by irritation but is fairly mild.	Rare in therapeutic dosage. Less likely to cause griping than some other irritant type cathartics.	Casanthranol contains cascara and glycyrrhiza.
Cascara sagrada tablets, N.F.	Dosage varies. Oral.				
Cascara sagrada aromatic fluid extract. U.S.P.	4-5 ml. Oral.				
Cascara sagrada elixir.	4 ml. Oral.				
Cascara sagrada extract, N.F.	300 mg. Oral.				
Cascara sagrada fluid extract, N.F.	1 ml. Oral.				
DANTHRON. *Synthetic from vegetable.*					
Danthron, N.F. (Dionone, Dorbane, Istizin, Modane) (dioxyanthraquinone, Danthrone [C]).	75-150 mg. h.s. Oral.	Use is much the same as for aloe.	Produces peristaltic stimulation of large bowel. Action occurs about 12 h. after ingestion.	Rare in therapeutic dosage.	May impart laxative qualities to breast milk.
SENNA. *Cassia acutifolia and C. angustifolia.*		Use is much the same as for aloe.	Resembles cascara but is more powerful.	Some griping may occur.	
Compound senna powder	4 Gm. Oral.				Compound senna powder contains senna, sulfur, fennel, glycyrrhiza.
Senna, N.F. (Aperens, Senokot).	600 mg.-2 Gm. Best given as a tea with manna. Oral.				

Name, Source, Synonyms, Preparations	Dosage and Administration	Uses	Action and Fate	Side Effects and Contraindications	Nursing Implications and Remarks
SENNA. (Continued)					
Senna fluid extract, N.F.	2 ml. Oral.				
Senna syrup, N.F.	8 ml. Oral.				
Sennosides A and B (Glysennid).	12 mg. Oral. These should be given at bedtime because of their action on the colon.				Sennosides A and B are the purified senna principles.
IRRITANT OILS					
CASTOR OIL. *(oleum ricini)* *Ricinus communis.*					
Castor oil, U.S.P.	15-60 ml. Oral.	Used to secure rapid catharsis. Especially valuable to remove toxic substances and to clear the intestinal tract before surgery or diagnostic tests.	Acts on the small intestine and produces soft watery stools within 2-3 hr. Castor oil is hydrolyzed in the intestine to glycerol and ricinoleic acid. This fatty acid is responsible for the irritating effect.	Nausea is not uncommon. Excessive purgation may occur. May cause constipation after catharsis. Contraindicated in patients with ulcerative bowel lesions, pregnant women and nursing mothers.	Has an unpleasant odor and taste. It is excreted in milk of nursing mothers. Emulsions or aromatic preparations somewhat mask the disagreeable taste. To avoid rancidity, store at temperatures below 40°C.
Castor oil, aromatic, N.F. (Neoloid).	15-60 ml. Oral. Usually given before breakfast in fruit juice or soft drinks. Ice held in the mouth before taking it will help prevent tasting the drug.				
MERCURIALS					
MERCURY. *Mineral.*					
Mercurous chloride, mild (Calomel).	120 mg. Usually given in divided doses, h.s. Oral.	Used to increase peristalsis and glandular secretions, especially bile. Also used as an intestinal antiseptic and to reduce edema.	Decreased absorption of food and food products. Causes soft, dark green stools.	Griping, colic, severe diarrhea, metallic taste, oliguria, anuria and hematuria may occur. Treatment: saline cathartics are given to remove drug. Treat for shock and treat symptoms. Dimercaprol (British Antilewisite, BAL) is used in chronic poisoning. Mercurial cathartics should be used with caution in anemia, cachexia, nephritis, pulmonary tuberculosis, scurvy,	May destroy needed intestinal bacteria. Mercurous chloride mild compound pills contain calomel and a number of drastic purgatives.

				dysentery, severe heart disorders or when iodides are being given.	
MISCELLANEOUS					
BISACODYL. *Synthetic.*					
Bisacodyl, U.S.P. (Dulcolax) (Bisacolax, Laco, Sopalax [C]).	5 mg. h.s. Oral. 10 mg. p.r.n. Suppositories.	A contact laxative for the relief of all types of constipation, even in patients with ganglionic blockage or spinal cord injury.	Acts as a stimulant to the mucosa of the colon and initiates a reflex peristalsis. No appreciable absorption. With oral administration, effects occur within 6-8 h., with rectal, in 15-60 min.	Abdominal cramping can occur.	Do not chew or crush tablets. Do not use orally within 1 hour of ingestion of an antacid or milk. Can be used by pregnant women and nursing mothers.
Biscacodyl Tannex (Clysodrast).	1 packet in 1 liter of water as enema.			The tannic acid present in bisacodyl tannex precipitates protein, and its astringent action decreases mucous secretion in the large intestine.	
DIOCTYL SODIUM SULFOSUCCINATE. *Synthetic.*					
Dioctyl calcium sulfosuccinate, N.F. (Surfak). Dioctyl sodium sulfosuccinate, N.F. (Colace, DioMedicone, Diosuccin, Doxinate, D.S.S., Duosol, Kosate, Laxinate, Parlax, Regutol, Revac) (Bantex, Constiban, Octyl-Softener, Regulex [C]).	50-240 mg. h.s. or more often p.r.n. Oral. 60-250 mg. As above. Oral. 100 mg. rectal suppository.	Used any time a laxative is indicated. Especially valuable when a soft stool is desired.	Acts as a wetting agent. Does not cause any intestinal irritation or increase in bulk, but makes stools soft. Effects occur within 1-3 days after oral administration.	Rare in therapeutic dosage, but may increase the risk of hepatotoxicity from other drugs, including some laxatives. Appears to do so by enhancing absorption of other oral drugs.	Preparations are available for infants and children.

DRUGS ACTING ON THE GASTROINTESTINAL SYSTEM (Continued)

CATHARTICS *(Continued)*

Name, Source, Synonyms, Preparations	Dosage and Administration	Uses	Action and Fate	Side Effects and Contraindications	Nursing Implications and Remarks
PHENOLPHTHALEIN. *Phenol and phthalic anhydride.* Phenolphthalein, N.F. (Thalinol) (Fractines, Laxatabs [C]).	60 mg. h.s. Oral.	Used as a purgative or laxative according to dosage.	Action is similar to that of the anthracene cathartics. Mildly irritating to mucous lining of both large and small intestines, especially the former. It is excreted in the bile, absorbed and resecreted and exerts action over a longer period than most purgatives.	Skin rashes, renal irritation, especially if taken over a period of time. Stop drug and treat symptoms.	This drug is the active ingredient found in many proprietary cathartic preparations.
POLOXALKOL. *Synthetic.* Poloxalkol (Alaxin, Magcyl, Polykol).	250-750 mg. h.s. Oral.	Similar to dioctyl sodium sulfosuccinate.	See dioctyl sodium sulfosuccinate.	Toxicity apparently low.	

Suppositories, especially glycerin, cause catharsis by irritation of the lower bowel. Also available for securing evacuation of the lower bowel are enema solutions such as sodium biphosphate and sodium phosphate (Phospho-Soda, Fleet), sodium dihydrogen phosphate (anhydrous) and sodium citrate (dihydrous) (Travad).

METABOLIC DRUGS

HORMONES

All hormones are secured from either animal or synthetic sources; all hormones are relatively nontoxic except in large doses; many hormones, especially new ones, are experimental. Many changes occur in the use, dosage, etc., of these drugs as their clinical significance and usefulness become better known. See also other biologic and metabolic drugs, such as vitamins, sera and drugs acting on the reproductive organs. See also Miscellaneous Drugs.

OVARIAN HORMONES

ESTROGENS. *Synthetic, animal.* Benzestrol, N.F. (Chemestrogen) Chlorotrianisene, N.F. (Tace). Dienestrol, N.F. (Dienestrol) (dienoestral, Willnestrol [C]). Diethylstilbestrol, U.S.P. (DES, Stilbestrol) (diethylstilbestrol, Honvol, Stilbilium [C]). Diethylstilbestrol dipropionate, N.F. (Orestrol [C]).	1-5 mg. Oral. 12-72 mg. Oral. 0.1-10 mg. Oral topical, as vaginal cream or suppository. 0.1-100 mg. Oral, I.M. or vaginal suppository. 0.5-5 mg. I.M. } synthetic sources	Estrogens are indicated for use in the following; atrophic vaginitis, kraurosis vulvae, female hypogonadism, female castration, primary ovarian failure, postpartum breast engorgement, relief of severe vasomotor symptoms of menopause, prostatic carcinoma and in breast cancer when the woman is at least 5 years postmenopausal and other therapy (surgery or irradiation) cannot be used.	Estrogens act as do the natural hormones. They tend to inhibit pituitary activity, cause hyperplasia of the endometrium and to bring about breast development. They also tend to cause closure of the epiphyseal-diaphyseal junction in youth; conversely, they cause bone development in adult women, thereby preventing and correcting osteoporosis. The estrogens have some tendency to cause sodium and fluid retention, but less than the adrenal hormones.	A statistically significant correlation between the use of estrogen-containing drugs and coronary thrombosis and neuro-ocular lesions has been shown. For this reason estrogens should be used only for those conditions that specifically warrant their use. Other side effects include nausea and vomiting, anorexia, G.I. symptoms, edema, breakthrough bleeding, breast tenderness and enlargement, amenorrhea, hypercalcemia, headache, allergic rash, pruritus, migraine aggravation, jaundice, blood pressure, cystitis-like syndrome, loss of hair, change in libido, fatigue, backache, malaise, erythema multiforme, increase in size of uterine fibromyomata, chloasma and melasma. Long-continued use may produce sclerosis of the ovaries, and may also disturb the calcium metabolism or cause increased blood sugar levels and decreased glucose tolerance. *(Continued on next page.)*	The time for the use of various estrogen substances varies widely according to condition of patient and use for which drug is given. Females exposed in utero to diethylstilbestrol have an increased risk of developing in later life a form of vaginal or cervical cancer (vaginal adenosis) that is ordinarily extremely rare. It should not be used routinely as a postcoital contraceptive.

Name, Source, Synonyms, Preparations	Dosage and Administration	Uses	Action and Fate	Side Effects and Contraindications	Nursing Implications and Remarks
ESTROGENS (Continued)					
Estradiol, N.F. (Aquadiol, Aquagen, Femogen).	10-25 mg. Implant. 1-10 mg. Parenteral (animal sources)			Because of possible adverse reaction on the fetus, the risk of estrogen therapy should be weighed against possible benefits when used during pregnancy or in patients who may become pregnant. The use of estrogens is contraindicated in known or suspected cancer of the breast (except where indicated, see column 3, p. 249), estrogen-dependent neoplasia, undiagnosed abnormal genital bleeding, thrombophlebitis or thromboembolic disorder or past history of same associated with previous estrogen use. Estrogens have been reported to increase the risk of endometrial cancer in postmenopausal women and also increase the incidence of gall bladder disease in these women.	
Estradiol benzoate, N.F.	1-2 mg. Oral. 1 mg. I.M. (animal sources)				

Estradiol cypionate, U.S.P. (Depo-Estradiol)	1-15 mg. I.M. synthetic.				
Estradiol dipropionate, N.F. (Ovocylin, Progynon) (Di-Ovocylin [C]).	1 mg. I.M. Pellets.				
Estradiol valerate, U.S.P. (Delestrogen, Femogen) (Femogen [C]).	10-40 mg. I.M.				In combination with progestational agents it can be used in habitual or threatened abortion or alone for breast engorgement.
Estrogens, esterized, U.S.P. (Evex-21, Amnestrogen, Estrifol, Menest, S.K.-Estrogens, Zeste).	0.3-2.5 mg. daily 3 to 4 weeks. Oral. (animal sources)				
Estrogens, conjugated, U.S.P. (Premarin).	0.3-2.5 mg. Oral. 25 mg. injection, 0.1% vaginal cream.				
Estrone, N.F. (Follestrol, Menagen, Menformon (A) suspension, Theelin) (ketohydroxyestrin, Femogen [C]).	0.2-1 mg. (in oil) I.M. 1-5 mg. (aqueous) I.M.				

Name, Source, Synonyms, Preparations	Dosage and Administration	Uses	Action and Fate	Side Effects and Contraindications	Nursing Implications and Remarks
ESTROGENS (Continued)					
Ethinyl estradiol, U.S.P. (Estinyl, Feminone) (Nadestryl [C]).	0.02-0.5 mg. Oral (synthetic)				
Hexestrol (dihydrodiethylstilbestrol).	2-3 mg. Oral or I.M. (synthetic)				
Piperazine estrone sulfate, N.F. (Ogen).	0.625-2.5 mg. Oral. Vaginal cream, topical. (synthetic)				
Promethestrol dipropionate (Methestrol [C]).	1 mg. Oral. (synthetic)				
PROGESTATIONAL HORMONES. *Animal or Synthetic.*					
Dydrogesterone, N. F. (Isopregnenone, Duphaston, Gynorest).	5-40 mg. Oral.	Used in the treatment of dysmenorrhea, menorrhagia, metrorrhagia and threatened abortion. But its use here lacks evidence of efficacy.	The natural hormone is secreted by the corpus luteum and is ineffective when given orally. Synthetic preparations are effective orally. It elicits to varying degrees the following: induction of secretory changes in the endometrium; increase in basal body temperature; histological changes in vaginal epithelium; relaxation of uterine smooth muscle; stimulation of mammary alveolar tissue; pituitary inhibition and production of withdrawal bleeding in presence of estrogen.	Side effects include breast tenderness, galactorrhea, prolonged postpartum bleeding, missed abortion, nervousness, insomnia, somnolence, fatigue, dizziness, thromboembolic phenomenon, sensitivity reactions, acne, alopecia, hirsutism, jaundice, breakthrough bleeding, melasma, chloasma and mental depression. They are contraindicated in thrombophlebitis, thromboembolic disorders, cerebral apoplexy or history of these conditions; liver dysfunction or disease, known or suspected malignancy of	Most progestational hormonal drugs are prepared synthetically, although originally they were obtained from animal corpus luteum or placenta. Time of administration varies according to purpose, use, duration of action of various products, and condition of patient.
Ethisterone (anhydrohydroxyprogesterone, Lutocylol, Progestolets, Progestoral [C]).	10 mg. Oral.				
Hydroxyprogesterone caproate, U.S.P. (Delalutin).	125-250 mg. I.M.	Used in secondary amenorrhea and in abnormal uterine bleeding due to hormonal imbalance in the absence of organic pathology.			
Medroxyprogesterone acetate, U.S.P. (Amen, Provera)(Depo-Provera [C]).	2-5-10 mg. Oral 50 mg. I.M. 400 mg./ml. for injection. I.M. To start, 400-1000 mg. weekly, then as little as 400 mg. per month.	Used for inoperable, recurrent and metastatic endometrial carcinoma.			

				breast or genital organs, undiagnosed vaginal bleeding and missed abortion.	
Norethindrone, U.S.P. (Norlutin, Norlutate) (Norethisterone [C]).	5-30 mg. Oral.	See also under Tissue-building hormones, page 277.			Norlutate is norethindrone acetate, U.S.P.
Pregnenolone (Natolone, Sharmone).	100 mg./cc. I.M.	Used in the treatment of rheumatoid arthritis.			
Progesterone (Gesterol, Lipo-Lutin, Proluton) (Luteinol, Progestilin [C]).	5-50 mg. Oral or parenteral.				
OTHER OVARIAN HORMONES. *Animal and synthetic.*					

There are several drugs similar to Norethynodrel used as oral contraceptives. They are all combined hormonal drugs. Some of the major ones are Demulen, Enovid, Norinyl, Norlestrin, Ortho-Novum, Ovral, Ovulen, Brevicon and Modicon.

Another type of oral contraceptive involves the use of a small amount of a progestational agent on a continual daily basis. There is a greater chance of pregnancy with this type. If two consecutive days are missed, the manufacturers state that other means of contraception should be employed until the next menstrual period.

It has been shown statistically that women on progestin-estrogen birth control pills have a higher incidence of the following serious reactions than women not taking the "pill": thrombophlebitis, pulmonary embolism and cerebral thrombosis.

Norethindrone, U.S.P. (Micronor).	0.35 mg./tablet One tablet daily on a continuous basis.	Contraceptive.	Effectiveness less than with the combination drugs.	Side effects, contraindications, etc., same as with the others.	Safety during pregnancy or lactation has not been established.
Norgestrel, U.S.P. (Ovrette).	0.075 mg. q.d. Oral.	Contraceptive.			

Name, Source, Synonyms, Preparations	Dosage and Administration	Uses	Action and Fate	Side Effects and Contraindications	Nursing Implications and Remarks
PANCREAS. (Islets of Langerhans).					
INSULIN. *Animal.* (Bovine, porcine and a mixture of bovine and porcine available.	All insulin in given in units. Actual dosage varies widely from 1-100 units. Insulin is given S.Q. Regular (unmodified) insulin is also given I.V.	Treatment of diabetes mellitus. Also used in cases of hyperglycemia not directly caused by diabetes mellitus.	Insulin is secreted by the beta cells (islets of Langerhans) of the pancreas. Stimulates carbohydrate metabolism by facilitating transport into the cell. In the liver, insulin facilitates phosphorylation of glucose to glucose-6-phosphate, which is converted to glycogen or further metabolized. Stimulates lipogenesis and inhibits lipolysis and release of free fatty acids from adipose cells. Also stimulates protein synthesis. Absorption is influenced by type of insulin, method of administration and presence of insulin-binding antibodies, which develop in all patients after 2-3 months therapy. Rapidly distributed throughout extracellular fluids and metabolized primarily in liver.	Excessive doses may cause hypoglycemia (insulin shock) with weakness, sweating, nervousness, anxiety, pallor, or flushing. Later symptoms of insulin shock include aphasia, convulsive seizures, coma and even death. Give soluble sugar orally or I.V. Orange juice, if given early, will relieve the symptoms. Hyperinsulinism results in hypoglycemia and may occur with brittle diabetes or in patients who have received an overdose of insulin, decreased or delayed food intake or an excess amount of exercise in relation to insulin dose. Hypoglycemic reactions have been reported in patients who were changed from beef to pork insulin. Atrophy or hypertrophy of subcutaneous fat tissue may occur at site of frequent injections. Prevent by rotating sites so that the same site is not used more than once q. 1-2 months. Resistance to insulin occurs infrequently and is associated with obesity, infection, trauma and other stress-producing conditions. Chronic resistance may	Since insulin is a protein molecule, it is destroyed by the digestive juices and hence must be given parenterally. Nonprotein hypoglycemic agents are available for specific uses. See pages 257–258. Insulin is stable at room temperature up to 1 month; however, avoid exposure to direct sunlight and extremes of temperature. Stock supply should be refrigerated. Injection of cold insulin should be avoided, since it can lead to reduced rate of absorption and local reactions, such as lipodystrophy. To avoid dosage errors, always use an insulin syringe that coordinates with the strength of insulin being administered. Insulin injection techniques reported to reduce lipodystrophy involve lifting the skin and fat away from the muscle, inserting a 5/8-7/8 in. needle at a 20-45° angle into the base of the fold, aspirating to verify avoidance of intravascular injection and injecting into pocket

				occur when insulin therapy is reinstituted after a period of withdrawal. Hypoglycemic action of insulin is increased by administration of alcohol, anabolic steroids, monoamine oxidase (MAO) inhibitors, guanethidine or salicylates. Addition of insulin to an I.V. infusion may result in adsorption of insulin to the container and tubing. This is highly variable and influenced by many factors. Insulin injection may be administered directly into a vein or I.V. tubing with no significant loss due to adsorption. Only regular insulin may be administered I.V.	between the fat and muscle layers. Apply pressure (without massage) to puncture site for 2-3 seconds after removal of the needle. Patient knowledge of the following is most important and should be incorporated into the plan of care: (1) nature of diabetes mellitus, (2) insulin action, administration, storage and drug interactions, (3) adjustments in insulin dosage, (4) urine testing and recording, (5) causes, symptoms, prevention and treatment of hypo- and hyperglycemia, (6) importance of adhering to prescribed diet and optimal weight, (7) exercise schedule, (8) personal hygiene, (9) importance of regular follow-up with the physician.

Name, Source, Synonyms, Preparations	Dosage and Administration	Uses	Action and Fate	Side Effects and Contraindications	Nursing Implications and Remarks
INSULIN (Continued)	**Type of Action**	**Onset of Action**	**Height of Action**	**Duration of Action**	
Insulin injection, U.S.P. (regular, unmodified) (Iletin).	Quickest acting.	20-30 minutes.	1-2 h.	5-8 h.	When mixed with other insulins (except Lente), time and duration can be affected.
Insulin zinc suspension, prompt, U.S.P. (Semi-Lente Iletin).	Quick acting,	50-60 minutes	4-6 h.	12-16 h.	Main use is for patients allergic to regular instilin.
Globin insulin with zinc, U.S.P.	Medium acting.	1-2 h.	6-10 h.	12-18 h.	
Insulin isophane, suspension, U.S.P. (NPH Iletin).	Medium acting.	2 h.	8-12 h.	18-24 h.	
Insulin zinc suspension, U.S.P. (Lente Iletin).	Medium acting.	2-4 h.	8-12 h.	18-24 h.	Lente insulins can be mixed with each other or with any insulin as their action depends on the size of the particle, rather than additives.
Insulin zinc suspension, extended. U.S.P. (Ultra-Lente Iletin).	Long acting.	4-6 h.	16-18 h.	24-36 h.	
Insulin protamine zinc suspension, U.S.P. (Protamine Zinc and Iletin).	Long acting.	4-6 h.	16-18 h.	24-36 h. or longer.	
Glucagon, U.S.P. (pancreatic polypeptide [C]). *Glandular extract.*	0.5-2 mg. Dosage individually adjusted. Parenteral.	For use in hypoglycemic coma resulting from any cause.	A crystalline polypeptide pancreatic extract. Causes increased blood glucose concentration by stimulating hepatic glycogenolysis through activation of phosphorylase. Intensity of hyperglycemia is dependent on hepatic glycogen reserve and presence of phosphorylase. Has positive inotropic and chronotropic action on the heart. Maximum effects achieved within 30 min.; blood glucose levels return to normal or hypoglycemic levels within 1-2 h. Metabolized primarily in the liver.	Carbohydrates should be administered orally as soon as the patient is alert, to prevent secondary hypoglycemic reactions. In deep coma, I.V. dextrose should be given. See Nursing Implications under insulin.	Failure of patients to respond to glucagon therapy may be a result of prolonged hypoglycemia or depletion of liver glycogen stores. Side effects rare when administered in usual dose for short periods. Most frequent are nausea and vomiting, but these may be due to hypoglycemia. Because of its protein nature, hypersensitivity reactions can occur.

NONHORMONAL DRUGS USED IN THE TREATMENT OF DIABETES MELLITUS: SYNTHETIC HYPOGLYCEMIC DRUGS.

Synthetic preparations used chiefly in treatment of older diabetics. Not usually recommended for juvenile or ketotic diabetics. All dosages are individually adjusted. The safe use of these drugs during pregnancy has not been established. Their use in women of child-bearing age should involve careful weighing by the physician of hazards against benefits.

The sulfonylurea compounds interact with a number of drugs. With phenylbutazone, oxyphenbutazone and sulfinpyrazone, there can be an increased hypoglycemic effect, and the dose of the sulfonylurea drug should be adjusted downward if given concurrently with any of these drugs. Chloramphenicol increases the half-life of the sulfonylurea compounds, and this can cause a hypoglycemic reaction. Patients who regularly take alcohol in quantity will metabolize tolbutamide at an accelerated rate and will require larger than usual doses.

Acetohexamide, U.S.P. (Dymelor) (Dimelor [C]).	250-500 mg. o.d. to q.i.d. Oral.	Used in stable, mild, adult diabetes. Occasionally used in moderately severe diabetes in conjunction with insulin.	A sulfonylurea drug; tends to increase the release of endogenous insulin. Half-life in body of 6-8 hours, with duration of action of 12-24 hours. Mechanism of long-term hypoglycemic effect of sulfonylurea agents has not been established.	Gastrointestinal disturbances, skin rash, headache, nervousness, etc. Jaundice has been reported infrequently. Hypoglycemia may appear in those patients who do not eat regularly or who exercise without caloric supplementation. Contraindicated in juvenile or severe diabetes and during pregnancy. Used with caution in debilitated patients or in patients known to have liver damage.	
Chlorpropamide, U.S.P. (Diabinese) (Chlorolase, Chloromide, Diazene, Novopropamide, Stabinol, Melinase [C]).	100-250 mg. Oral. Up to 750 mg. daily for maintenance.	Use and indications similar to those for tolbutamide.	See tolbutamide. Rapidly absorbed. Is bound to plasma proteins. Is slowly excreted by the kidneys largely unchanged. Half-life is about 36 hours.	Similar to tolbutamide. Contraindicated in patients with impairment of hepatic, renal or thyroid function.	
Tolazamide, U.S.P. (Tolinase).	Individually adjusted. Oral. If more than 500 mg. is required daily, it should be divided 250 mg. b.i.d. More than 1000 mg. per day will probably not result in better control.	Used to treat stable or maturity onset diabetes.	Appears to act as the other sulfonylurea type drugs. Has half-life of 7 hours and a duration of 10-14 hours.	Contraindicated in juvenile diabetes, severe trauma, impending surgery, ketosis, acidosis, coma or history of these complications.	Available in 100-250 mg. tablets. Not recommended for patients with concurrent liver, renal or endocrine disease or during pregnancy.

Name, Source, Synonyms, Preparations	Dosage and Administration	Uses	Action and Fate	Side Effects and Contraindications	Nursing Implications and Remarks
Tolbutamide, U.S.P. (Orinase) (Chem-Butamide, Glycemex, Hypoglymol, Mallitol, Mobenol, Neo-Dibetic, Novobutamide, Oramide, Tolbugen, Tolbutol, Tolbutone, Wescotol, Wilbutamide [C]).	0.5-3 Gm. Oral.	Used in the treatment of diabetes mellitus in the adult whose condition is stabilized.	Appears to stimulate the beta cells to secrete insulin, hence is valuable only in patients who retain some functioning cells. It is chemically related to the sulfonamide drugs. Rapidly absorbed from gastrointestinal tract; peak concentration in 3-5 hours. Bound to plasma proteins and metabolized. Half-life in body about 5 hours.	Nausea and other gastric disturbances and skin eruptions. Reduce dosage or stop drugs and treat symptoms. Contraindicated in juvenile or severe diabetes mellitus.	

DRUGS USED IN THE TREATMENT OF HYPOCALCEMIA

Name, Source, Synonyms, Preparations	Dosage and Administration	Uses	Action and Fate	Side Effects and Contraindications	Nursing Implications and Remarks
Dihydrotachysterol, U.S.P. (Hytakerol).	750 mcg. -2.5 mg./d. Oral. Dose individualized to maintain normal blood calcium levels.	Treatment of hypocalcemia associated with postoperative or idiopathic hypoparathyroidism and pseudohypoparathyroidism.	Similar to ergocalciferol (Vit. D) and parathyroid hormone but with weak antirickitic activity. Elevates serum calcium by increasing its intestinal absorption and possibly by enhancing urinary excretion of inorganic phosphate. Phosphaturia is accompanied by mobilization of calcium and phosphate from bone. Large doses enhance osteoclastic and osteocytic resorption. Maximum hypercalcemic effects occur within 4-6 weeks. Effects occur faster with a loading dose. Metabolized by liver; majority is	Toxic effects are those of hypercalcemia. Narrow margin of safety. Dose must be carefully titrated. Early symptoms of hypercalcemia include weakness, lethargy, vertigo, headache, anorexia, abdominal cramps, nausea, vomiting, diarrhea or constipation, tinnitus, ataxia (especially of lower extremities), exanthema. Later and more serious symptoms include impairment of renal function, osteoporosis, weight loss, anemia, convulsions. Fatalities due to overdose have occurred. Treatment of mild hypercal-	Frequent blood calcium levels must be done during therapy. Patient must be advised of dangers and symptoms of toxicity. Some recommend forcing fluids to produce large urine volume and thus minimize formation of renal stones in patients with hypercalciuria. Capsules should be stored at 20-25°C., since colder temperatures may cause cracking and leakage of the drug. Limit phosphorous intake (including milk). Calcium may need supplementing.

			probably excreted in bile and feces. Has been reported excreted also in breast milk.	cemia includes discontinuance of drug, lots of fluids, low calcium diet, and use of a laxative. Given to patients with renal stones only when benefits outweigh possible risks. Contraindicated in patients with hypercalcemia and those with hypocalcemia associated with renal insufficiency. Safe use in pregnancy not established. If administered to nursing mothers, the infant may be at risk of hypercalcemia.	
PARATHYROID. *Animal.* Parathyroid injection, U.S.P. (Para-Thor-mone).	25-50 U. o.d. Parenteral.	Short term treatment of acute hypocalcemic tetany secondary to hypoparathyroidism.	Parathyroid hormone raises the blood calcium level from a tetanic level of 5-7 mg./100 ml. of blood to the normal of 10-12 mg./100 ml. in about 9-18 hours. However, this effect lasts only 12-36 hours. Well absorbed from parenteral sites. Partly excreted in urine.	Hypercalcemia is the most common and serious hazard. See above. S.Q. injection may produce moderate inflammation.	Since increase in serum calcium is delayed after injection, I.V. calcium must be given until the effects of parathyroid hormone occur.

Name, Source, Synonyms, Preparations	Dosage and Administration	Uses	Action and Fate	Side Effects and Contraindications	Nursing Implications and Remarks
PITUITARY *ANTERIOR. Animal and synthetic.*					
Several hormones secreted by this gland control growth and development, stimulation of the various other glands and general regulation of many body functions.					
Cosyntropin (Cortrosyn).	0.25-0.75 mg. I.M. or I.V.	For a rapid screening test of adrenal function and can be used to differentiate between some types of primary and secondary insufficiency.	Cosyntropin exhibits the full corticosteroidogenic activity of natural ACTH. Cosyntropin contains 24 of the 39 amino acids of natural ACTH starting from the N terminus. In activity, 0.25 mg. of cosyntropin has the activity of 25 units of natural ACTH. It also possesses the extra-adrenal effects of natural ACTH which include increased melanotropic activity, increased growth hormone secretion and an adipokinetic effect. It has been shown that with the 24 amino acid chain length there is much less antigenicity then with the 39 chain natural substance.	It has slight immunologic activity and is not completely devoid of hypersensitivity reactions. There have been only three such reactions, and in all three cases, the patients had a pre-existing allergic disease and/or a previous reaction to natural ACTH.	
Corticotropin injection, U.S.P. (adrenocorticotropin, ACTH, Acthar, Acton-X, Cortrophin [C]).	10-100 U. o.d. I.M., S.Q. or I.V.	Corticotropin is used to test for adrenal function. Can be used as adjunct therapy in: arthritis, collagen, allergic, ophthalmic, pulmonary, neoplastic or edematous states; in trichinosis with neurologic or myocardial involvement and in hematologic disorders.	Corticotropin stimulates the adrenal cortex to secrete its hormones. It is useful only if the adrenal cortex is able to respond to the stimulation.	Use of corticotropin may result in a rounded contour of the face, mild hirsutism, mental disorders, transient retention of salt and water with edema, restlessness, insomnia, euphoria and hyperglycemia. Contraindicated in scleroderma, systemic fungal infections, congestive heart	Corticotropin depresses the activity of the anterior pituitary substance, with atrophy from prolonged use. For interactions, see under suprarenal, page 266.
Corticotropin injection repository, U.S.P. (Acthar-Gel-HP, ACTH-Gel, Corticotropin-Gel, Cortropin-Gel) (Duracton [C]).	10-80 U. U.S.P. units. o.d. Entire daily dose may be given at one time. Individually adjusted. The gel				

	delays absorption and prolongs the action. I.M.			failure, hypertension, ocular herpes simplex, active or latent peptic ulcer, osteoporosis, severe hypertension and thromboembolic phenomena.	
Corticotropin zinc hydroxide suspension, U.S.P. (Cortrophin-Zinc).	40-80 U.S.P. units. o.d. Dosage individually adjusted. I.M.				
Chorionic gonadotropin, U.S.P. (Antuitrin-S, A.P.L., Follutein, Pregnyl, Riogon).	4000 U. I.M. Two or three times weekly (q. 2-3 s.). 10,000 U. I.M. following menotropin.	Chorionic gonadotropin is used to stimulate gonadal secretion of sex hormones in treatment of cryptorchidism, hypogonadism. Also in conjunction with menotropin in treatment of anovulatory women who have low levels or absence of gonadotropins.	A polypeptide hormone produced by the human placenta. In males, stimulates differentiation of Leydig cells of testes, androgen production, and differentiation and early maturation of the seminiferous tubular lining cells. In women of childbearing age with normally functioning ovaries, causes ovulation in follicles that have been stimulated by FSH and promotes development of corpus luteum. It has no known effect on fat mobilization, appetite or sense of hunger.		These preparations have properties similar to those of anterior pituitary hormone. They are placental hormones obtained from urine of pregnant women.
CLOMIPHENE CITRATE. *Synthetic.*					
Clomiphene citrate, U.S.P. (Clomid).	50 mg. o.d. oral for 5 days. May increase to 100 mg. o.d. for 5 days if 50 mg. is not effective. Increasing dose or duration of therapy beyond 100 mg. for 5 days should not be done. Three courses of 5 days each constitutes an adequate trial and treatment. Use beyond this is not recommended.	Used to induce ovulation in appropriately selected cases. (See brochure.)	Action appears to be mediated through increased output of pituitary gonadotropins, which in turn stimulates the maturation and endocrine activity of the ovarian follicle and the subsequent development and function of the corpus luteum. The pituitary role is indicated by increased urinary excretion of gonadotropins and the response of the ovary is shown by increased urinary estrogen excretion.	Contraindications: pregnancy, liver disease, abnormal bleeding of undetermined origin, ovarian cyst. Side effects: visual symptoms (if they occur, stop drug and have complete ophthalmologic evaluation), multiple births, ovarian enlargement. Also hot flashes and abdominal discomfort.	Great care should be taken in the selection of the patients to be put on this drug. (See brochure.) This drug is not a hormone, but is placed here because it appears to act on the pituitary gland.

Name, Source, Synonyms, Preparations	Dosage and Administration	Uses	Action and Fate	Side Effects and Contraindications	Nursing Implications and Remarks
SOMATOTROPIN					
Somatotropin (Asellacrin).	2 I.U. or 0.05-0.1 I.U./kg. 3 times weekly with a minimum of 48 h. between doses. I.M.	Promotes linear growth in patients with growth failure caused by a deficiency of endogenous growth hormone.	Elicits the responses produced by endogenous human growth hormone. The magnitude and duration of response is greater in patients with deficient growth hormone than in patients with normal levels. Exerts anabolic effect on all body tissues. 90% is metabolized in the liver. Does not cross the placenta.	Low order of toxicity. Discomfort, swelling and pain may occur at injection site. Hypercalciuria occurs frequently but is not sustained for more than 2-3 months. Lipoatrophy, lipodystrophy, myalgia and early morning headache reported rarely. Circulating antibody has developed in 30-40% but in general has not interfered with clinical response except in about 5% of patients. Allergic reactions and hypersensitivity are possible. Contraindicated in patients with progressive intracranial lesions. Thyroid hormones and androgens promote accelerated maturation of bone and may precipitate epiphyseal closure. Corticosteroids may diminish growth response to somatotropin but act synergistically in increasing blood glucose levels and decreasing sensitivity to exogenous insulin.	Patient progress should be monitored by physician for bone age progression as well as for blood and urine levels. Treatment is discontinued when patient reaches a satisfactory adult height, upon closure of epiphysis and/or when patient fails to exhibit growth response.
POSTERIOR PITUITARY. *Animal and synthetic.*					
Desmopressin acetate (DDAVP).	0.1-0.4 ml. daily in single or divided doses. Intranasally. Individually adjusted.	Antidiuretic replacement therapy in management of cranial diabetes insipidus and for temporary polyuria and polydipsia associ-	Synthetic analogue of 8-arginine vasopressin. Provides prompt onset of antidiuretic action with long duration after each	At high doses, has caused slight elevation of blood pressure, which is eliminated with reduced dose. Use with caution in pa-	Instruct patient to insert one end of plastic tube into nostril, then blow the other end to force drug deep into nasal cavity. Tube has grad-

		ated with trauma and/or surgery in the pituitary region. Ineffective in treatment of nephrogenic diabetes insipidus.	dose. Decreased vasopressor activity and decreased action on visceral smooth muscle so that therapeutic doses are below threshold effects on vascular and visceral smooth muscle.	tients with coronary artery insufficiency and/or hypertensive cardiovascular disease. Patients on high doses have reported transient headache, nausea, nasal congestion, rhinitis, flushing, mild abdominal cramps, and vulval pain. Symptoms disappear with dose reduction. In very young and in elderly patients, fluid intake should be adjusted to decrease the potential of water intoxication and hyponatremia. Contraindicated in patients with hypersensitivity to the drug.	uation marks for 0.2, 0.1, and 0.05 ml. Response to therapy is estimated by adequate duration of sleep and adequate, not excessive, water turnover.
Lypressin. *Synthetic.* (Diapid).	Nasal spray (one spray approximately 2 U.S.P. posterior pituitary [pressor] units) (0.185 Gm./ml. equivalent to 50 units). 1-2 sprays in one or both nostrils q.i.d. and h.s. If patient needs more than this, results are better if the time interval is reduced rather than increasing the number of sprays per dose.	Used for the control of diabetes insipidus due to a deficiency of endogenous posterior pituitary antidiuretic hormone.	This is a synthetic product that takes the place of the endogenous antidiuretic hormone. Absorption is fairly good from the nasal mucosa. It is not effective orally. Duration of action is 3-8 hours. Lypressin increases the rate of renal reabsorption of water by making the epithelium of the distal renal tubules more permeable to water, resulting in an increased urine osmolality and decrease in water clearance.	Cardiovascular effects are minimal when used nasally as directed. But it should be used with caution in patients in whom such effects are undesirable. Large doses may cause coronary artery constriction.	This drug is synthetic lysine-8-vasopressin. The effectiveness may be lessened with nasal congestion, allergic rhinitis and upper respiratory infection. For best results in administration, the container should be held upright and the nozzle inserted into the nostril with the patient's head in a vertical position.

Name, Source, Synonyms, Preparations	Dosage and Administration	Uses	Action and Fate	Side Effects and Contraindications	Nursing Implications and Remarks
POSTERIOR PITUITARY. (Continued) *Animal and Synthetic.* Oxytocin injection, U.S.P. (Pitocin, Syntocinon, Uteracon).	0.3-1 ml. p.r.n. S.Q. I.V. or I.M.	An oxytocic agent. Drug of choice to induce and maintain labor. Given post-partum to prevent or control hemorrhage and to correct uterine hypotonicity.	Oxytocin is specifically oxytocic and is devoid of most pressor activity.	Premature ventricular contractions, fetal bradycardia and cardiac arrhythmias have been seen. Water intoxication can occur after prolonged I.V. infusion. Should not be used early in labor as trauma to mother or child may result. Contraindications include cephalopelvic disproportion, malpresentation, central placenta previa, breech presentation with small pelvis, uterine scar from previous "C" section, hysterotomy or myomectomy.	
	Nasal spray 40 U./ml.	To promote milk ejection but has no galactopoietic properties.			
Oxytocin citrate (Pitocin citrate).	200-400 U. in parabuccal spaces q. 30 min.	Until desired uterine response is obtained or a total of 3000 U. has been given.	Same as injection but absorption is unpredictable and less reliable than I.V. route.		
Sparteine sulfate (Tocosamine) (Tocine [C]).	75-150 mg. up to a total not to exceed 600 mg. I.M.	Oxytocic for the induction of labor and for the treatment of uterine inertia.	Oxytocic.	Contraindications: heart disease, normal labor, when there is evidence of hypertonic or tumultuous uterine contractions, cephalopelvic disproportion, previous abdominal deliveries, abdominal	WARNING: This drug, as with other oxytocic agents, may cause tetanic uterine contractions and in multiparous patients can cause uterine rupture. If drug is not effective and oxytocin

				scar, placenta previa, abruptio placentae, grand multiparity, elective induction of labor when obstetrical conditions are not favorable.	is to be used, several hours should elapse between drugs because of their synergistic action. Sparteine sulfate is not a hormone, but is placed here because of its similarity in use and action to oxytocin.
Posterior pituitary Posterior pituitary injection (Infundin, Pituitrin).	5-20 mg. Snuffed, p.r.n. 3-10 U. S.Q. 3 to 4 times daily.	Used to treat diabetes insipidus and to stimulate smooth muscle tissue.	See oxytocin and vasopressin.	Tremors, sweating, vertigo, pounding in head, abdominal cramps, nausea, vomiting, urticaria, bronchial constriction, anaphylaxis. Use cautiously in presence of epilepsy, migraine, asthma, heart failure or any state where rapid addition to extracellular water may produce a hazard.	Contains complete posterior pituitary hormone.
Vasopressin injection, U.S.P. (Pitressin).	0.3-1 ml. p.r.n. S.Q. or topically to nasal mucosa.	As above.	Vasopressin is a vasopressor and an antidiuretic agent. It raises blood pressure and stimulates smooth muscle contraction of the G.I. tract and all parts of the vascular bed, especially capillaries, small arterioles and venules.	As above. Lithium, large doses of epinephrine, heparin, demeclocycline and alcohol block the antidiuretic activity of vasopressin; chlorpropamide, urea and fluorocortisone potentiate antidiuretic effects.	Vasopressin injection has been used to treat actute G.I. bleeding and bleeding of esophageal varices. To avoid side effects, give doses just sufficient to elicit response. Patient must be monitored closely. To improve response and reduce side effects, 1-2 glasses of water may be given with the drug. I.M. vasopressin tannate has a cumulative effect, and response cannot be determined for several days. Therapy adjusted to maintain urine specific gravity at 1.005 or greater.
Vasopressin tannate (Pitressin in Oil).	1.5-5 U. q. 2-3 d., preferably h.s. I.M. dose individually adjusted.	As above.			

Name, Source, Synonyms, Preparations	Dosage and Administration	Uses	Action and Fate	Side Effects and Contraindications	Nursing Implications and Remarks
SUPRARENAL (Adrenal)					
CORTEX					
Adrenal cortex (Eschatin, Recortex).	2-10 ml. (50 dog U./ml.) Parenteral. 0.5-1 U. Oral	They are probably used for the greatest number of purposes of any group. One or all of the drugs are indicated for the treatment of Addison's disease and endocrine disorders, rheumatic disorders, collagen diseases, dermatologic diseases, allergic states, ophthalmic diseases, respiratory diseases, hematologic disorders, neoplastic diseases, edematous states, cerebral edema and certain G.I. disease states.	The adrenal glands appear to be concerned mainly with stress conditions: the medulla with acute stress, the cortex with chronic or prolonged stress. There are several active steroids secreted by the adrenal cortex. Aldosterone and desoxycorticosterone are concerned primarily with electrolyte balance. They tend to increase the retention of sodium and the excretion of potassium. These are sometimes called mineral corticoids. Cortisone and hydrocortisone are concerned primarily with glucose metabolism and are called glucocorticoids. Aldosterone and hydrocortisone have more selective action. Cortisone and desoxycorticosterone have more general action. Most of the synthetic products are used for their anti-inflammatory properties, both systemic and local.	Same contraindications and toxicity as those listed under corticotropin. Toxicity of individual preparations may vary somewhat in kind and extent. Also contraindicated in systemic fungal infections. Safe use of these drugs during pregnancy has not been established. Interactions: phenytoin, barbiturates and antihistamines decrease the pharmaceutical and physiological effect of the steroids by enzyme induction. Salicylates and phenylbutazone displace the steroids from plasma protein binding sites and give enhanced steroid effects so that lower doses will be effective. Steroids antagonize the hypoglycemic action of the oral agents and insulin, because of their gluconeogenic and glycogenolytic activity in the liver. Side effects of topical corticosteroid therapy include acneiform eruptions, pruritus, hypertrichosis, burning sensation, folliculitis and hypopigmentation.	Many of these preparations are combined with other drugs such as the antibiotics, especially the topical preparations. Check blood pressure frequently and watch for edema. High dose therapy for short duration may be reduced and discontinued quite rapidly; however, withdrawal following long-term therapy should be gradual. Dose of glucocorticoids may need to be adjusted during periods of stress.
Betamethasone, N.F. (Celestone) (Betnelan, Betnesol, Betnovate [C]).	0.6 mg. Oral.	The betamethasone series of compounds is used in most instances mentioned above.			The dose range is very great. Strengths shown are those available and do not necessarily constitute actual dosage administered.
Betamethasone acetate, N.F.	Intrabursal, intralesional, periarticular, I.M. or intradermal. (Constituent of Celestone Soluspan.)				
Betamethasone benzoate (Benison, Uticort).	0.025% cream and gel. Topical.				Topical steroids usually do not provoke physical evidence of absorption unless applied to large areas, covered with occlusive dressings and/or applied over prolonged periods.
Betamethasone dipropionate, U.S.P. (Diprosone).	0.05% cream, lotion and ointment, 0.1% aerosol.				
Betamethasone sodium phosphate, N.F. (Celestone Phosphate).	4 mg./ml. Parenteral				
Betamethasone 17 valerate, N.F. (Valisone) (Celestoderm [C]).	0.1% cream, ointment lotion, 0.15% aerosol. Topical.				

Cortisone acetate, N.F. (Cortone acetate) (Novocort [C]).	5-25 mg. Oral or I.M. 0.25-2.5% ointment. Topical.	Cortisone primarily affects protein, fat and carbohydrate metabolism. Used in the treatment of a variety of conditions, such as asthma, other allergies, some infections, arthritis, etc. Primary use is replacement therapy in chronic adrenocortical insufficiency.	Most appear to be readily absorbed. Metabolized primarily in the liver and excreted in the urine.		
Desonide (Tridesilon).	0.05% ointment. Topical.	Same as other topical steroids.	This is a nonfluorinated corticosteroid. Same as other topical steroids.	Same as other topical steroids.	
Desoxycorticosterone acetate, N.F., U.S.P. (Cortate, Deoxycortone acetate, DOCA-acetate, Percorten) (desoxycortone [C]).	2-5 mg. Buccal or parenteral. 75-125 mg. Tablet implants.	Desoxycorticosterone primarily affects water and salt metabolism. Used for replacement therapy for primary and secondary insufficiency in Addison's disease and for treatment of salt-losing adrenogenital syndrome.			WARNING: Do not administer more than 10 mg. desoxycorticosterone acetate in oil at any one time.
Desoxycorticosterone pivalate, N.F. (Percorten trimethylacetate).	25 mg. I.M.				Repository form.
Desoximetasone (Topicort).	0.25% cream b. or t.i.d.	Relief of inflammatory manifestations of corticosteroid-responsive dermatoses.		Burning, itching, irritation, striae, skin atrophy, secondary infection, dryness, folliculitis, hypertrichosis, acneiform eruptions and hypopigmentation.	
Dexamethasone, U.S.P. (Decadron, Deronil, Dexameth, Gamma-corten, Hexadrol, Maxidex).	0.5-4 mg. Oral 0.1% ophthalmic solution.	Anti-inflammatory and immunosuppressant therapy.	A synthetic glucocorticoid. Almost devoid of any mineralocorticoid effects.		
Dexamethasone acetate (Decadron LA).	8 mg./ml. Doses individualized I.M., intralesional, intro-articular, soft tissue injection.				

Name, Source, Synonyms, Preparations	Dosage and Administration	Uses	Action and Fate	Side Effects and Contraindications	Nursing Implications and Remarks
SUPRARENAL (Continued)					
Dexamethasone phosphate sodium, U.S.P. (Decadron phosphate, Hexadrol) (Dexamethadrone, Maxidex, Novo-Methasone [C]).	4-100 mg. I.M. or I.V. 0.8-8 mg. Intra-articular. 0.05-0.1% solution.				
Dichlorisone acetate (Diloderm).	0.18-0.25% Aerosol and cream. Topical.	Used for treatment of allergic or pruritic inflammations.			
Flumethasone pivalate, N.F. (Locorten) (Locacorton [C]).	0.03% cream. Apply 3 to 4 times a day. Topical.	A topical corticosteroid. Used as others of this group.	As with others of this group.	As with others of this group. Contraindications: as with others and hypersensitivity—vaccinia and varicella.	
Fluocinolone acetonide, U.S.P. (Fluonid, Synalar) (Synamol [C]).	0.01-0.2% cream. Topical. 0.1% suspension for eyes.				
Fluocinonide, U.S.P. (Lidex, Topsyn).	0.05% cream, ointment. Topical.	As adjunct therapy for relief of inflammatory manifestations of acute and chronic corticosteroid responsive dermatoses.			21 acetate ester of fluocinolone acetonide.
Fludrocortisone acetate, U.S.P. (Cortef-F acetate, Florinef acetate) (Fluorocortone [C]).	0.1 mg. Oral.	Mainly used for its effect on electrolytes, as in Addison's disease and any salt-losing form of congenital adrenogenital syndrone.	Glucocorticoid with potent mineralocorticoid properties.	Edema, hypertension, hypokalemia and cardiac hypertrophy.	
Fluorometholone, N.F. (Oxylone).	0.025% cream or ointment. Topical.				
Fluorometholone, N.F. (FML).	0.1% solution. Topical in eyes. 1-2 gtts. b.i.d. to q.i.d. May be used as much as gtt. q. 2 h.	For inflammation of palpebral and bulbar conjunctiva, cornea and anterior segment of the globe.	Same as others of this group.	As with others of this group.	
Fluprednisolone. (Alphadrol).	0.75-1.5 mg. Oral.	Anti-inflammatory and immunosuppressant therapy.	Minimal mineralocorticoid properties.	Edema and hypertension rarely occur.	

Flurandrenalide, U.S.P. (Cordran) (Drenison [C]).	0.025-0.05% cream, lotion or ointment. Topical. 4 mcg./sq. cm. tape. Topical.			Contraindicated with tubercular or secondary bacterial skin infections.	
Halcinonide (Halog).	0.1% cream. Topical. b. or t.i.d.	As other topical steroids.		As other topical steroids.	
Hydrocortamate hydrochloride (Ulcort) (ethamicort [C]).	0.5% ointment. Topical.	As for cortisone.			
Hydrocortisone, U.S.P. (Cort-Dome, Cortril, Cortef, Domolene-HC, Heb-Cort, Hydrocortone) (Bio-Cort, Cortanal, Corticreme, Cortiment, Cortiphate, Manticor [C]).	5-20 mg. Oral. Also prepared for topical and rectal use.	Uses same as for cortisone.	Same therapeutic and metabolic effects as cortisone. Concerned primarily with glucose metabolism and participates in physiological reactions under stress conditions.		
Hydrocortisone acetate, U.S.P. (Cortef acetate, Cortril-A, Hydrocortone Acetate) (Emo-Cort, Hytone, Ipso-Hydrocortisone, Microcort, Novohydrocort, Sterocort, Surfa-Cort, Texacort, Unicort, Wincort [C]).	5-20 mg. Intra-articular. 1-2.5% solution or ointment. Topical.				
Hydrocortisone sodium phosphate.	50-500 mg. Parenteral.				
Hydrocortisone sodium succinate, U.S.P. (Solu-Cortef).	500-1000 mg. Parenteral. Also available in preparations for topical use.				
Medrysone, U.S.P. (HMS).	1% solution eye drops. One drop in conjunctival sac q.i.d.	Used for allergic conjunctivitis, episcleritis and epinephrine sensitivity.	Has topical anti-inflammatory and antiallergic action.	Transient burning and stinging on instillation. Contraindications: untreated purulent ocular infections, acute herpes simplex keratitis, viral diseases of conjunctiva and cornea, ocular tuberculosis and fungal diseases of the eye.	This is an anti-inflammatory agent related to progesterone.
Meprednisone, N.F. (Betapar).	4 mg. Oral.	Anti-inflammatory and immunosuppressant therapy.	Synthetic glucocorticoid with minimal mineralocorticoid activity.		There is less sodium retention than with some others, such as prednisone.
Methylprednisolone, N.F. (Medrol, Wyacort).	2-16 mg. Oral.				

Name, Source, Synonyms, Preparations	Dosage and Administration	Uses	Action and Fate	Side Effects and Contraindications	Nursing Implications and Remarks
SUPRARENAL (Continued)					
Methylprednisolone acetate, U.S.P. (Depo-Medrol, Medrol, Wyacort).	20-40 mg. I.M. 20-120 mg. Intra-articular.				For long-term therapy with short-acting steroids (prednisone, prednisolone and methylprednisolone), oral dose should be on an alternate day and morning regimen. This simulates natural circadian rhythm of corticosteroid secretion, providing for relief of symptoms while minimizing adrenal suppression, protein catabolism and other adverse effects. Following long-term therapy, drugs should be withdrawn slowly.
Methylprednisolone sodium succinate, U.S.P. (Solu-Medrol).	10-1000 mg. I.M. or I.V.				
Paramethasone acetate, U.S.P. (Haldrone, Stemex).	1-2 mg. Oral. Also prepared for aerosol use.	Use and action similar to those of prednisolone and derivatives.			
Prednisolone, U.S.P. (Delta-Cortef, Meticortelone, Paracortol, Prednis) (metacortandrolone, Cormalone, Inflamase, Isopto-prednisolone [C]).	1-5 mg. Oral. 0.5% cream. Topical. 0.1-1.0% ophthalmic suspension.	These are cortisone derivatives with greater activity than cortisone, thus allowing lower dosage and less toxicity.	Synthetic glucocorticoid with minimal mineralocorticoid activity.		
Prednisolone acetate, U.S.P. (Nisolone, Sterane acetate).	25 mg. I.M., intra-articular, soft tissue.	Used topically for anti-inflammatory action, as are many corticosteroids.			
Prednisolone tertiary tabutate (Hydeltra-T.B.A.).	4-30 mg. S.Q. or intrasynovial.				
Prednisolone sodium phosphate, U.S.P. (Hydeltrasol, PSP I.V.).	2-30 mg. S.Q. I.M., intrasynovial, I.V. 0.25-0.5% cream. topical.				
Prednisolone sodium succinate, U.S.P. (Meticortelone Soluble).	50 mg. injection.				
Prednisone, U.S.P. (Delta-Dome, Deltasone, Deltra, Meticorten). (metacortandracin, Colisone, Decortancyl, Prednisol, Wescopred, Winpred [C]).	1-80 mg. Oral.	Probably the most widely used oral preparation in this class.			
Triamcinolone acetonide, U.S.P. (Aristocort-acetonide, Aristoderm, Kenalog) (Triamalone [C]).	0.025-0.05% cream, ointment or lotion. Topical.		As above.		
Triamcinolone diacetate, N.F. (Aristocort, Diacetate).	2-4 mg. liquid. Oral. 10-25 mg. Intra-articular or intralesional.				

Triamcinolone, N.F. (Aristocort, Kenacort).	1-16 mg. Oral.	A fluorinated derivative of prednisolone that is said to have fewer side effects.			
Triamcinolone hexacetonide, U.S.P. (Aristospan).	5-10 mg. injection.				
MEDULLA					
For use of the adrenal medullary hormone, refer to Drugs Acting on the Autonomic Nervous System–Epinephrine. (See Page 69).					
TESTICULAR HORMONES					
Animal, Synthetic.	Times for all these drugs vary with the use and the condition of the patient.				
Fluoxymesterone, U.S.P. (Halotestin, Ora-Testryl, Ultrandren) (Oratestin [C]). *(A halogenated androgen similar to testosterone, but more potent.)*	4-10 mg. Oral.	Used in the treatment of male hypogonadism, climacteric and cryptorchidism. Also used to treat symptoms of menopausal state in females, menorrhagia and other gynecologic conditions. Can be used for their anabolic properties and to treat certain refractory anemias.	The secretion of the testes, whose primary function is the maintenance of the secondary male characteristics. Performs the same function in the male as estrogen does in the female. Androgens exert an effect on erythropoiesis by stimulating production of erythropoietin. Other systemic effects include nitrogen retention and effects on skin, muscle, bone and organs.	Patient should be watched for elevated blood calcium, exacerbation of condition being treated, edema, flushing or acne of face, and—in the female—hirsutism and deepening of voice as well. Reduce or stop drug. In males, the following post-pubertal adverse reactions have occurred: inhibition of testicular function, testicular atrophy, oligospermia, impotence, chronic priapism, gynecomastia, epididymitis and bladder irritation. Contraindicated in patients with severe liver damage and in male patients with prostate or breast cancer. Also in patients with nephrosis or the nephrotic phase of nephritis.	Fluoxymesterone is also used as an anabolic agent. Contraindicated in female patients during pregnancy and lactation.

Name, Source, Synonyms, Preparations	Dosage and Administration	Uses	Action and Fate	Side Effects and Contraindications	Nursing Implications and Remarks
TESTICULAR HORMONES (Continued)					
Methyltestosterone, N.F. (Metandren, Neo-Hombreol-M, Oreton-M) (Andrhormone, Testostelets [C]).	5-25 mg. Oral.	Also used to treat metastatic breast carcinoma in female.			
Testosterone Cypionate, U.S.P. (Depo-Testosterone).	50-200 mg. I.M.				A long-acting form of testosterone.
Testosterone enanthate, U.S.P. (Delatestryl, Reposo-TE) (Melogex [C]).	100-200 mg. in oil. I.M.				
Testosterone pellets, N.F. (Oreton micro pellets).	75 mg. Subcutaneous implants.				
Testosterone propionate, U.S.P. (Androlin, Neo-Hombreol, Oreton) (Andrhormone, Perandren, Testavirol [C]).	50-100 mg. in oil. I.M. 10 mg. buccally.				
Testosterone suspension, N.F. (Andronaq, Malestrone, Neo-Hombreol-F, Oreton Sterotate).	50 mg. aq. I.M.				
Calusterone (Methosarb).	50 mg. q.i.d. (range 150-300 mg./day).	Only for palliative therapy of inoperable or metastatic carcinoma of the breast in postmenopausal women when hormonal therapy is indicated.	Biochemical mechanism by which calusterone produces its effects is at present unknown. May act in manner similar to testosterone but does not stimulate erythropoiesis. Has been reported to stimulate platelet production.	Side effects: hypercalcemia may occur; drug related edema, PSP retention and increases in SGOT have been observed. Others are those usually seen with the androgen drugs: deepening of voice, acne, facial hair growth. Nausea or vomiting is also a common side effect. Said to produce less virilization than other androgens. Contraindicated in carcinoma of the male breast and premenopausal women.	Should be given a minimum of 3 months to evaluate the response unless there is active progression of the disease. A synthetic steroid chemically related to testosterone.

Danazol (Danocrine).	400 mg. b.i.d. Oral. Therapy should continue uninterrupted for 3-6 months but may extend to 9 months.	Only for the treatment of endometriosis amenable to hormonal management in those patients who cannot tolerate or do not respond to other drug therapy.	Danazol is a synthetic androgen derived from ethisterone. It inhibits the output of gonadotropins from the pituitary gland. The only other hormonal effect is a weak androgenic activity that is dose related.	Mainly androgenic effects, such as acne, mild hirsutism, etc., and hypoestrogenic manifestations such as flushing, sweating, vaginitis, and so on. Others include rashes, dizziness, headache, sleep disorders, fatigue, paresthesia in extremities, visual disturbances, changes in appetite, changes in libido, elevations in BP and, rarely, pelvic pain.	Safe use in pregnancy has not been established, and if patient becomes pregnant during therapy, the drug should be stopped.
Dromostanolone propionate (Drolban).	100 mg. 3 times weekly I.M.	Palliation of advanced or metastatic carcinoma of breast in women who are inoperable, are 1-5 years post-menopause when diagnosed or have demonstrated a hormone-dependent cancer.	Synthetic steroid, a variant of testosterone. Induces retention of nitrogen, potassium and phosphorus; increase in protein anabolism and decrease in amino acid catabolism. Lower incidence of androgenic side effects than testosterone propionate.	Most frequent side effects are deepening of voice, acne, facial hair growth, increased libido and enlargement of clitoris. Edema may occur and necessitate diuretic treatment. Severe hypercalcemia and acceleration of disease contraindicate continued use.	At least 8-12 weeks of therapy may be necessary before any conclusions regarding effectiveness can be made.

Name, Source, Synonyms, Preparations	Dosage and Administration	Uses	Action and Fate	Side Effects and Contraindications	Nursing Implications and Remarks
THYROID HORMONE					
Animal, Synthetic					
Calcitonin-Salmon (Calcimar).	50-100 MRC units q.d. or q.o.d. I.M. or s.q.	Treatment of Paget's disease of bone. (Has been effective in patients with moderate to severe disease characterized by polyostotic involvement with elevated serum alkaline phosphatase and urinary hydroxyproline excretion.)	Calcitonin is a polypeptide hormone secreted by the parafollicular cells of the thyroid gland in mammals and by the ultimobranchial gland of birds and fish. This is a synthetic compound with the same configuration as that found in calcitonin of salmon origin. Acts on bone to lower serum calcium concentration. Also has direct renal effects and actions on the G.I. tract. Its action on bone and its role in normal human bone physiology are still incompletely understood.	Contraindicated with allergy to salmon calcitonin or its gelatin diluent. Side effects include nausea, vomiting in about 10% of patients, local inflammatory reactions at site of injection in about 10% and facial flushing in about 2%. Hypersensitivity reactions are possible because of its protein nature.	Do not administer to nursing mothers as it does inhibit lactation in animals. Has adverse effect on animal fetus (2 species), and data in humans is not available to exclude a possible adverse effect on human fetus.
Etidronate disodium (Didronel, EHDP).	5 mg./kg./day not to exceed 6 mos. Oral.	Treatment of symptomatic Paget's disease.	Acts primarily on bone. Slows rate of bone turnover (bone resorption and new bone secretion) in Pagetic bone lesions and in normal remodeling process. Can modify the crystal growth of hydroxyapatite by chemisorption onto the crystal surface. Depending on concentration, may inhibit either crystal resorption or growth. These actions are reflected in increased excretion of hydroxyproline and	Increased or recurrent bone pain at existing Pagetic sites and/or appearance of pain at previously asymptomatic sites. Risk of fractures occurs at doses above 20 mg./kg./d. in excess of 3 mos. If fractures occur, drug is stopped. Complaints of loose stools and diarrhea, and of nausea increase in some patients with doses above 5 mg./kg./d. Drug should be withheld in patients with enterocolitis. Use with	Tablets are given u.i.d., 2 h. a.c. since food may reduce absorption, especially if high in calcium. May give with water or fruit juice. Urinary hydroxyproline excretion and/or serum alkaline phosphatase levels should be monitored during therapy. More advantageous than calcitonin-salmon in that it permits oral administration, does not cause antibody formation and is more economical.

			increased serum levels of alkaline phosphatase. Etidronate is not metabolized. Within 24 h. about 50% excreted in the urine. Remainder is chemically adsorbed on bone and slowly eliminated in feces.	caution in patients with renal function impairment. Etidronate should be given only when clearly needed to women who are or may become pregnant. Breast feeding should not be undertaken. No data to support use in children.	Advise patients to maintain adequate nutritional status with particular attention to calcium and vitamin D. Response to therapy is slow and may persist for months after discontinuing.
Protirelin (Thypinone) (Thyrotropin-releasing hormone).	200-500 mcg. I.V. while patient is in a supine position. Children: 7 mcg./kg. of body weight. A blood sample is drawn just prior to injection and another in exactly 30 minutes. TSH levels are measured in each.	Adjunctive agent in the diagnostic assessment of thyroid function. Testing may yield useful information about pituitary or hypothalamic dysfunction.	Protirelin increases the release of TSH from the anterior pituitary. Prolactin release is also increased, but there is no significant effect on the release of other pituitary hormones. After I.V. administration the mean plasma half-like in normal subjects is 5 minutes. TSH levels rise rapidly and reach a peak at 20-30 minutes after injection. They approach baseline levels after 3 hours.	Transient changes in blood pressure occur so patient should be in supine position. Increases in systolic and diastolic pressures have been observed more often than decreases. About 50% of those tested have had minor side effects that generally persisted for only a few minutes. In lactating women it has caused breast engorgement and leakage that lasted up to 2 or 3 days.	Elevated serum lipid levels may interfere with test, so fasting or a low-fat meal is recommended prior to the test. Patients receiving thyroid preparations should be taken off them 7-14 days before testing for thyroid function. Chronic administration of levodopa has been reported to inhibit TSH response to protirelin. An interval of 7 days is recommended before re-testing. See package brochure for further information and interpretation of results.

Name, Source, Synonyms, Preparations	Dosage and Administration	Uses	Action and Fate	Side Effects and Contraindications	Nursing Implications and Remarks
THYROID HORMONE (Continued)					
Sodium levothyroxine, U.S.P. (Letter, Synthroid) (Eltroxin [C]). Sodium liothyronine, U.S.P. (Cytomel, Trionine) (Tertroxin [C]). Thyroglobulin (Endothyrin Proloid, Thyroprotein). Thyroid, U.S.P. (Thyronol [C]).	0.025-0.5 mg. Oral. 0.5 mg. injection. 5-50 mcg. Oral. 15-300 mg. Oral. 15-300 mg. daily. Oral.	Used as a specific in hypothyroidism, which produces conditions such as goiter, myxedema (adult) or cretinism (child), mental and physical retardation, gonadal disorders and obesity.	The thyroid hormone is reciprocal with the thyrotropic hormone of the anterior pituitary. An increase in one causes a decrease in the other. The thyroid hormone is also related to the normal functioning of the gonads, the involution of the thymus, carbohydrate metabolism and proper calcium level. There are, perhaps, other functions. It increases the rate of body metabolism.	Thyroid preparations may cause excessive weight loss, tachycardia, excessive nervousness, tremors, visual disturbances, hypertension and other symptoms of excessive metabolism. May have cumulative action. Interactions: thyroid appears to enhance the effects of the tricyclic antidepressants, especially in patients with depressed or abnormal thyroid function. Thyroid absorption is hindered by the concurrent administration of cholestyramine. It is recommended that 4 to 5 hours should elapse between oral doses of these two drugs. Patients treated with thyroid compounds will require a lower dose of oral anticoagulants when the drugs are given concurrently.	Skipping an occasional day's dosage is advised by some physicians. All doses of thyroid preparations are individually adjusted. Total dose may be taken at one time (o.d.) or in divided doses. It should not be given too late in the day as it may cause insomnia.
Thyrotropin (Thytropar) (Thyrotron [C]).	5-10 U. I.M. or S.Q.	Diagnostic and therapeutic agent. Thyrotropic hormone from anterior pituitary (TSH).	Acts to stimulate the thyroid gland.		
dl-Triiodothyronine sodium (dl-Liothyronine, Trinone).	5-50 mcg. Oral.		See thyroid.		
Sodium dextrothyroxine, N.F. (Choloxin) (d-thyroxine sodium [C]).	1.0-2.0 mg. o.d. Oral first day. Increase 1.0-2.0 mg. and hold this daily dose 2.0-4.0 mg. for one month. Increase in this manner until controlled. Do not increase beyond 6.0-8.0 mg. daily. Maintenance dose is	Used to treat hypercholesteremia in euthyroid patients. May also be used to treat hypothyroidism in patients with cardiac disease who cannot tolerate other types of thyroid medication. Main use is to lower blood cholesterol.	Thought to stimulate normal catabolism of cholesterol and its degradation products in the body with subsequent increase in excretion of cholesterol and its degradation products via the biliary route. Absorbed orally, metabolized by body. Small amounts	Contraindications: known organic heart disease, hypertensive states, advanced liver or kidney disease, pregnancy, during lactation, history of iodism. Side effects: mainly those of increased metabolism: insomnia, nervousness, tremors, palpitation, loss	This drug may potentiate the effect of anticoagulants. Dose should be reduced by one third on initiation of therapy and readjusted on the basis of prothrombin times. Has been shown to decrease concentration of blood factors VII, VIII and IX

	usually 4.0-8.0 mg. daily. Children: 0.05 mg./kg. daily. May increase 0.05-0.1 mg. monthly per kg. to 4.0 mg. daily if needed to control.		not metabolized are excreted in urine and feces in about equal amounts.	of weight, lid lag, sweating, flushing, hyperthermia, loss of hair, diuresis, menstrual disorders, abdominal disorders.	and platelet activity in some people.
TISSUE-BUILDING HORMONES *These are semisynthetic or synthetic preparations.*		Used to promote growth and repair of body tissues in senility, chronic illness, convalescence, and prematurity.	Tissue-building steroids. May also stimulate erythropoiesis in certain types of anemia. All are weak androgens.	Toxicity low, but edema may occur in malnourished patients with cardiac or renal impairment. The following adverse effects have been seen with the use of anabolic steroids: increased or decreased libido, flushing of the face, acne, habituation, excitation, sleeplessness, chills, leukopenia and bleeding in patients on concomitant anticoagulant therapy. These drugs are used with caution, if at all, in prostatic cancer and severe renal and hepatic disorders, some cardiac disorders and during pregnancy. Menstrual disturbance may occur during therapy.	Methandrostenolone potentiates warfarin and indandione anticoagulants, so prothrombin time should be closely monitored. Methandrostenolone and norethandrolone are said to be free of gonadal action. Adequate dietary protein is required when anabolic agents are used.
Ethylestrenol (Orgabolin, Maxibolin).	2-8 mg. Daily. (0.1 mg./kg. to start, increasing as required). Oral.				
Methandrostenolone, N.F. (Dianabol) (methandienone, Danabol [C]).	5 mg. q.d. Oral.				
Methandriol (Stenediol, Methyltestediol [C]).	10-15 mg. Oral five times weekly.				
Nandrolone decanoate, N.F. (Deca-Durabolin)	50-100 mg. Monthly. I.M.				
Nandrolone phenpropionate, N.F. (Durabolin).	25-50 mg. Once a week. I.M.				
Norethandrolone (Nilevar).	30-50 mg. q.d. Oral or I.M.				
Norethindrone, U.S.P. (Norlutin, Norlutate, Norethisterone).	5 mg. Up to 20 mg. q.d. daily. Oral.	Also used for gynecological symptoms associated with pregnancy and menstruation.	Synthetic progesterone with androgenic, anabolic and antiestrogenic properties. See progesterone classification for details.		Norethindrone is similar to norethandrolone in structure and action.
Oxandrolone, N.F. (Anavar) (Protivar [C]).	5-10 mg. daily. Two to four times daily. Oral.	Anabolic agent.			
Oxymetholone, N.F. (Anadrol, Adroyd tablets) (Anapolon [C]).	5-10 mg. Given in divided doses for 4-6 week period. Oral.				
Stanozolol, N.F. (Winstrol).	2 mg. t.i.d. Oral.	Used for debilitated, underweight and catabolic patients.	A steroidal anabolic agent used to produce positive nitrogen balance.	As above. Increased retention of sulfobromophthalein has been reported.	Androgenicity low; mild virilizing effects may occur with long use, especially in young women.

Name, Source, Synonyms, Preparations	Dosage and Administration	Uses	Action and Fate	Side Effects and Contraindications	Nursing Implications and Remarks
FAT-SOLUBLE					
	Since vitamins A and D are usually found in the same preparations, they will be listed together. Petroleum oil should not be given with the fat-soluble vitamins as it delays or prevents absorption of some of them. Dosages of vitamins vary according to purpose. In most cases, dosage given is average daily dosage. May be divided or given at one time according to circumstances.				
VITAMIN A. Precursors are carotene (alpha, beta, gamma) and cryptoxanthin. *Preformed vitamin A is secured from animal sources (fish liver oil, milk, fortified margarine, liver, egg yolk). Precursors are secured from vegetables (yellow fruits and vegetables and dark green vegetables). Only about 50% of the precursors taken are absorbed.*		Used to treat xerophthalmia, nyctalopia, retarded growth and susceptibility of the mucous membranes to infection.	Deficiency produces xerophthalmia, nyctalopia, hyperkeratosis of the skin, and increased susceptibility to colds, influenza and similar conditions. Vitamin A is readily absorbed from gastrointestinal tract. Most carotenes are changed to vitamin A in the intestinal wall and absorption is incomplete. It is widely distributed but stored in the liver. Almost completely metabolized to carbon dioxide, fatty acids and water-soluble derivatives.	Hypervitaminosis A (occurs only if amounts much in excess of R.D.A. are taken) may cause anorexia, weight loss, pruritus, cracking and bleeding of lips, fatigue, abdominal discomfort, ostealgia, arthralgia, pseudotumor cerebri, insomnia, alopecia, menstrual irregularities, hyperostoses and premature closure of epiphyses. Most conditions improve in about a week after withdrawal of vitamin A.	U.S. R.D.A.:* Infants, 1400-2000 U. Children under 4 years, 2000 U. Adults and children over 4 years, 2500-5000 U. Pregnant women, 5000 U. Lactating women, 6000 U.
Vitamin A, U.S.P. (Oleovitamin A) (Alphalin, Anatola, Vi-Alpha) (Afraxin, Aret-A, Viatate [C]).	25,000-100,000 U. Oral.				
Vitamin A water-miscible, U.S.P. (Acon, Aquasol, A-Visol, Sol-A-Caps, Vi-Dom-A) (Arovite, Win-Vite-A [C]).	25,000-50,000 U. Oral. 50,000 U. I.M.				
Tretinoin, U.S.P. (retinoic acid Vitamin A acid) (Retin-A, Aberel [C]).	Topical application to skin lesions once daily for 2-3 weeks or as long as 6 weeks. Then dose usually may be reduced.	Treatment of acne vulgaris when comedones and pustules predominate. Not effective in severe cases with pustules and deep cystic nodules.	Results may be seen in 2-3 weeks, but may not be optimal until 6 weeks. This drug may enhance the cancer-causing effects of the sun on the skin. FDA recommends warning patients using tretinoin of this potential.	During early treatment exacerbation may occur, but is due to revealing of deep pustules not previously seen. Can cause severe local erythema and peeling at site of application. If severe enough, use should be discontinued. Contraindicated for patients with eczematous skin.	Should not be used with other agents containing peeling agents such as sulfur, resorcinol, benzoyl peroxide or salicylic acid. If these drugs have been used, it is best to wait for their effects to subside before using tretinoin.

*These data based on Recommended Dietary Allowances, U.S. Department of Agriculture Home and Garden Bulletin, No. 72, Rev. April, 1977.

Beta-carotene (Solatene).	Adults: 30-300 mg. q.d. Children under 14 years 30-150 mg. q.d. preferably with meals. Several weeks' therapy are needed to allow accumulation in the skin before increasing exposure to the sun. The palms and soles appear yellow first (from 2 to 6 weeks).	To ameliorate the photosensitivity in patients with erythropoietic protoporphyria.	Exact mode of action is unknown. In spite of elevated blood carotene levels, vitamin A levels do not rise above normal. Patients become carotenemic and may have slightly yellow skin pigmentation. The sclerae do not become yellow, in contrast to patients with icterus.	This compound can cause loose stools. It should be used with caution in patients with impaired renal or hepatic function.	Safe use in pregnancy has not been established.
VITAMIN D. Precursors are ergocalciferol, D_2, 7-dehydrocholesterol (irradiated D_3). *Fish liver oil, egg yolk, ergosterol.* Ergocalciferol, U.S.P. (Deltalin, Deratol, Drisdol, Ertrone) (Ostoforte, Ostogen, Radiostol [C]).	50,000 U. Oral. 10,000 U./ml. liquid. Oral.	Used to treat rickets, bone fracture (especially in older people), infantile tetany, osteomalacia, arthritis, diarrhea, psoriasis and lupus vulgaris (the last four conditions with varying degrees of success).	Deficiency produces rickets, infantile tetany, osteomalacia, and other conditions in which bone and tooth development is delayed or abnormal. Vitamin D is absorbed from the gastrointestinal tract. Widely distributed; some is stored in the liver. Slowly metabolized and excreted, mostly by kidneys.	Excessive vitamin D may cause nausea, vomiting, diarrhea, lassitude and urinary infrequency in adults. It may also cause untoward symptoms in children.	Dosage of vitamin D should be carefully regulated to suit the individual, and the patient should be under the care of the physician at all times. U.S., R.D.A. Infants, 400 U. Children under 4 years, 400 U. Children over 4 years, and adults, 400 U. Pregnant and lactating women, 400 U.

Name, Source, Synonyms, Preparations	Dosage and Administration	Uses	Action and Fate	Side Effects and Contraindications	Nursing Implications and Remarks
VITAMIN D. (Continued)					
Calcitriol (Rocaltrol).	0.25 mcg./d. increased at 2-4 wk. intervals to 0.5-1 mcg./d. Oral.	Management of hypocalcemia in patients undergoing chronic renal dialysis.	The most active form of vitamin D_3 in stimulating intestinal calcium transport. Thus it can overcome the vitamin D resistant state arising in uremic patients. By increasing calcium absorption, it effectively raises serum calcium levels. Rapidly absorbed from G.I. tract with peak serum concentrations after 4 h. Vitamin D metabolites are transported in blood bound to specific plasma proteins. Pharmacologic activity is about 3-5 days.	Similar to those from excessive vitamin D intake. Early signs of vitamin D toxicity are associated with hypercalcemia and include: weakness, headache, somnolence, nausea, vomiting, dry mouth, constipation, muscle pain, bone pain, and metallic taste. Later signs include polyuria, polydipsia, anorexia, weight loss, nocturia, conjunctivitis, pancreatitis, photophobia, rhinorrhea, pruritus, hypothermia, decreased libido, elevated BUN, albuminuria, hypercholesterolemia, increased SGOT and SGPT, ectopic calcification, hypertension, cardiac arrhythmias, and rarely overt psychoses. Contraindicated in patients with hypercalcemia or vitamin D intoxication. Magnesium-containing antacids should not be used concomitantly because they can lead to development of hypermagnesemia. Cholestryramine may impair absorption. No studies of use of calcitriol in pregnancy, lactation or in children.	Advise patients about importance of compliance with dosage regimen, adherence to diet, calcium supplementation and avoidance of unapproved nonprescription drugs. Patients should also be informed of symptoms of hypercalcemia. Use aluminum carbonate or hydroxide gel to control serum phosphate levels in patients undergoing dialysis. Serum calcium, magnesium, and alkaline phosphatase and 24 h. urinary calcium and phosphorus should be determined periodically. During initial phase of therapy, serum calcium is determined at least twice weekly.

VITAMIN E. Tocopherol (alpha, beta, gamma). *Wheat germ, vegetable oils, leafy vegetables, milk, eggs, whole grains, legumes.*		Effective in treatment and prevention of vitamin E deficiency, which occurs rarely. Used to treat macrocytic megaloblastic anemia in some children with kwashiorkor, hemolytic anemia in premature infants, autohemolysis of red blood cells in vitro from patients with genetic low density lipoprotein deficiency.	Deficiency in animals produces sterility, loss of embryo, muscular dystrophy, paralysis and signs of nervous disorders. Research has not shown specific results of deficiency in man. Has antioxidant properties and is an essential nutrient, apparently having an important function in the synthesis of heme. Requirement for vitamin E increases with the increased intake of polyunsaturated fats. Readily absorbed from the gastrointestinal tract via lymph. Widely distributed. Very slowly excreted. Excretion is in bile and urine. Some is metabolized; some is excreted unchanged.	Rare in therapeutic usage.	U.S., R.D.A. Infants, 4-5 U. Children under 4 years, 7 U. Children over 4 years and adults, 9-15 U. Pregnant and lactating women, 15 U. 1 international unit equals 1 mg.
dl-alpha-Tocopherol (Alfacol, Aquasol E, Denamone, Ecofrol, Eprolin, Epsilan-M).	10-200 mg. Oral.				
Tocopherols, mixed concentrate (Eprolin Gelseals, Tofaxin, Vitamin E Concentrate).	10-200 mg. Oral or I.M.				
d-alpha-Tocopheryl acetate concentrate, N.F. (Ecofrol, Econ, E-Ferol, Natopherol-A_2, Tocopherox, Tocopherol, Tokols, Vi-E).	10-200 mg. Oral or I.M.				
d-alpha-Tocopheryl acetate.	10-200 mg. Oral or I.M.				
d-alpha-Tocopheryl acid succinate, N.F. (E-Ferol Succinate).	10-200 mg. Oral.				
(Canadian trade names for various vitamin E preparations: Daltose, Ephynal, Eprolin, Phytoferol, Tocopherex, Tofaxin, Vita-E).					

Name, Source, Synonyms, Preparations	Dosage and Administration	Uses	Action and Fate	Side Effects and Contraindications	Nursing Implications and Remarks
VITAMIN K. *Pork liver, green vegetables, cereals, vegetable oils, synthetic.*		Used to treat hemorrhagic conditions, especially when associated with low prothrombin, liver and biliary disturbances, or both.	Deficiency produces delayed bleeding time, low prothrombin, delayed clotting time. Most commonly seen with disturbances of the liver and biliary tract. Recommended daily allowance has not been established. Natural forms absorbed from gastrointestinal tract via lymph, water-soluble forms via blood. Not stored to any great extent. Completely metabolized by the body. The vitamin K found in stools is apparently produced by intestinal bacteria.	Toxicity generally considered low, but menadione should be used with caution during pregnancy and in newborn infants.	
Menadiol sodium diphosphate, N.F. (Kappadione, Synkayvite) (Vitamin K_4, Synkavite [C]).	5 mg. Oral. 5-75 mg. Parenteral.				
Menadione, N.F. (menaphthone [C]).	1 mg. Oral.			Nausea, vomiting and headache have occurred after 5 mg. oral doses of menadione.	
Menadione sodium bisulfite, N.F. (Hykinone) (Vitamin K_3 [C]).	2-5 mg. Oral. or parenteral.				
Phytonadione, U.S.P. (Vitamin K_1) (AquaMephyton, Konakion, Mephyton) (phytomenadione [C]).	1-100 mg. I.V. or S.Q. 5 mg. Oral.	A recognized antidote for Dicumarol or warfarin toxicity.		Hypersensitivity reactions may occur.	Phytonadione is the drug of choice for prevention of hemorrhagic disease of newborn. It will not hemolyze red cells in individuals deficient in glucose-6-phosphate dehydrogenase (especially in premature infants), as the menadiones will.

WATER-SOLUBLE

Since vitamin B consists of many different factors that have different uses, each factor will be considered as a separate vitamin. It is common practice to give two or more factors at the same time; often the entire B-complex is given because deficiency in one B-fraction is usually associated with deficiency in other B-fractions. It is often wise not to give one factor alone, since this produces a lessening of the absorption of the other B-fractions from the food. Research is being done on many B-factors whose therapeutic value has not been established. Among these are biotin (vitamin H), choline and inositol.

B COMPLEX. *Liver, yeast and other foods as listed under the various B-factors.*		Used to treat all the conditions listed under the various factors and to aid in building the body generally (as a "tonic").	See various individual fractions. Recommended daily allowances are listed under the various factors. B-vitamins are essential for general health, especially concerned with nerve functioning and cell metabolism.	Rare.	There are numerous proprietary B-complex preparations.
Brewer's yeast.	10 Gm. Oral.				
Yeast, dried, N.F.	Dosage varies. Oral.				
Liver B-vitamin concentrate.	Dosage varies. Oral or parenteral.				
CYANOCOBALAMIN, VITAMIN B_{12}. *Mainly from liver, organs and muscles of animals and commercially from Streptomyces fermentation.*		Used to treat pernicious anemia, other macrocytic anemias and sprue. Used in Schilling's test for pernicious anemia.	Deficiency produces pernicious anemia; other conditions produced by deficiency not yet satisfactorily determined. Oral absorption, except in extremely high doses, is dependent upon gastric intrinsic factor. Readily absorbed from parenteral sites. Bound to plasma proteins; fairly widely distributed. Some stored in the liver.	Usually nontoxic, even in large doses; however, mild transient diarrhea, peripheral vascular thrombosis, itching, transitory exanthema, urticaria, feeling of swelling of entire body, anaphylaxis and death have been reported. Absorption from the G.I. tract may be decreased by aminoglycoside antibiotics, colchicine, extended release potassium preparations, aminosalicylic acid and its salts, anticonvulsants, cobalt irradiation of the small bowel and by heavy alcohol intake lasting more than 2 weeks. It has been reported that concurrent administration with chloramphenicol may result in antagonism of the hematopoietic response to vitamin B_{12} in B_{12}-deficient patients.	Combinations of vitamin B_{12} with "intrinsic factor" are available. Radiocyanocobalamin, U.S.P., also available for diagnosis of pernicious anemia. U.S., R.D.A. Infants, 0.3 mcg. Children under 4 years, 1 mcg. Adults and children over 4 years, 1.5-3 mcg. Pregnant and lactating women, 4 mcg.
Vitamin B_{12}, U.S.P. (Cyanocobalamin) (cobalamin, cobalamine) (Berubigen, Betalin-12, Bevidox, Docibin, Dodecavite, Dodex, Ducobee Hepcovite, Redisol, Rubramin, Sytobex, Vi-Twel) (Anacobin, Bedox Cyanabin, Duodebex, Nova-Rudi, Pinkamin, Rubion [C]).	10 micrograms to 1 mg. Oral or parenteral.				
Hydroxocobalamin, N.F. (alpha-Redisol, Sytobex-H) (Vitamin B_{12a} [C]).	10 micrograms-1 mg. I.M.				

Name, Source, Synonyms, Preparations	Dosage and Administration	Uses	Action and Fate	Side Effects and Contraindications	Nursing Implications and Remarks
WATER-SOLUBLE (Continued)					
FOLIC ACID, VITAMIN M. *Yeast, liver and organs and muscles of animals.*		Used to treat sprue, macrocytic anemia, megaloblastic anemias of infancy and pregnancy.	Deficiency produces macrocytic anemia; other conditions produced by deficiency not yet established. Pregnant women should receive a prophylactic dose of 1 mg./day.	Folic acid is usually given in combination with other drugs. It alone is not sufficient to control pernicious anemia. It may mask symptoms of pernicious anemia until nerve damage has occurred.	U.S., R.D.A. Infants, 50 mcg. Children under 4 years, 100 mcg. Adults and children over 4 years, 200-400 mcg. Pregnant women, 800 mcg. Lactating women, 600 mcg.
Folic acid, U.S.P. (Folvite, L. casei factor, Pteroylglutamic acid, vitamin Bc) (Novofolacid [C]).	1-5 mg. p.r.n. Oral.				
Folate sodium (Folvite solution).	5 mg. Parenteral.				
NICOTINIC ACID. *Yeast, liver, organs and muscles of animals, rice polishings and bran.*					
Aluminum nicotinate (Nicalex). Niacin, N.F. (Naotin, Nicosode, Nicotinic acid, Efacin, Nico-Span) (Nioforte [C]).	500 mg.-7.5 Gm. daily. 20-50 mg. Oral or parenteral. Three to 10 times daily. 1.5-6 Gm. daily.	Used to treat pellagra, dermatitis, glossitis and gastrointestinal and nervous system disturbances, and to aid in the treatment of many other diseases and conditions. Used to treat hyperlipoproteinemias, except type I. Also used for peripheral vasodilation.	Deficiency produces pellagra, dermatitis, glossitis and gastrointestinal and nervous system disturbances. Readily absorbed, widely distributed. Most is metabolized, excess excreted by the kidneys, as are the metabolites.	Large doses of nicotinic acid cause transitory flushing and other unpleasant symptoms.	U.S., R.D.A. Infants, 5-8 mg. Children under 4 years, 9 mg. Adults and children over 4 years, 12-20 mg. Pregnant women, 15-18 mg. Lactating women, 17-20 mg.
Niacinamide, U.S.P. (Aminicotin, Dipegyl, Nicamindon, Nicotamide, Nicotilamide, Nicotinic acid amide, Pelonin Amide.)	50 mg. Oral or parenteral.	Does not produce flushing.			
PANTOTHENIC ACID. *Yeast, liver, rice, bran, wheat germ, organs and muscles of animals, tikitiki (rice polishings).*		Essential nutrient for man. Forms part of coenzyme A. No proven cases of spontaneously occurring clinical deficiency have been seen.	Deficiency symptoms not determined. Readily absorbed. Wide distribution with highest concentrations in the liver. Excreted unchanged, about 70% in urine, 30% in feces.	Rare. Contraindicated in hemophilia.	U.S., suggested R.D.A. Infants, 3 mg. Children under 4 years, 5 mg. Adults and children over 4 years, 10 mg. Pregnant and lactating women, 10 mg.
Calcium pantothenate, U.S.P. (Pantholin).	20-100 mg. Oral.				

Dexpanthenol (Cozyme, Ilopan, Intrapan, Pantonyl) (Motilyn, Panthoderm [C]).	250-500 mg. q. 6 h. for 2-3 days. I.M.	Treatment of postoperative abdominal distention and paralytic ileus.	Insufficient evidence to base recommended daily dietary intakes on.		
VITAMIN B_1. *Egg yolk, bran and wheat germ, whole grains and tikitiki (rice polishings). Synthetic.* Thiamine hydrochloride, U.S.P. (anuerin hydrochloride, thiamine, thiamine chloride, vitamin B_1) (Apatate, Betalin S, Bethiamin, Bewon) (Betaxin [C]). Thiamine mononitrate (Thiamine nitrate).	1-100 mg. Oral or I.M. 1-15 mg. Oral.	Used to treat beriberi, gastrointestinal disturbances, visual phenomena, polyneuritis (especially that associated with alcoholism), pregnancy, pellagra and arrested growth in infancy and childhood. It produces a feeling of well-being and is helpful in many diseases and conditions.	Deficiency produces beriberi, gastrointestinal disturbances, visual phenomena, polyneuritis of alcoholism, pellagra, arrested growth in children. Poorly absorbed from gastrointestinal tract, but large doses allow for ample absorption of required amounts. Widely distributed with highest concentration in liver, brain, kidneys and heart. Some is split by the body to pyrimidine. This and excess thiamine are excreted by the kidneys.	Rare, but anaphylactoid reactions have occurred after I.V. administration of large amounts of thiamine in sensitive patients.	Rarely given alone; more often with other B-fractions. U.S., R.D.A. Infants, 0.3-0.5 mg. Children under 4 years, 0.7 mg. Adults and children over 4 years, 0.9-1.5 mg. Pregnant and lactating women, 1.3-1.5 mg.
VITAMIN B_2. *Yeast, liver, organs and muscles of animals, eggs, some vegetables, whole grains. Synthetic.* Riboflavin, U.S.P. (lactoflavin, vitamin B-2, vitamin G, Riboderm) (Flamotide [C]).	1-5 mg. Oral. 1-10 mg. Parenteral.	Used to treat cheilosis, glossitis, seborrheic lesions, loss of weight and photophobia.	Deficiency produces cheilosis, glossitis, seborrheic lesions, loss of weight, and photophobia. Good absorption and wide distribution with highest concentration in kidneys, liver and heart. Very little is stored. With normal intake only about 9% is excreted in urine. Fate of remainder is not known.	Rare.	U.S., R.D.A. Infants, 0.4-0.6 mg. Children under 4 years, 0.8 mg. Adults and children over 4 years, 1.1-1.8 mg. Pregnant women, 1.5-1.7 mg. Lactating women, 1.7-1.9 mg.

Name, Source, Synonyms, Preparations	Dosage and Administration	Uses	Action and Fate	Side Effects and Contraindications	Nursing Implications and Remarks
WATER-SOLUBLE (Continued)					
VITAMIN B_6. *Yeast, liver, lean meats, whole grains, legumes, egg yolk and fish.* Pyridoxine hydrochloride, U.S.P. (Bedoxine, Beesix, Hexa-Betalin, Hydoxin) (Hexavibex, Winvite-6 [C]).	5-100 mg. Oral or parenteral.	Used in treatment of deficiency states, in infants with epileptiform convulsions and hypochromic anemias due to familial B_6 deficiency. For prevention or treatment of peripheral neuritis caused by certain drugs such as isoniazid, penicillamine and hydralazine.	Deficiency produces gastrointestinal disturbances and neuromuscular pains, seborrhea, intertrigo, dermatitis, cheilosis, glossitis, stomatitis. Readily absorbed. Well distributed. Metabolized in liver and degradation products excreted by the kidneys.	Rare.	U.S., R.D.A. Infants, 0.3-0.4 mg. Children under 4 years, 0.6 mg. Adults and children over 4 years, 0.9-2.0 mg. Pregnant and lactating women, 2.5 mg.
VITAMIN C. *Oranges, lemons, limes, tomatoes, raw cabbage, onions, peppers, turnips, grapefruit.* Ascorbic acid, U.S.P. (cevitamic acid) (Cecon, Cevalin, C-Quin, Ce-Vi-Sol, Lequi-Cee) (Adenex, C-Vita, C-Vite, Erivit-C, Redoxon, Scortab, Vitascorbol [C]). Ascorbic acid injection, U.S.P. (Ascorbin, Cantaxin, Cenolate, Cevalin, Vicin).	100 mg.-1 Gm. Oral. 100 mg.-1 Gm. Parenteral.	Used to treat and prevent scurvy and similar conditions. Valuable in any condition in which there is an increased tendency to bleed or tendency toward capillary fragility. Essential for wound healing and beneficial in severely traumatized patients, especially persons with severe burns. Also used to acidify the urine.	Deficiency produces scurvy, defective teeth and prescorbic conditions. Readily absorbed from gastrointestinal tract. Widely distributed. Most is utilized by body. Excretion via urine, occurs mainly when there is excess intake.	Rare.	U.S., R.D.A. Infants, 35 mg. Children under 4 years, 40 mg. Adults and children over 4 years, 40-45 mg. Pregnant women, 60 mg. Lactating women, 80 mg.

There are too many multivitamin compounds to permit all of them to be considered here. Many combinations of two or three vitamins are available, as well as innumerable preparations that include most of the known vitamins. Vitamin preparations also often include essential minerals.

MINERALS

Certain minerals are used directly to change body metabolism. These are usually considered with the metabolic drugs. Other minerals are used to treat specific conditions alone or in various combinations; these are discussed with the areas involved. Considerable attention is now focused on the so-called trace elements—those elements that occur in the body in minute amounts but seem to play a very important part in body metabolism. As research in this field continues there will, no doubt, be significant developments.

CALCIUM AND PHOSPHORUS. *Mineral.* Calcium carbonate, U.S.P. (Calabarb [C]). Calcium Chloride, U.S.P. Calcium glubionate (Neo-Calglucon) Calcium gluconate, U.S.P. (Calglucon) (Glucaloids [C]).	1 Gm. q.i.d. Oral. 1 Gm. p.r.n. I.V. 1-3 Gm. t.i.d. Oral. 1 Gm. I.V. p.r.n. 5 Gm. t.i.d. Oral. 1 Gm. p.r.n. I.V.	Source of calcium cation in treatment and prevention of calcium depletion in patients in whom dietary measures are or may be inadequate. Administration of calcium salts does not preclude use of other measures to correct the underlying cause of the depletion.	Calcium and phosphorus are essential elements. Calcium is essential for maintenance of functional integrity of nervous, muscular and skeletal systems, cell membrane and capillary permeability. It is an important activator in many enzyme reactions. It is essential to physiological processes, such as transmission of nerve impulses; contraction of cardiac, smooth, and skeletal muscles; respiration; blood coagulation; and renal function. Calcium has a regulatory role in uptake and binding of amino acids, in absorption of vitamin B_{12}, in gastrin secretion, in release and storage of neurotransmitter and hormones. Actively absorbed in small intestine to varying degrees, depending on a variety of factors.	Rare in therapeutic dosage. Low calcium may produce relaxation of the heart, while excess may cause a prolonged state of contraction. Stop drug and treat symptoms. Interactions: an increase in plasma calcium concentration markedly enhances the action of digitalis and a decrease diminishes its effect. This fact should be remembered when giving calcium I.V. to patients on digitalis therapy. For interaction with the tetracyclines see page 29.	When administered I.M. or I.V., calcium salts are irritating to tissues and cause mild to severe local reactions. Should be administered slowly I.V. to avoid too rapid an increase in serum calcium as well as vasodilation, decreased blood pressure, bradycardia, cardiac arrhythmias, syncope and cardiac arrest. Orally administered calcium may be irritating to G.I. tract, especially the chloride salt, which has been reported to cause G.I. bleeding. 1.395 Gm. dibasic calcium phosphate is equivalent to 1.0 Gm. calcium gluconate.

METABOLIC DRUGS (Continued)
MINERALS *(Continued)*

Name, Source, Synonyms, Preparations	Dosage and Administration	Uses	Action and Fate	Side Effects and Contraindications	Nursing Implications and Remarks
CALCIUM AND PHOSPHORUS (Continued)					
Calcium glycerophosphate.	0.3 Gm. Usually given in solution up to q.i.d. Oral.		Following absorption, enters extracellular fluid and then is incorporated into skeletal tissues. Crosses the blood-brain barrier and placenta. Excreted primarily in feces as unabsorbed calcium.		U.S., R.D.A. C = calcium P = phosphorus Infants, C 360-540 mg. P 240-400 mg. Children under 4 years, C 800 mg. P 800 mg. Adults and children over 4 years, C 800 mg.-1.2 Gm. P 800 mg.-1.2 Gm. Pregnant and lactating women, C 1.2 Gm. P 1.2 Gm.
Calcium lactate, N.F. (Novocalcilate [C]).	5 Gm. t.i.d. or q.i.d. Oral.				
Compound hypophosphites syrup.	8 ml. t.i.d. Oral.				
Dibasic calcium phosphate, N.F. (Calphate, DCP).	1-5 Gm. daily. Oral.				
IODINE. *Seaweed.*		Used for various conditions such as disorders of the thyroid gland, as a specific and as an antiseptic. For the last two usages see page 228 and page 2. Also used to cause liquefaction and aid removal of abnormal tissue.	The primary function of iodine in the body is in the production of thyroglobin. However, iodine performs many medicinal functions (see uses). Potassium iodide increases protective secretions of bronchi, thus soothing inflamed areas.	Adverse effects rare, but the following may occur: "brassy taste," sore gums, salivation, rhinitis, adenitis, edema of eyelids, frontal headache, rash, gastric and pulmonary irritation. Hypersensitivity reactions have been reported. Acute poisoning: vomiting, abdominal pain, diarrhea, gastroenteritis.	Iodobrassid is also used in cough medications. U.S., R.D.A. Infants, 35-45 mcg. Children under 4 years, 60 mcg. Children over 4 years, adults, 80-150 mcg. Pregnant women, 125 mcg. Lactating women, 150 mcg.
Iodobrassid (Lipodine, Lipiodine).	300-600 mg. Up to q.i.d. Oral.				
Potassium-iodide, U.S.P. (KI-N-tabs).	300 mg. Up to q.i.d. Oral.				
Sodium iodide, U.S.P.	100-300 mg. Up to q.i.d. Oral. 1 Gm. I.V. every other day.				
Strong iodine solution, U.S.P. (Lugol's solution, capu-Lugols, Lugol Caps).	0.1-1 ml. Up to t.i.d. Give in a bland medium.	Used to prepare patients for thyroid surgery.			

POTASSIUM. *Mineral.* Potassium acetate, bicarbonate, and citrate (Potassium Triplex Elixir). Potassium chloride, U.S.P. (Kadelex, Kaochlor, Kay Cel, K-10, Slow-K). Potassium gluconate, N.F. (Kaon, K-G, Kalinate).	15-30 ml. daily. Oral. 1 Gm. Up to t.i.d. Oral. 250 mg.-2 Gm. p.r.n. given slowly. I.V. 15-30 ml. daily. Oral. 5 mEq. tablets, 8 daily. Oral.	Prevention and treatment of potassium depletion in patients in whom dietary measures are inadequate. Used prophylactically in conditions in which there is an additional need for potassium, as after surgery, prolonged thiazide or steroid therapy, especially if patient is digitalized.	A major constituent of intracellular fluid. Essential for maintenance of acid-base balance, isotonicity and electrodynamic characteristics of the cell. An important activator of many enzyme reactions. Essential to physiological processes, such as transmission of nerve impulses, gastrin secretion, renal function, contraction of cardiac, smooth and skeletal muscle, tissue synthesis and carbohydrate metabolism. Well absorbed from G.I. tract, with absorption varying with preparations. Enters extracellular fluid and transported to cells. Excreted primarily by kidneys.	Nausea, vomiting, diarrhea and abdominal cramps may occur. Small bowel ulcerations have been reported with enteric-coated tablets. Mouth ulcerations have occurred when patients have sucked rather than swallowed the wax matrix tablets. Pain at site of injection and phlebitis may occur during I.V. administration of solutions containing 30 mEq. or more potassium per liter of fluid. Most serious hazard is hyperkalemia. Signs and symptoms include: paresthesia of extremities, listlessness, mental confusion, weakness or heaviness in legs, flaccid paralysis, cold skin, pallor, fall in blood pressure with peripheral vascular collapse, cardiac arrhythmias, heart block and cardiac arrest. Patients on thiazide diuretics, furosemide, ethacrynic acid or digitalis should be closely followed. Contraindicated in renal disorders.	Since exact measurement of potassium deficiency is not possible, I.V. supplements should be administered slowly and with caution. Adequate renal function must be confirmed. Frequent monitoring of patient's clinical status, serum potassium levels and periodic ECG should be made. Whenever possible, potassium supplements should be given orally, since slow absorption prevents sudden large increases in plasma potassium levels. Oral liquid preparations are best administered with or after meals with a full glass of water or tomato juice to minimize possible gastric irritation and a saline cathartic effect. Normal adult daily requirement is 40-80 mEq. Potassium chloride is available in various forms: liquids 10-20%, effervescent tablets and powders. 5.0 ml. of a 10% solution of potassium chloride = 6.7 mEq. of potassium.

Name, Source, Synonyms, Preparations	Dosage and Administration	Uses	Action and Fate	Side Effects and Contraindications	Nursing Implications and Remarks
SODIUM. *Mineral.* Sodium fluoride (Flura, Flursol, Karidium, Luride, Pediaflor, Pergantene, So-Flo) (Fluordrops, Fluorotabs, Pre-Care [C]).	0.25-0.5 mg. daily. Oral. Dosage is adjusted to suit fluoride content of drinking water. 2% solution applied topically.	Prophylaxis against dental caries.	Fluoride decreases the formation of dental caries. Readily and almost completely absorbed from G.I. tract. Stored in long bones and teeth and released to allow low levels of fluoride in the body. Excreted primarily in urine.	In patients hypersensitive to fluoride, skin reactions such as eczema, dermatitis and urticaria may occur.	Do not use if drinking water contains more than 0.7 parts of fluoride per million. 2.2 mg. of sodium fluoride = 1.0 mg. of fluoride.

NUTRIENTS

There are many preparations containing amino acids, easily absorbed carbohydrates, vitamins and needed minerals. These are available in various combinations for oral or intravenous administration. They are especially valuable in debilitating diseases and during convalescence.

Name, Source, Synonyms, Preparations	Dosage and Administration	Uses	Action and Fate	Side Effects and Contraindications	Nursing Implications and Remarks
Balanced diet. *Low residue.* (Jejunal, Vivonex, W-T Low Residue).	Varies with requirements of the patient. Oral.	To provide nutrients for patients on low residue diets. To aid in preventing or overcoming a negative nitrogen balance.	Provides calories, essential amino acids and other nutrients such as carbohydrates, fats, vitamins and minerals.	May cause nausea and/or diarrhea. Adjustment of dosage and/or times of administration usually is all that is required.	Consult manufacturer's brochure before administering these products. Osmolality of the various preparations and flavors varies considerably, and some patients react unfavorably (diarrhea).

Medium chain triglycerides oil (MCT). *A lipid fraction of coconut oil.*	15 ml. 3 or 4 times daily. Oral.	Special dietary supplement for use in nutritional management of children and adults who cannot efficiently digest and absorb long chain food fats.	Consists of medium length (C-6 to C-8) chains of fats. 15 ml. weighs 14 grams and contains 115 K calories.	In persons with advanced cirrhosis of the liver, large amounts of medium chain triglycerides in the diet may result in elevated blood and spinal fluid levels. These elevated levels have been associated with pre-coma and hepatic coma in some patients.	
METHIONINE. *Synthetic.* Methionine, N.F. (Amurex, Meonine, Oradash, Pedameth, Uracid) (dl-methionine, Methurine, Ninol [C]).	3-6 Gm. daily. Oral.	Used to provide needed amino acid. Adjunct in treatment of liver diseases. Used orally to treat diaper rash when it is thought to be due to ammoniacal urine.	An essential amino acid for which lipotropic activity has been suggested. Acts by lowering the pH of urine in treatment of diaper rash.		
PROTEIN HYDROLYSATE. *Water and protein products.* Protein hydrolysate, U.S.P. (Amigen, Aminogen, Aminonat, Aminosol, Lofenalac).	5% solution. 250-1500 ml. I.V. 15 Gm. In easily assimilated form. Oral.	Used to replace body proteins when depleted for any reason. To provide protein when intake, digestion, or absorption is interfered with, as after operation or in severe illness.	To provide a readily available source of amino acids.	Rare in therapeutic dosage. With I.V. administration of more than 5 days, patient may experience nausea, vomiting, abdominal pain, hyperpyrexia, vasodilation, edema and convulsions. Phlebitis and thrombosis may occur at I.V. site.	Use with extreme caution in patients with acute renal impairment.
Crystalline amino acid mixture (Freamine 8.5% solution, Veinamine 8% solution). *Isolated and purified from edible soybean hydrolysate or synthesized.*	Varies with requirement of patient. Parenteral hyperalimentation.	As an adjunct in prevention of nitrogen loss or in the treatment of negative nitrogen balance, when oral alimentation is not feasible and/or there is impaired gastrointestinal absorption of protein.	Provides all essential nutrients when given with sufficient dextrose.	Contraindicated in anuria or hepatic coma.	Consult manufacturer's brochure before administering this product.

Name, Source, Synonyms, Preparations	Dosage and Administration	Uses	Action and Fate	Side Effects and Contraindications	Nursing Implications and Remarks
FAT EMULSION I.V. Fat emulsion 10% (Intralipid).	First daily dose not over 500 ml. Then dose should not exceed 2.5 Gm./kg. of body weight and should make up no more than 60% of the total caloric intake of the patient. (Carbohydrates and amino acids should make up the remaining 40%.) In children do not exceed dose of 4 Gm./kg. of body weight per day. I.V.	As a source of calories and essential fatty acids for patients needing parenteral nutrition and as a source of essential fatty acids when a deficiency occurs. 1 ml. = 1.1 calories	A source of calories. The patient must be able to clear the lipemia from the circulation between daily infusions.	Liver function tests should be performed with long-term therapy. Platelet counts should be done, especially in neonatal patients.	Caution must be observed in patients with liver damage, pulmonary disease, anemia or coagulation disorders or in patients in whom there is danger of fat embolism.

DRUGS ACTING ON THE RESPIRATORY SYSTEM

STIMULANTS

Name, Source, Synonyms, Preparations	Dosage and Administration	Uses	Action and Fate	Side Effects and Contraindications	Nursing Implications and Remarks
CARBON DIOXIDE. *Gas.* Carbon dioxide with oxygen, U.S.P. (Carbogen) (carbon dioxide 5%, oxygen 95%).	Dosage varies. Inhalational.	Used to increase depth and rate of respiration in such conditions as asphyxia, postanesthesia, carbon monoxide poisoning.	Direct stimulant to the respiratory center in the medulla. Other effects include pulmonary hyperventilation and increased muscle tone.	Rare in therapeutic dosage, but excessively deep and rapid respirations may occur. Stop drug and give oxygen. Carbon dioxide is contraindicated in pulmonary edema, cardiac decompensation, and pulmonary collapse (except for very brief administration).	Hyperventilation may be treated by breathing into a closed space (a paper or plastic bag) for 5 minutes.
DOXAPRAM. *Synthetic.* Doxapram hydrochloride, N.F. (Dopram).	0.5-1.0 mg./kg. I.V. Maximum daily dose 24 mg./kg.	Used to stimulate respiration in patients with postanesthetic respiratory depression or apnea other than that due to muscle relaxant drugs.	Acts as a respiratory stimulant. Stimulates all levels of the C.N.S., augmenting descending C.N.S. impulses. Rapidly metabolized. Metabolites and unchanged drug distributed throughout	Contraindications: Epilepsy and other convulsive states, incompetence of the ventilatory mechanism due to muscle paresis, flail chest, pneumothorax, airway obstruction, extreme dyspnea,	Narrow range of safety. Early signs of toxicity include increases in blood pressure, tachycardia, dyspnea and arrhythmias, skeletal muscle hyperactivity,

			the tissues and excreted in urine.	severe hypertension and cardiovascular accidents. Not recommended for children under 12 years of age or for women during pregnancy.	increased deep tendon reflexes, muscle spasticity and involuntary movements. Monitoring of blood pressure, heart rate and deep tendon reflexes is recommended during treatment.
LOBELIA. *Lobelia inflata.* Alpha lobeline hydrochloride (Lobeline).	3-10 mg. Parenteral.	Used to increase the depth and the rate of respiration. Especially used in emergencies when respiration is failing. It is sometimes used in asphyxia neonatorum.	Acts as carotid sinus stimulant.	Nausea, vomiting, collapse, convulsions, Cheyne-Stokes respirations. Treat symptoms.	Rarely used now, as it is unreliable and toxic symptoms occur from therapeutic doses.
Lobeline sulfate (Lobelcon, Kiloban, No-Kotin) (Fumaret [C]).	1 mg. Oral.	Used to help reduce or stop smoking.	As above.	As above.	

Name, Source, Synonyms, Preparations	Dosage and Administration	Uses	Action and Fate	Side Effects and Contraindications	Nursing Implications and Remarks
SMOOTH MUSCLE RELAXANTS (BRONCHIAL DILATORS) (See also Sympathomimetics.)					
AMINOPHYLLINE (theophylline ethylenediamine). *Synthetic.* Aminophylline, U.S.P. (Aminocardol, Ammophyllin, Cardophyllin, Carena, Diophyllin, Genophyllin, Inophylline, Metaphyllin, Phyllidon, Rectalad-Amino-phylline, Theolamine, Theophyldine) (Aminophyl, Corophyllin, Ethophylline [C]). Aminophylline injection, U.S.P. Aminophylline suppositories, U.S.P. (neutraphylline) (Suppophylline [C]).	100-200 mg. t.i.d. or q.i.d. Oral. 200-500 mg. I.M. or I.V. Given very slowly, often added to I.V. infusions. 250-500 mg. Rectal suppository usually h.s.	Aminophylline is indicated for relief of bronchial asthma, pulmonary emphysema, chronic bronchitis and other pulmonary diseases. It is used as an adjunct in acute pulmonary edema or paroxysmal nocturnal dyspnea associated with left-sided heart failure. May help Cheyne-Stokes respiration.	Aminophylline relaxes smooth muscle, notably bronchial muscle, stimulates the CNS, acts on the kidneys to cause diuresis and stimulates cardiac muscle to increase output. On a cellular level it is said to act by inhibiting the phosphodiesterases that metabolize cyclic AMP. The drug is erratically absorbed orally so if available, theophylline serum levels may be helpful to prevent dangerously high blood levels that may occur. Metabolized by the liver. Individuals metabolize the drug at different rates. Unchanged drug and metabolites excreted primarily in urine. Small amounts found unchanged in feces. Secreted in human milk in concentrations of about 70% that found in plasma.	Causes G.I. irritation, with anorexia, nausea, vomiting, epigastric pain, abdominal pain and rarely diarrhea. C.N.S. stimulation causes headache, irritability, restlessness, nervousness, insomnia, dizziness, convulsions. Cardiovascular side effects include mild, transient palpitations, sinus tachycardia and increased pulse rate. Severe toxic reactions manifested by vomiting, agitation and sometimes convulsions may occur. With I.V. administration watch for signs of cardiovascular distress. I.M. administration is not advised since drug is irritating to the tissues. Theophylline increases excretion of lithium carbonate. May enhance sensitivity and toxic potential of cardiac glycosides. May exhibit synergistic toxicity with ephedrine and other sympathomimetics. Excreted in breast milk and as it is not readily excreted by newborns, nursing by	Aminophylline is synthetic theophylline. It is one of the xanthine preparations. The others are caffeine, used mainly as a central nervous system stimulant, and theophylline and theobromine. All these drugs cause central nervous system stimulation, increased urinary output and smooth muscle relaxation. However, degree of action varies with each drug. Aminophylline is widely used for so many conditions that it could be placed in many categories. Oral preparations should be given p.c. with a full glass of water with an antacid to minimize local G.I. irritation. To minimize side effects, I.V. doses should be administered slowly. Rapid I.V. injection may produce dizziness, faintness, palpitation, precordial pain, syncope, flushing, bradycardia, severe hypotension and cardiac arrest. Theophylline has a low therapeutic index; therefore, patients receiving I.V.

				mothers on this drug should probably be avoided.	therapy should be monitored closely. Oral combinations with ephedrine frequently used in asthma.
THEOPHYLLINE. *Active principle of Thea sinensis. Synthetic.*		As above.	As above.	As above.	See remarks for aminophylline.
Dyphylline (Neothylline) (diprophylline, Protophylline, Coeurophilline, Dilin, Neuphylline, Neutraphylline [C]).	100-200 mg. t.i.d. Oral.				
Oxtriphylline, N.F. (Choledyl) (choline theophyllinate [C])	100-400 mg. t.i.d. or q.i.d. Oral.				
Theophylline, U.S.P. (Acrolate, Elixophyllin, Theocin) (Theofin [C]).	200-300 mg. t.i.d. or q.i.d. Oral.				
Theophylline and calcium salicylate (Phyllicin) (Theocalcin [C]).	200-300 mg. t.i.d. or q.i.d. Oral.				
Theophylline sodium acetate, N.F.	200-300 mg. t.i.d. or q.i.d. Oral.				
Theophylline monethanolamine (Clysmathane).	100-200 mg. three to six times a day. Oral. 400-800 mg. daily in divided doses. Oral.	For heart conditions. For asthma.			
Theophylline sodium glycinate, N.F. (Synophylate, Theoglycinate) (Corivin, Theocyne [C]).	300 mg.-1 Gm. q. 4-6 h. Oral. 870 mg. q. 4-6 h. Rectal. 400 mg. in 10 ml. slowly p.r.n. I.V.				

Name, Source, Synonyms, Preparations	Dosage and Administration	Uses	Action and Fate	Side Effects and Contraindications	Nursing Implications and Remarks
NEBULAE AND SPRAYS					
For others, see also Hormones (suprarenal and those acting on the nervous system).					
ACETYLCYSTEINE. *Synthetic.* Acetylcysteine, N.F. (Mucomyst) (Airbron, NAC [C]).	10%-20% or more dilute solution by inhalation. Loading dose of 140 mg./kg. then 50 mg./kg. q. 4 h. for 17 doses. If vomiting occurs within 1 h. after dose, repeat that dose. Oral.	Adjunct therapy in broncho-pulmonary disorders when mucolysis is desirable. Treatment of acetaminophen intoxication due to overdose.	Acts by breaking the disulfide bonds of the mucus and in this way reduces the viscosity and facilitates its removal.	Untoward reactions are rare. Warning: after administration the liquefied secretions must be removed. If cough is inadequate to clear the airway, mechanical suction might be indicated.	If bronchospasms in asthmatic patients progress, this drug should be discontinued.
Beclomethasone dipropionate (Beclovent, Vanceril).	Metered dose aerosol. 50 mcg. dose per actuation. 12-16 inhalations per day and adjust downward as tolerated. Not more than 20 inhalations per day. In children not more than 10 per day.	For patients who require chronic treatment with corticosteroids for control of bronchial asthma symptoms. *Not indicated in:* Asthma that can be controlled by bronchodilators and other nonsteroidal medication, patients who require steroids only infrequently, and in nonasthmatic bronchitis.	Precise mechanism is not understood, but glucocorticoids result in a reduction in inflammation and constriction of blood vessels, reduce edema and relax bronchial smooth muscle.	Adrenal insufficiency following transfer to beclomethasone from systemic corticosteroids has resulted in death. Beclomethasone can suppress the HPA (hypo-thalamic-pituitary-adrenal) function. Mouth, throat and larynx infections with *Candida albicans* or *Aspergillus niger* have been seen. Beclomethasone is teratogenic in rodents.	Not indicated for an acute asthmatic attack. If patient is receiving bronchodilators by inhalation, it is best to use the bronchodilator first, then follow with the beclomethasone several minutes later to help absorption of the beclomethasone.
Tyloxapol (Alevaire, Macilose-Super, Superinone, Triton-WR).	Dosage varies. Given through nebulizer or with a stream of oxygen. Inhalational.	Used to aid liquefaction and removal of mucopurulent material from the respiratory tract.	A detergent, used to help liquefy mucus.	Rare in therapeutic dosage. However, patients should be watched for signs of pulmonary edema. Treatment: none is usually required, but if signs of edema develop, stop drug and treat symptoms.	

GASES USED MEDICINALLY

(See also General Anesthetics and Respiratory Stimulants.)

HELIUM. *Gaseous element.* Helium, U.S.P.	Dosage varies, p.r.n. Inhalational.	Used as a vehicle for the administration of other gases. It is especially useful with oxygen in the treatment of laryngeal stridor, acute pulmonary edema, emphysema and pulmonary fibrosis. Helium is also used as a vehicle for general anesthetics.	An inert gas which, because of its lightness, allows greater distribution of the other gases than does the atmospheric nitrogen.	None when administered with oxygen.	Helium 75-80% and oxygen 20-25% is the combination most frequently used.
OXYGEN. *Gaseous element.* Oxygen, U.S.P. (Lif-O-Gen, Oxy Swig).	Dosage varies. p.r.n. Inhalational.	Used in any case of anoxemia, such as pulmonary edema, cardiac disorders, carbon monoxide poisoning, asthma, lung collapse, migraine headache, shock and many other conditions. It effects a general improvement in the patient's condition, as all the organs receive more oxygen.	Oxygen by inhalation increases the available amount of oxygen to the blood. Relieves anoxia when processes for oxygen absorption, conveyance, and utilization are not unduly impaired.	None in therapeutic dosage. However, should be used with caution in the premature infant to avoid retrolental fibroplasia.	Widely used in the treatment of many disorders. The exact method of administration varies greatly.

Name, Source, Synonyms, Preparations	Dosage and Administration	Uses	Action and Fate	Side Effects and Contraindications	Nursing Implications and Remarks
	COUGH MEDICATIONS (ANTITUSSIVE AGENTS)				
	Many preparations could be considered under the heading "cough medications." Three groups will be discussed: (1) demulcents and emollients; (2) expectorants; (3) sedatives. See also nervous system drugs. Many cough preparations include two or more of the different groups of cough drugs. Since it is impossible to include all the ingredients, only the important main constituents will be considered.				
DEMULCENTS AND EMOLLIENTS					
	Demulcents and emollients are usually combined with other drugs. Preparations such as vegetable oils, psyllium seeds, flaxseed, methylcellulose, tragacanth and similar substances are used in combination with other drugs in various cough medications as demulcents or emollients.				
ACACIA. *Acacia senegal.* Acacia. Acacia mucilage.	Dosage varies. p.r.n. Oral or topical. 15 ml. p.r.n. Oral	Used to reduce cough.	A demulcent that coats and protects the mucous membranes.	None in therapeutic dosage.	
GLYCERIN. *Synthetic.* Glycerin, U.S.P. (Glyrol [C]).	Dosage varies. p.r.n. Oral. 2-3 ml./kg. body weight. Oral.	As above. Used presurgically in glaucoma to help to lower intraocular pressure.	An emollient used to coat and protect the mucous membrane.	As above.	
GLYCYRRHIZA. *Glycyrrhiza glabra.* Glycyrrhiza.	Dosage varies. p.r.n. Oral.	Used to reduce cough.	A demulcent used to coat and protect the mucous membrane.	As above.	
EXPECTORANTS					
		Drugs that aid in the removal of respiratory secretions and excretions.			
AMMONIA. *Mineral.* Ammonium carbonate. Ammonium chloride, N.F. (Amchlor, Ammoneric).	300 mg. Oral. 300 mg.-1 Gm. Oral.	Used to treat acute and chronic bronchitis and similar conditions.	Increases the liquefaction and removal of mucus from the lungs.	Rare in therapeutic dosage, but nausea may occur. Treatment: none usually required.	

BALSAM. *Myroxylon sp.*		Used to treat irritated or denuded conditions of skin and mucous membranes.	These induce repair of mucous membranes, reduce inflammation and decrease bronchial secretions. They act as irritants, astringents and to a certain extent as antiseptics.	Rare in therapeutic dosage.	
Benzoin, U.S.P.	30% tincture p.r.n. Topical. 10% compound tincture p.r.n. Topical.	Used topically to increase the rate of healing and to cover denuded areas.			
Peruvian balsam.	Dosage varies. Oral Topical.	An ingredient in many cough syrups. To aid in the healing of wounds or lesions.			
Tolu balsam.	Dosage varies. Oral	Same as above.			
CREOSOTE (Creosols, phenols). *Wood.*		Used to treat coughs from many causes.	See above.	Rare in therapeutic dosage.	
Creosote.	0.25 ml. p.r.n. Oral.	Ingredients in many cough syrups.			
Creosote carbonate.	1 Gm. p.r.n. Oral.				
Guaifenesin, N.F. (Dilyn, Glycotuss, Robitussin) (methphenoxydiol, glyceryl, guaiacol ether, Resyl, Balminil, Motussin, Pectus-Sachets, Tussanca [C]).	100 mg. in 5 ml. of syrup p.r.n. Oral.	Antitussive agent.		With guaifenesin, nausea and drowsiness occur, but rarely.	Formerly known as glyceryl guaiacolate.
EUCALYPTUS. *Eucalyptus globulus.*					
Eucalyptol.	0.3 ml. p.r.n. Oral.	See above.	See above.	Rare in therapeutic dosage.	
Eucalyptus oil.	0.5 ml. p.r.n. Oral.				
IODIDES. *Seaweed, minerals.*					
Hydriodic acid syrup (Hyodin).	5 ml. Oral.		Exact mode of action not determined.	Rare in therapeutic dosage. Contraindicated in thyroid disturbances or tuberculosis, and not advised in acute inflammatory conditions.	Hydriodic acid syrup should be diluted to avoid injury to the teeth. Potassium iodide solution's unpleasant taste may be masked if diluted in milk.
Potassium iodide solution, N.F.	0.3 Gm. Oral.	Used as an expectorant. Potassium and sodium iodide are also used in hyperthyroidism.			
Sodium iodide, U.S.P.	0.3 Gm. Oral.				

Name, Source, Synonyms, Preparations	Dosage and Administration	Uses	Action and Fate	Side Effects and Contraindications	Nursing Implications and Remarks
SQUILL. *Urginea maritima (sea-onion).*					
Squill compound syrup.	2 ml. p.r.n. Oral.	Used mainly as an expectorant.	Aids in removal of mucus.	Rare in therapeutic dosage.	Has been used for the same purpose as digitalis but is not as reliable.
Squill fluid extract.	0.1 ml. p.r.n. Oral.				
TURPENTINE. *Pine tree.*					
Rectified oil of turpentine.	0.3 ml. p.r.n. Oral.	See creosote.			
Terpin hydrate, N.F.	Dosage varies, q. 4 h. p.r.n. Oral.		Induces repair of mucous membrane, reduces inflammation and decreases bronchial secretions. It acts as an irritant, astringent and to a certain extent as an antiseptic.	Rare in therapeutic dosage.	Usually given in combination with other drugs. Not a true expectorant since it does not increase secretion.
Terpin hydrate elixir, N.F.	5 ml. q. 4 h. p.r.n. Oral.				
Terpin hydrate and codeine elixir, N.F.	5 ml. q. 4 h. p.r.n. Oral.				
Terpin hydrate and dextromethorphan elixir, N.F.	5 ml. q. 4 h. p.r.n. Oral.				
SEDATIVES					
	These are all synthetic preparations unless otherwise noted. These preparations aid in reducing the tendency to cough.				
Benzonatate, N.F. (Tessalon) (benzononatine [C]).	50-100 mg. t.i.d. Oral. Capsules should not be allowed to dissolve in mouth.	Used to treat coughs from many causes.	A selective antitussive agent which depresses cough without depressing respiration.	Mild drowsiness, nausea, nasal congestion, dizziness have been reported. Decrease dosage.	
Caramiphen ethanedisulfonate (ingredient in Dondril and Tuss-Ornade).	10-20 mg. p.r.n. Oral.	See carbetapentane citrate.	Antitussive agent similar to carbetapentane.	Rare in therapeutic dosage. Contraindicated in glaucoma.	
Carbetapentane citrate, N.F. (Loucarbate) (clofedanol, Ulone [C]).	15-30 mg. Usually given t.i.d. Oral.	For acute cough associated with upper respiratory infections.	An antitussive agent. Also has slight atropine-like antisecretory action.	A low order of toxicity is claimed. Contraindicated in glaucoma.	
Chlophedianol hydrochloride (Bayer-BL 86, Detigon, ULO).	10-25 mg. Syrup. t.i.d. Oral.	Used to suppress excessive and undesirable coughing.	A non-narcotic cough depressant.	Rare in therapeutic dosage, but drowsiness, dizziness, nausea and vomiting may occur.	

Dimethoxonate hydrochloride (Cothera).	25 mg./5 ml. syrup. 5-10 ml. t.i.d. p.r.n. Oral.	Used like other antitussive agents.	Depresses cough.	Drowsiness and nausea have been reported. Treatment: none usually required.	
Pipazethate hydrochloride (Theratuss).	10 mg. Oral.	A non-narcotic antitussive agent for suppression of cough from various causes.	Thought to depress cough centers in medulla without any sedative effect, and is nonaddicting.	Nausea and vomiting occur, but rarely. Not given to children under 7 years of age.	
CODEINE. *Active principle of opium.*					
Codeine syrups (Broncho-Tussin, Cheracol, Citro-Cerose, Citro-Codea, Cobenzil, Codahist, Cotussis, Daldrin, Ephedrol, Histussin, Prunicodeine, Respi-Sed, Senodin, Tussadine, Tussi-Organidin).	5 ml. q. 4-6 h. Oral. (Usually contain 10 mg. of codeine per 5 ml.)	Narcotic antitussive.	Has sedative action on the cough reflex.	Rare in therapeutic dosage but similar to opium if they occur. Treatment: if required, same as that for opium.	All contain several other ingredients. Other opium derivatives are also used in various cough preparations.
HYDROCODONE. *Synthetic codeine derivative.*					
Hydrocodone bitartrate syrup, N.F. (Dicodethal, Dicodid, Dicodrine, Hycodan, Mercodinene, Stodcodon) (dihydrocodeinone bitartrate [C]).	5 ml. Not more than q. 4 h. Oral.	See codeine.	See codeine.	None, though some depression may occur. Reduce dosage.	
Levopropoxyphene napsylate, N.F. (Novrad).	50-100 mg. t.i.d. p.r.n. Available in 50-100 mg. capsules and syrup 50 mg./5 ml. Oral.	For the control of cough in acute, chronic and allergic respiratory tract diseases and various conditions causing cough.	An antitussive agent.	Nausea, drowsiness, dizziness, and skin rash or urticaria have been reported.	
NOSCAPINE. *Isoquinolin alkaloid of opium.*					
Noscapine, N.F. (Nectadon) (narcotine, Oscotabs [C]).	15-30 mg. Oral.	Used as a cough suppressant in acute and chronic respiratory disorders.	Action similar to that of papaverine; smooth muscle relaxant and antitussive agent. Primarily used for antitussive effect.	Rare in therapeutic dosage.	Formerly called narcotine.
Noscapine hydrochloride (Nectadon-H).	15-30 mg. Oral.				

There are any number of drugs used in cough medications. Space does not permit the inclusion of all these preparations.

ACIDIFIERS—ALKALINIZERS

These drugs increase the general acid or alkaline content of the body but they are usually given to increase the acidity or alkalinity of the urine. Many foods also increase the body acids or alkalis. See also Drugs Acting on the Gastrointestinal System and Drugs Acting on the Circulatory System. Some of these are also diuretic in action.

Name, Source, Synonyms, Preparations	Dosage and Administration	Uses	Action and Fate	Side Effects and Contraindications	Nursing Implications and Remarks
INORGANIC ACIDS AND SALTS. *Mineral, synthetic.*	Most of these drugs are best given after meals to prevent gastric irritation. All the purely acid preparations should be given well diluted through a straw or tube. Rinse mouth with an alkaline solution after use.	Used to replace the acid in the gastric juice and to increase general body and urine acidity. The diuretic effect of acid-producing salts depends upon large doses. These salts are usually used with other diuretics to enhance their action.	Acid-producing salts cause a shift in the acid base equilibrium to the acid side and the specific action of the acid radical. The nitrate radical has the most marked diuretic effect; the chloride radical produces the most marked shift in acid-base balance to the acid side.	Rare in therapeutic dosage. May cause local burning sensation. Excessive dosage may cause acidosis. Stop drug and give alkalinizer.	Diluted nitrohydrochloric acid, phosphoric acid and sulfuric acid have been largely replaced by other preparations.
Ammonium chloride, N.F. (Amchlor, Ammoneric).	1 Gm. q.i.d. Oral.	Ammonium chloride is also used as an expectorant. Diluted hydrochloric acid is mainly used to increase gastric acidity. Calcium chloride, sodium biphosphate and sodium phosphate are mainly used to acidify urine.		Use ammonium chloride with caution in patients with renal, hepatic or pulmonary insufficiency.	
Calcium chloride.	1 Gm. q.i.d. Oral or I.V.				
Hydrochloric acid, diluted.	0.3-4 ml. Oral.				
Nitrohydrochloric acid, diluted.	1 ml. Oral.				
Phosphoric acid, diluted.	1 ml. Oral.				
Potassium chloride, U.S.P. (Hypomal, Kaochlor, K-lyte, Kluride, K-Ciel, Slow-K [C]).	1 Gm. Up to six times daily. Oral.	Should always be given well diluted.			
Potassium nitrate (Crataganite).	1 Gm. Up to nine or 12 times daily. Oral.				
Diluted Sulfuric acid.	0.3-4 ml. Oral.				
Sodium biphosphate (Betaphos).	600 mg. q.i.d. Oral.				

ORGANIC ACID SALTS. *Various plants.*		Used mainly when an alkaline urine is desirable.			
Potassium acetate.	1 Gm. Up to q.i.d. Oral. 2-4 Gm. q.i.d. Oral.	To give an alkaline urine. As diuretic.	Most alkaline metal and alkaline earth metal salts of organic acids act as alkalinizers after absorption and various metabolic processes.	Rare in therapeutic dosage. Excessive use may cause mild adverse symptoms, but this is rare. Stop drug and treat symptoms.	
Potassium citrate.	1 Gm. t.i.d. Oral.	To alkalinize the urine.			
Sodium acetate.	1.5 Gm. Oral. q.i.d. 2.4 Gm. Oral. q.i.d.	As above. As diuretic.			
Sodium citrate, U.S.P.	1 Gm. Oral. q.i.d.	To alkalinize the urine. Also used to prevent coagulation of blood for indirect transfusions.			

ANTISEPTICS

(See also general anti-infective drugs.)

ETHOXAZENE HYDROCHLORIDE. *Synthetic.*					
Ethoxazene hydrochloride (Serenium) (Diamazol, Diaphenyl [C]).	100 mg. q.i.d. Usually given in enteric-coated tablets. Oral.	Used as urinary analgesic and antiseptic in nephritis, pyelitis and cystitis.	Action similar to that of phenazopyridine.	Low, but gastrointestinal disturbances may occur. Contraindicated or used with caution in pyelonephritis of pregnancy, severe liver disease, uremia or parenchymatous nephritis with poor renal function.	Colors urine orange to red.
MANDELIC ACID. *Synthetic.*		Used as a urinary antiseptic in nephritis, pyelitis, and cystitis. Especially valuable in enterococcal infections.	This is a keto acid that is bacteriostatic. It is excreted unchanged in the urine.	Nausea, vomiting, diarrhea, dysuria, hematuria and ringing in ears with lessened auditory acuity may occur. Stop drug, force fluids and treat symptoms.	Effective only in strongly acid urine, therefore fluids are restricted and an acidifying agent given. Citrus fruits may be restricted. Urine should be tested regularly.
Ammonium mandelate.	300-500 mg. q.i.d. Oral.				
Ammonium mandelate syrup (Amdelate).	5 ml. q.i.d. Oral.				
Calcium mandelate (Urisept).	4 Gm. q.i.d. Oral.				
Mandelic acid.	2-3 Gm. q.i.d. Oral.				

Name, Source, Synonyms, Preparations	Dosage and Administration	Uses	Action and Fate	Side Effects and Contraindications	Nursing Implications and Remarks
METHENAMINE. *Synthetic compound of ammonia and formaldehyde.*		Used as a urinary antiseptic in nephritis, pyelitis and cystitis.	A compound of ammonia and formaldehyde. The latter is liberated in an acid medium and acts as a bacteriostatic agent. Readily absorbed and rapidly excreted by kidneys.	Rare in the therapeutic dosage but G.I. discomforts, skin rashes, dysuria, hematuria, bladder pain and albuminuria may occur. Stop drug and treat symptoms.	Effective only in acid urine. An acidifying drug should be given with this and the urine tested regularly. Adequate fluid intake should be maintained.
Methenamine, N.F. (Cystamin, Cystogen, Uritone, Urotropin) (hexamine, Uroformine [C]).	500 mg.-1.5 Gm. q.i.d. Oral.				
Methenamine anhydromethylene-citrate (Formanol, Helmitol, Neo-Urotropin, Uropurgol).	600 mg.-1 Gm. Oral.				
Methenamine and sodium biphosphate, N.F. (Hexosed).	300 mg. q.i.d. Oral.				
Methenamine with ammonium chloride (Uro-Chor).	1-1.3 Gm. q.i.d. Oral.				
Methenamine hippurate (Hiprex).	1 Gm. b.i.d. Oral.	See methenamine mandelate.	Same as others of this group.		
Methenamine mandelate, U.S.P. (Mandelamine) (Mandelurine, Methadine, Sterine [C]).	250 mg.-1 Gm. q.i.d. Oral.	Effective against *E. coli, S. aureus, S. albus* and some streptococci. Effectiveness approximately that of the sulfonamides or streptomycin.	Readily absorbed and rapidly excreted by the kidneys.		Methenamine mandelate, U.S.P., yields methenamine and mandelic acid and requires an acid urine to be effective.
NALIDIXIC ACID. *Synthetic.*					
Nalidixic acid, N.F. (NegGram).	250 mg.-1 Gm. q.i.d. Oral.	Used for the treatment of acute and chronic infections caused by one or more species of susceptible organisms. Most effective in gram-negative infections of the genitourinary tract.	Anti-infective effective against *E. coli, Enterobacter aerogenes, Klebsiella pneumoniae, Shigella flexneri* and *Salmonella typhimurium.* Good oral absorption and rapid excretion by kidneys.	Gastrointestinal disturbances, occasional drowsiness, fatigue, pruritus, rash, urticaria and a mild eosinophilia have occurred.	Blood levels are increased when drug is given at least 1 h. a.c. See below.
Oxolinic acid (Utibid).	750 mg. b.i.d. Oral. For at least 14 days.	Treatment of initial or recurring nonobstructive urinary tract infections caused by susceptible gram-negative organisms.	Structurally related to nalidixic acid. Believed to inhibit DNA synthesis of bacteria. Rapidly absorbed from G.I. tract. No data available on distribution. Metabolized by the liver and possibly by the kidneys. Both active and inactive metabolites excreted	Most common side effects are G.I. and CNS in nature and include nausea, nervousness, headache, insomnia, dizziness. Less frequent side effects include abdominal pain, vomiting, weakness, drowsiness, pruritus, diarrhea or constipation. Contraindicated in infants	Safe use in pregnancy and children under 12 years has not been established. To minimize bacterial resistance, the patient should be advised not to omit any doses of the drug. Use for periods longer than 28 days has not been established.

			primarily in urine.	and nursing mothers, in hypersensitivity and in patients with a history of convulsive disorder. It is possible that oxolinic acid may enhance effects of warfarin or Dicumarol. It may also be additive to CNS stimulants.	
NITROFURANTOIN. *Synthetic.* Nitrofurantoin, U.S.P. (Cyantin, Furadantin, N-Toin) (Furanex, Furanite, Furantine, Nephronex, Novofuran, Nifuran, Urex, Urofuran [C]).	50-100 mg. q.i.d. Best given with or following ingestion of food. Oral.	Used as a urinary antiseptic in nephritis, pyelitis and cystitis.	A nitrofurantoin derivative with a wide range of antibacterial activity against both gram-negative and gram-positive organisms. It is both bacteriostatic and bactericidal. It is not effective against viruses or fungi. Rapidly and almost completely absorbed from the G.I. tract, but nitrofurantoin macrocrystals are absorbed more slowly. Widely distributed, crossing the blood-brain barrier and the placenta. Degraded by many body tissues. About 30-50% is excreted unchanged in the urine. Some excreted in the bile and may appear in small amounts in the feces and the milk.	Usually mild, but nausea, vomiting and skin sensitivity may occur. Reduction of dosage is usually sufficient for these. Hemolytic anemia and neuropathies have been reported. When used in patients on probenecid there is increased renal clearance of nitrofurantoin, and this may lead to nitrofurantoin toxicity and decreased efficacy as urinary tract anti-infective owing to lower levels of drug in urine.	Tints the urine brown. Nitrofurantoin macrocrystals are less irritating to gastrointestinal tract. Use with caution, if at all, during pregnancy and lactation and in women of child-bearing age. Not used for infants under 1 year. Safe use for these patients has not been established.
Nitrofurantoin sodium.	180 mg. b.i.d. I.M. or I.V. for patients 120 lb. and over. 3 mg./kg. b.i.d. I.M. or I.V. for patients under 120 lb. Should not be used longer than 5 days when given I.M.				
Nitrofurantoin macrocrystals (Macrodantin).	50-100 mg. q.i.d. Oral.	As above.			

Name, Source, Synonyms, Preparations	Dosage and Administration	Uses	Action and Fate	Side Effects and Contraindications	Nursing Implications and Remarks
PHENAZOPYRIDINE. *Synthetic coal tar derivative.* Phenazopyridine hydrochloride, N.F. (Phenylazo, Pyridium).	100-200 mg. q.i.d. Usually given in enteric-coated tablets. Oral.	Used as urinary antiseptic in nephritis, pyelitis and cystitis. It also has an analgesic effect upon the urinary mucosa.	An azo dye, it is mildly antiseptic. Exerts a definite analgesic effect upon the urinary mucosa.	Low toxicity, but sensitivity may occur. Contraindicated in conditions producing poor renal function, in severe hepatitis, pregnancy and nursing mothers.	Causes orange-colored urine.
Trimethoprim (Combined with sulfamethoxazole in the preparations Septra and Bactrim).	80 mg. in each tablet. Usual dose 2 tablets q. 12 h. Each tablet also contains 400 mg. sulfamethoxazole. Oral.	Used to treat chronic urinary tract infections due to Klebsiella-Enterobacter group, *Proteus mirabilis, vulgaris* and *morganii.* Also in treatment of *Pneumocystis carinii* in children with reduced host defenses, and of shigellosis as an alternative to tetracycline or ampicillin.	Trimethoprim blocks production of tetrahydrofolic acid from dihydrofolic acid by binding to and reversibly inhibiting the required enzyme dihydrofolate reductase. Body half-life is 16 hours. Excreted mainly by kidneys. Peak blood levels reached 1 to 4 hours after oral dose.	Refer to sulfonamides. Trimethoprim has been reported to interfere with hematopoiesis in some patients. Frequent blood tests are advised. If blood changes occur, drug should be stopped.	

DIURETICS

Diuretics are drugs used to reduce the volume of extracellular fluid by increasing the output of water and certain electrolytes, mainly sodium, but also chloride and potassium. The various compounds differ in the amount and kinds of electrolytes excreted. Patients on long-term use of diuretics should have serum electrolyte determinations at intervals during therapy.

Diuretics are contraindicated in most renal disorders, except the nephrotic syndrome, since they would increase the severity of the condition. One of the most important functions of diuretics is in the control of edema accompanying cardiac disorders, especially cardiac decompensation. They are also used in the management of certain types of hypertension, but during pregnancy they should be used only when the edema is caused by a pathological problem. Diuretics do not prevent the development of toxemia of pregnancy, and there is little satisfactory evidence that they are useful in its treatment.

The interaction of diuretics with other medicinal agents will vary somewhat with the specific diuretic drug, but some are the same for most of the drugs. Some of the more important interactions include the following.

1. When diuretics are given to patients taking any of the digitalis glycosides, there can be an increase in the possibility of digitalis toxicity, owing to lower levels of serum potassium and higher levels of calcium. The higher levels of calcium are seen especially when the thiazide diuretics are being given.

2. The thiazide compounds as well as ethacrynic acid and furosemide may, because of their hypoglycemic effect, result in loss of control in the diabetic patient using the oral hypoglycemic agents. Those requiring insulin may need to increase the amount of insulin used.

3. With the nondepolarizing muscle relaxants, the hypokalemia produced by most diuretics may result in loss of deep tendon reflexes and can progress to paralysis.

4. When diuretics are given concurrently with antihypertensive agents such as methyldopa, guanethidine or a ganglionic blocking agent, orthostatic hypotension can result. The dose of the antihypertensive drugs should be lowered to avoid this possibility.

5. The use of ethacrynic acid or furosemide with any of the aminoglycoside antibiotics, especially if given intravenously, should be avoided, because of the increased possibility of ototoxicity seen with such combinations. With cephaloridine and these diuretics, there may be nephrotoxicity due to additive action.

6. The thiazide diuretics can cause an elevation of the serum level of uric acid. This can disrupt the control of the patient with gout or gouty arthritis who is being treated with probenecid or sulfinpyrazine. It can also increase the uric acid level in other patients.

7. Diuretics can replace warfarin from plasma protein binding sites, and this may require an adjustment of the dosage of the anticoagulant agent.

Name, Source, Synonyms, Preparations	Dosage and Administration	Uses	Action and Fate	Side Effects and Contraindications	Nursing Implications and Remarks
THIAZIDE DIURETICS *Thiazide Series. Synthetic.*	Dosage individually adjusted.	The thiazides are used to treat hypertension either as the sole agent or in combination with other drugs. They are also used in the management of conditions involving retention of fluid: congestive heart failure, renal edema, edema associated with hepatic disease, corticosteroid and estrogen therapy and fluid retention occurring in premenstrual tension and obesity. They can also be used in various forms of renal dysfunction, such as nephrotic syndrome, acute glomerulonephritis and chronic renal failure.	Enhances the excretion of sodium, chloride and potassium. Onset of action following oral administration is usually within 2 hours, with maximal effects in 6 to 12 hours. The thiazides are rather rapidly absorbed from the gastrointestinal tract. Diuretic effect may appear in as little as 1 hour. Widely distributed in the extracellular fluid. They are concentrated only in the kidneys. Excretion is usually complete in 6 hours. Some are excreted unchanged, others are metabolized. Mechanism by which these agents lower blood pressure is not understood. It may be related to extracellular volume depletion, a negative sodium balance or even to direct effect on vascular smooth muscle.	Side effects include the following: early signs of electrolyte imbalance such as dryness of mouth, thirst, weakness, lethargy, drowsiness or restlessness, muscle pains or cramps, muscular fatigue, hypotension, oliguria, gastrointestinal disturbances, azotemia, hyperglycemia and glycosuria. Thrombocytopenia, leukopenia, agranulocytosis and aplastic anemia have been reported as rare side reactions. Photosensitivity, purpura, rash and other dermatologic manifestations have been reported. Contraindicated in patients with anuria or oliguria.	Patients using these diuretics should have a serum electrolyte determination in order to protect against a possible depressed potassium or other electrolyte imbalance. Hypochloremic alkalosis or hypokalemia may occur. Potassium supplements should be administered during use in digitalized patients and in patients with cardiac arrhythmias or if secondary aldosteronism is suspected. The thiazide compounds should be used with caution during pregnancy and lactation since these drugs cross the placental barrier and also appear in the milk. This may result in fetal or neonatal hyperbilirubinemia, thrombocytopenia, altered carbohydrate metabolism and possibly other adverse reactions that have been seen in the adult patient.
Bendroflumethiazide, N.F. (Naturetin) (benzydroflumethiazide [C]).	2.5-5 mg. o.d. Oral.				
Benzthiazide, N.F. (Edenex, Exna, NaClex) (ExNa [C]).	25-100 mg. o.d. Oral.				
Chlorothiazide, U.S.P. (Diuril) (Chlorthiazidex [C]).	250 mg.-1 Gm. o.d. Oral.				
Chlorothiazide sodium, N.F. (Lyovac Diuril).	0.5 Gm. o.d. or p.r.n. I.V.				
Cyclothiazide, N.F. (Anhydron).	1-2 mg. daily. Oral.				
Hydrochlorothiazide, U.S.P. (Aquarius, Esidrix, Hydro-Diuril, Oretic) (Edemol, Fluvin, Hydrozide, Hydril, Hydrite, Hydrodiuretic, Hydrosaluret, Hydro-Aquil, Manuril, NeoCodema, Novohydrozide, Urozide [C]).	25-100 mg. o.d. Oral.				
Hydroflumethiazide, N.F. (Saluron).	50 mg. o.d. Oral.				
Methyclothiazide, N.F. (Enduron) (Duretic [C]).	2.5-5 mg. o.d. Oral				
Polythiazide, N.F. (Renese) (Lotense [C]).	1-4 mg. o.d. Oral.				
Trichlormethiazide, N.F. (Flutra, Metahydrin, Naqua).	2-4 mg. o.d. Oral.				
OSMOTIC DIURETICS					
Dextrose, U.S.P.	10-50% solution. p.r.n. I.V.	Dextrose (glucose) is also used to treat cerebral edema as well as other edema.			

Mannitol, U.S.P. (Osmitrol).	5-10-20% concentration. p.r.n. I.V. infusion.	Used to increase urinary output in oliguria, anuria, edema, ascites, intoxications and to aid in lowering intraocular pressure in acute glaucoma prior to surgery.	Mannitol increases the osmotic pressure in the urinary tubules, thus preventing reabsorption of water. Diuresis occurs within 1-3 h. Remains confined to extracellular fluid. Metabolized slightly, if at all, to glycogen in the liver. About 80 % excreted unchanged in urine.	Most serious side effects are fluid and electrolyte imbalance. Mannitol may produce such side effects as thirst, headache, chills, constrictive feeling in chest. At large dosage, patients may show signs of water intoxication, including pulmonary edema. Contraindicated in severe renal impairment and some cases of metabolic edema.	Avoid infiltration. To avoid circulatory overload, mannitol should not be administered until the adequacy of renal function and urine flow are established. The cardiovascular status of the patient should also be established.
Urea, U.S.P. (Urevert, Ureaphil).	60 gtts. of a 30% sol. per minute I.V.	Used to reduce intracranial pressure.	A normal constituent of blood resulting from the deaminization of amino acids. It is excreted along with water. Osmotic effect causes diuresis.	Most frequent side effects are nausea, vomiting, and headache. Others include dizziness, syncope, agitation, confusion, hypotension, nervousness, tachycardia and ECG changes. Contraindicated in impaired renal function.	Urevert is a solution of urea 90 Gm. in 210 ml. of 10% invert sugar solution. Pain, phlebitis, thrombosis may occur at I.V. site; use a large vein for injection site.
MERCURIAL DIURETICS *Mineral, vegetable, synthetic.*					
Mercaptomerin sodium, U.S.P. (Thiomerin sodium) (40 mg. mercury). Merethoxylline procaine (Dicurin Procaine) (39.3 mg. mercury/ml.).	1 ml. o.d. Irritating if given too deeply. S.Q. 2 ml. o.d. S.Q. or I.M.	Mainly used to reduce edema in cardiac decompensation. Also used to treat ascites associated with liver disorders, nephrotic edema and occasionally in certain related cases of subacute and chronic nephritis. Most effective if given with a xanthine diuretic–usually theophylline–and with simultaneous use of acid-producing salts such as ammonium chloride.	These preparations act by irritation of the renal tubules. This is a toxic effect and may be too severe. It prevents the reabsorption of certain electrolytes, especially the chloride ion, and thus increases the excretion of sodium chloride and water. Rapid absorption from parenteral sites, but absorption from gastrointestinal tract is slow and unpredictable. Excreted by kidneys, 50% within 3 hours, 95% within 24 hours.	May produce profound diuresis with resultant fluid and electrolyte depletion and possible hypovolemia. May cause stomatitis, gingivitis, salivation, diarrhea, nausea, vomiting, albuminuria, hematuria and cardiac failure. For mild symptoms no treatment is required. For severe symptoms stop drug and treat as indicated by symptoms.	Mercaptomerin appears to be less toxic than other mercurial diuretics.

Name, Source, Synonyms, Preparations	Dosage and Administration	Uses	Action and Fate	Side Effects and Contraindications	Nursing Implications and Remarks
CARBONIC ANHYDRASE INHIBITORS. *Synthetic.*		Most of these are given o.m. to avoid interference with sleep.			
Zolamide Series. Acetazolamide, U.S.P. (Diamox). Acetazolamide sodium, U.S.P. (Diamox sodium).	250-500 mg. o.d. Oral. Tablets and Spansules. 250-500 mg. o.d. I.M. or I.V.	Used primarily as adjuncts in treatment of open-angle glaucoma not controlled by miotics alone, and in secondary glaucoma. Also used to lower intraocular pressure prior to certain types of eye surgery. Use as a diuretic is very limited.	Inhibit the action of the enzyme carbonic anhydrase which acts to convert carbon dioxide and water to carbonic acid. Some of these drugs also appear to have diuretic action in addition to carbonic anhydrase inhibition. These drugs decrease the reabsorption of sodium and chloride ions and to a lesser extent that of potassium. Decrease formation of aqueous humor, thus lowering intraocular pressure in both normal and glaucomatous eyes. They do not increase the facility of aqueous outflow. These effects are independent of the diuretic effect. Acetazolamide and ethoxzolamide have anticonvulsant activity. Readily absorbed orally. Peak plasma levels in approximately 2 hours. Tightly bound to carbonic anhydrase, especially in the erythrocytes and renal cortex. It is excreted unchanged within 24 hours.	Usually slight, but with continued use patient should be watched for signs of electrolyte imbalance. Potassium depletion may occur. There may be drowsiness, mild paresthesia (especially with the "zolamide" preparations), confusion, loss of appetite, urticaria, melena, hematuria, glycosuria, hepatic insufficiency or convulsions. Contraindicated in renal hyperchloremic acidosis, Addison's disease, when severe sodium or potassium loss has been previously encountered, or in conditions with low sodium or potassium blood levels.	Most of these drugs are chemically related to the sulfonamides. Some may not be carbonic anhydrase inhibitors technically, but all have similar action. All dosages are individually adjusted for maintenance. Acetazolamide should not be used during pregnancy, especially in the 1st trimester, unless the physician feels that the benefits outweigh possible adverse effects.
Dichlorphenamide, U.S.P. (Daranide, Oratrol).	100-200 mg. Initial dose o.d. Oral. 25-50 mg. maintenance o.d. Oral.				
Ethoxzolamide, U.S.P. (Cardrase, Ethamide).	62.5-125 mg. o.d. Oral	Used mainly in edema, glaucoma or epilepsy.			
Methazolamide, U.S.P. (Neptazane).	50 mg. o.d. Oral.	Used mainly in glaucoma.			

XANTHINES (See also caffeine, under Central Nervous System Stimulants and theophylline, under Bronchial Dilators.)					
THEOBROMINE. *Active principle of Theobroma cacao.* Theobromine sodium salicylate. Theobromine calcium gluconate. Theobromine calcium salicylate (Theocalcin) (contains theobromine, calcium, and calcium salicylate).	500 mg.-1 Gm. Oral. 500 mg.-1 Gm. Oral. 500 mg.-1 Gm. Oral.	Used to increase the flow of urine, especially when edema is present, as in cardiac and renal insufficiency.	Decreases the reabsorption of water in the renal tubules. It tends to dilate the coronary vessels and to improve the general circulation, giving all the organs a better blood supply. Also stimulates cardiac and skeletal muscles. The action of theobromine is weaker than that of theophylline or aminophylline, but its effects are more lasting.	Toxicity low, but gastric and urinary irritation, fullness in the head and headache all have been reported. If symptoms persist, reduce dosage or stop drug and treat symptoms. Tolerance may develop after several days of therapy but will disappear after a rest period.	
MISCELLANEOUS These are all synthetic preparations unless otherwise stated. Aminometradine (Nictine, Mincard).	200-800 mg. o.d. Oral.	A nonmercurial diuretic used mainly in edema due to mild cardiac decompensation, cirrhosis of the liver, nephrosis, pregnancy and for premenstrual tension.	Mode of action not entirely clear, but apparently due to lessened reabsorption of the sodium ion.	Little toxicity has been noted. Not recommended in severe congestive heart failure.	
Chlorazinil hydrochloride (Daquin).	150 mg. Oral.	Similar to the thiazide drugs.	Similar to the thiazide drugs.	Rare in therapeutic dosage. Watch for signs of potassium depletion.	
Chlorthalidone (Hygroton) (Chlorphthalidone, Uridon [C]).	25-100 mg. daily or three times weekly. Oral.	Same as the thiazides.	Structurally and pharmacologically similar to the thiazides.	See the thiazides.	See thiazides for side effects, contraindications and warnings.

Name, Source, Synonyms, Preparations	Dosage and Administration	Uses	Action and Fate	Side Effects and Contraindications	Nursing Implications and Remarks
MISCELLANEOUS (Continued)					
COPAIBA. *Balsam of Copaifera officinalis* and *C. langsdorffi.* Copaiba.	1 ml. Oral.	Used mainly in chronic urinary conditions.	Is a diuretic with some antiseptic action.	May cause anorexia, colic, diarrhea and occasionally skin rash. Stop drug and treat symptoms.	Copaiba is an ingredient in some nonprescription (OTC) diuretic preparations. Similar products include buchu, from a species of *Barosma* and juniper, from *Juniperus communis.*
Ethacrynic acid, U.S.P. (Edecrin).	Dosage varies with situation and condition of patient. Refer to manufacturer's brochure for details. 25-50 mg. Oral or I.V.	Congestive heart failure, acute pulmonary edema, renal edema, hepatic cirrhosis with ascites and edema due to other causes. Useful in children with nephrotic syndrome and congenital heart disease when a diuretic is indicated. Not recommended for infants.	Acts on the proximal and distal tubules and on the ascending limb of the loop of Henle. Readily absorbed. Accumulates only in the liver. Some excreted in bile. Some undergoes degradation. The acid and metabolites are excreted in urine.	Hyperuricemia and decreased urinary urate excretion. May produce profound diuresis with resultant fluid and electrolyte depletion and possible hypovolemia, hyponatremia, hypokalemia, hypochloremia, hypocalcemia and hypomagnesemia. Signs and symptoms of electrolyte imbalance include weakness, fatigue, dizziness, faintness, mental confusion, lassitude, headache, muscle cramps, paresthesia as well as G.I. complaints. With prolonged therapy, blood dyscrasias may occur. See introduction to diuretics. Use in pregnancy and lactation is not recommended.	Can precipitate an attack of gout. Drug may augment effects of alcohol. Dosage of coadministered antihypertensive drugs may require adjustment. Frequent serum CO_2, electrolyte and blood urea nitrogen checks are desirable. Use of this drug I.V. with kanamycin or other aminoglycosides should be avoided. See kanamycin.

Furosemide, U.S.P. (Lasix) (frusemide [C]).	40-80 mg. b.i.d. Oral. 20-80 mg. o.d. Depending upon response a second dose may be given 4-6 hours later. Oral. 20-100 mg. parenterally. Dosage may be titrated up to 600 mg. daily, and higher doses are under investigation. Dose in infants and children: 2-6 mg./kg. as a single dose individually adjusted.	Indicated in the treatment of hypertension either alone or with other agents, in edema associated with congestive heart failure, cirrhosis of the liver, renal disease, the nephrotic syndrome and acute pulmonary edema.	Primarily inhibits the reabsorption of sodium in the proximal and distal tubule and in the loop of Henle. Action is independent of any inhibitory action of carbonic anhydrase and aldosterone. Onset of action, 1 hour; height, 1-2 hours; duration, 6-8 hours. Appears to have a blood pressure lowering effect similar to the thiazides. About 60% of the oral dose is absorbed, and 95% is bound to plasma proteins. Crosses the placenta. Metabolized in the liver and excreted in the urine.	Contraindications: anuria, or if azotemia and oliguria increase during use in renal disease, drug should be stopped, or in hepatic coma or in a state of electrolyte imbalance. Increase in blood glucose and alteration of glucose tolerance tests have been reported with the use of furosemide. Contraindicated during pregnancy, lactation and in women of child-bearing potential because of possible teratogenic effects. Side effects: skin rashes, pruritus, paresthesia, blurred vision, postural hypotension, nausea, vomiting, diarrhea, fatigue, weakness, lightheadedness, dizziness, muscle cramps, thirst, urinary frequency.	Excessive diuresis may cause dehydration and reduction in blood volume with circulatory collapse. In patients taking digitalis, excessive potassium loss may precipitate digitalis toxicity. Serum electrolyte, CO_2 and blood urea nitrogen should be checked frequently, especially during first few months of therapy.
Metolazone (Diulo, Zaroxolyn).	5-10 mg. daily. 5-20 mg. daily. 2.5-5 mg. daily. Oral.	For edema of congestive heart failure. For renal disease. For mild to moderate hypertension.	Interferes with tubular reabsorption of electrolytes. Exact mechanism not known. Does not inhibit carbonic anhydrase. Therapeutic dosage approximately equal to thiazides in action. Effect begins in about 1 hour, peak level in about 2 hours, lasts 12 to 24 hours. Antihypertensive effect appears in 3 to 4 days, but does not reach peak effect for about 3 weeks. It can be effective even in patients with a low glomerular filtration rate.	Shares toxic effects of thiazides. Contraindications: anuria, hepatic coma, allergy, sensitivity to drug. Safe use during pregnancy has not been established. Appears in milk of mothers.	Periodic determination of serum electrolytes, BUN, uric acid and glucose levels should be done during therapy.

Name, Source, Synonyms, Preparations	Dosage and Administration	Uses	Action and Fate	Side Effects and Contraindications	Nursing Implications and Remarks
MISCELLANEOUS (Continued)					
Quinethazone, U.S.P. (Hydromox) (Aquamox [C]).	50 mg. q.d. or b.i.d. Oral.	Used to treat edema and hypertension.	Action is similar to that of the thiazide diuretics and metolazone.	Increase in serum uric acid, photosensitivity, skin rash, and gastrointestinal disorders. Hypokalemia may require potassium supplementation.	Drug not related chemically to the thiazide series but shares the toxic effects.
Spironolactone, U.S.P. (Aldactone).	25-200 mg. in divided doses. Oral. Individually adjusted depending on condition being treated.	Used in conditions in which excess aldosterone is produced, such as nephrotic syndrome or hepatic cirrhosis with ascites. Also used as an adjunct to prevent hypokalemia and in treatment of essential hypertension where other therapy is inappropriate or inadequate.	Spironolactone competitively inhibits the action of aldosterone in the renal tubules, thus increasing excretion of sodium and chloride; at same time retards excretion of potassium and may even cause hyperkalemia.	Contraindicated in anuria. Electrolyte imbalance, dehydration and hyponatremia may occur. Drowsiness, gynecomastia in males, ataxia and skin rashes have been reported with high dosage. Spironolactone has been shown to be tumorigenic in chronic toxicity studies in rats.	Patients with impaired renal function should be checked for hyperkalemia.

Triamterene, U.S.P. (Dyrenium).	100 mg. Up to b.i.d. Oral. Total daily dose should not exceed 300 mg.	Used in edema associated with congestive heart failure, cirrhosis of the liver, nephrotic syndrome, late pregnancy, steroid-induced edema, idiopathic edema and edema due to secondary hyperaldosteronism. May be used with other diuretics for its potassium-conserving potential.	Triamterene acts directly on the tubular transport by inhibiting reabsorption of sodium and chloride. Potassium excretion not affected. Net effect seen with triamterene resembles that seen with spironolactone. Diuresis begins in 2 hours and peak effect occurs in 4-8 hours, but maximum therapeutic effect may not be seen for several days.	Nausea, vomiting, gastrointestinal distress, weakness, headache, dry mouth, rash and electrolyte imbalance, mainly hyperkalemia.	It has been theorized that withdrawal of triamterene may result in rebound kaliuresis so the drug should be withdrawn slowly.

MISCELLANEOUS DRUGS

DRUGS USED FOR ALCOHOLISM

Name, Source, Synonyms, Preparations	Dosage and Administration	Uses	Action and Fate	Side Effects and Contraindications	Nursing Implications and Remarks
DISULFIRAM. *Synthetic.* Disulfiram, N.F. (Alcophobin, Antabuse).	2 Gm. first day (do not give in divided doses). 1.5 Gm. second day. 1 Gm. third day. 500 mg. fourth through eighth days. Oral. 125-500 mg. maintenance. Oral.	Used to discourage the intake of alcohol so that supportive treatment and psychotherapy can be given.	Disulfiram alone has no effect, but in the presence of alcohol it produces very distressing symptoms. Disulfiram blocks the oxidation of alcohol at the acetaldehyde stage. This accumulates in the body, producing unpleasant symptoms. As small an amount as ½ ounce of whiskey will produce any or all of the following: flushing, palpitation, dyspnea, hyperventilation, tachycardia, nausea and vomiting, cyanosis, lowered blood pressure and occasionally profound collapse. Readily absorbed. It tends to accumulate in the fat. Action is relatively slow. Reaches peak in about 12 hours. Some is oxidized by liver and some excreted unchanged by the kidneys.	Rare in absence of alcohol: mild drowsiness, fatigue and headache may occur. Treat symptoms. Many drug interactions with this drug occur since it decreases the rate at which some drugs are metabolized. Examples: phenytoin blood level is increased; with the oral anticoagulants, the prothrombin time is increased; patients on isoniazid should be closely observed for changes in gait or marked changes in mental status due to increased serum levels of isoniazid. This drug should be used with caution in patients with the following conditions: diabetes mellitus, hyperthyroidism, epilepsy, cerebral damage, chronic or acute nephritis, hepatic cirrhosis or insufficiency. Its safe use during pregnancy has not been established.	Disulfiram may potentiate the effects of barbiturates and other CNS depressants.

ANTIRHEUMATIC DRUGS

(See also Analgesic Drugs, especially salicylates and phenylbutazone.) These are all synthetic drugs, except as indicated.

Allopurinol, U.S.P. (Zyloprim) (Bloxanth [C]).	100-200 mg. up to q.i.d. For children: 6-10 yrs. 100 mg. t.i.d. Oral. Under 6 years 50 mg. t.i.d. Oral.	Indicated in treatment of gout, either primary or secondary, due to hyperuricemia seen with blood dyscrasias and their therapy. Also in primary and secondary uric acid nephropathy, recurrent uric acid stone formation, prophylactic treatment to prevent tissue urate deposition, renal calculi or uric acid nephropathy in patients with malignancies receiving chemotherapy. Used only for children if hyperuricemia is secondary to malignancy.	Inhibits uric acid production, reducing both serum and urinary uric acid levels. Said to prevent the formation of tophi in gout and the reduction in size of tophi already present. Acts on purine catabolism without disrupting the biosynthesis of purines. It does this by inhibiting the enzyme xanthine oxidase. About 80% of oral dose is absorbed and metabolites are excreted primarily in urine.	Contraindications: Not used for other types of hyperuricemia than those listed. Give to children only as indicated. Not advised for women of child-bearing age or during pregnancy. Side effects include skin rashes; exfoliative, urticarial and purpuric lesions, as well as Stevens-Johnson syndrome and, rarely, a generalized vasculitis that may lead to irreversible hepatotoxicity; G.I. disturbances; occasionally chills, fever and blood dyscrasias. Allopurinol should be discontinued at the first sign of skin rash or any sign of adverse reaction.	Should not be given with iron salts or if the immediate relatives of patient have idiopathic hemochromatosis. Maintenance doses of colchicine should be used when allopurinol is started to prevent increased attacks of gout. Fluid intake should assure at least 2 liters of urine per day. The urine should be kept neutral or slightly alkaline. Liver and kidney function tests should be done early in therapy. If Purinethol is being given, dosage should be reduced by one fourth to one third.
Probenecid, U.S.P. (Benemid, Probalan, Prebenimead, Robenecid).	0.5-1 Gm. one to three times daily. Oral.	Used mainly in the treatment of hyperuricemia associated with gout and gouty arthritis. Also used to delay the excretion of penicillin, ampicillin, methicillin, oxacillin, cloxacillin and nafcillin so as to maintain higher blood levels of these antibiotics.	Depresses renal secretion of certain organic compounds. Well absorbed orally. Body half-life 6 to 12 hours. Largely bound to plasma proteins. Excreted in urine. More rapidly excreted in alkaline than in acid urine.	Rare, but skin rashes have occurred. Stop drug or reduce dosage and treat symptoms. Interactions: probenecid competes with various drugs for the same renal tubular excretory mechanism and can potentiate the effect of these drugs, sometimes requiring a reduction in the dose of the drug. Examples include indomethacin, sulfonamides, aminosalicylic acid and dapsone. (For others see column 3.) For interaction with nitrofurantoin, see page 305.	Should not be used with the salicylates as their action is antagonistic. Contraindicated in children under 2 years of age. Daily urine output should be kept at a minimum of 2-3 liters.

Name, Source, Synonyms, Preparations	Dosage and Administration	Uses	Action and Fate	Side Effects and Contraindications	Nursing Implications and Remarks
Sulfinpyrazone (Anturane) (Sulphinpyrazone, Anturan [C]).	100-200 mg. b.i.d. Individually adjusted. Administer with food or milk in case of gastrointestinal disturbance. Oral. Doses as high as 800 mg. may be used.	For treatment of chronic gout, especially with joint involvement.	Interferes with the tubular transport of uric acid and thereby increases the excretion of uric acid. Not useful in relieving an acute attack of gout. Has the ability to reduce platelet aggregation. Readily absorbed. Highly bound to plasma proteins. Most excreted unchanged by the kidneys.	May include upper gastrointestinal disturbance and skin rash. Patient's blood picture should be watched. Citrates and salicylates are contraindicated since they antagonize its ability to increase renal excretion of uric acid, and they can reduce renal clearance of nitrofurantoin and lead to toxic blood levels while decreasing the effectiveness of the anti-infective agent in urinary tract infections. Caution: do not give to patients with peptic ulcers. Interactions same as for phenylbutazone.	Insure adequate fluid intake and alkaline urine to prevent urolithiasis or renal colic. Safety in pregnancy not established.
GOLD. *Mineral.*		Used in treatment of rheumatoid arthritis.	Mechanism unknown. Water soluble salts are rapidly absorbed from intramuscular sites. If suspended in oil, absorption is much slower. It is bound to plasma proteins and is very slowly excreted by the kidneys.	Incidence of side effects is high. They generally occur during the 2nd or 3rd month of therapy but may occur any time and up to several months after therapy is discontinued. Most reactions respond favorably to discontinuation of the drug. Most frequent effects involve skin and mucous membranes. Skin reactions range from simple urticaria to severe exfoliative dermatitis with alopecia. Mucous membrane reactions range from stomatitis, gastritis, proctitis and vaginitis. A metallic taste	All dosages individually adjusted; usually started low and increased gradually. Before therapy is started, baseline hematologic studies and urinalysis are performed. Before each injection, the patient should be quizzed as to presence of possible side effects. Patient should be advised that therapeutic effects occur slowly and at least 6-8 weeks of therapy are necessary before improvement may be seen.
Aurothioglucose, U.S.P. (Gold thioglucose, Solganal).	25-50 mg. weekly I.M.				
Gold sodium thiomalate (Myochrysine) (sodium authiomalate [C]).	25-50 mg. weekly I.M.				
Gold sodium thiosulfate (Auricidine, Aurocidin, Aurolin, Aurosan, Auropin, Novacrysin, Solfocrisol, Thiochrysine).	25-50 mg. weekly I.M.				

				may precede oral mucosal reactions. Most serious side effects are hematologic and although rare, include thrombocytopenia, agranulocytosis and leukopenia. May be nephrotoxic and hepatotoxic. Anaphylaxis has also been reported.	

DRUGS USED FOR BIOLOGICAL DEBRIDEMENT

BROMELAINS. *Plant proteolytic enzyme from pineapple.* Bromelains (Ananase, plant protein concentrate).	50,000-100,000 U. Oral.	Used to relieve symptomatology related to episiotomy. May help reduce inflammation and edema in postoperative tissue reaction and accidental trauma.	A proteolytic enzyme that tends to dissolve fibrin. Reduces inflammation.	Rare, but sensitivity may be a factor. Used with caution in blood clotting disorders and renal or hepatic disease.	Safety in pregnancy not established.
COLLAGENASE. Derived from *Clostridium histolyticum.* Collagenase (Santyl).	250 units of collagenase per gram ointment. Topical. Apply once a day.	Used for debriding of dermal ulcers and burned areas.	Has ability to digest native collagen as well as denatured collagen. Optimal pH range for enzyme is 7-8.	Enzymatic action is adversely affected by detergents, hexachlorophene, heavy metal ions and by acidic solutions such as Burow's solution.	The action of the enzyme may be stopped by application of Burow's solution (pH 3.6 to 4.4). The commercial brochure should be consulted before using this product.

Name, Source, Synonyms, Preparations	Dosage and Administration	Uses	Action and Fate	Side Effects and Contraindications	Nursing Implications and Remarks
Dextranomer (Debrisan).	Topical application of 3 mm. thickness to wounds. About 4 Gm. to an area 1½ × 1½ in. Dressing changed p.r.n.	Cleansing secreting lesions, such as venous stasis ulcers, infected traumatic and surgical wounds, infected burns, cratered decubitus ulcers.	Consists of spherical beads that allow substances with a molecular weight of less than 1000 to enter freely. When applied to the surface of secreting wounds, can remove various exudates and particles that tend to impede tissue repair. Higher molecular weight components, as plasma protein, fibrinogen, etc., are found between the swollen beads. This retards eschar formation and keeps the lesion soft and pliable. Rapid and continuous removal of exudates results in reduced inflammation, edema and pain. Appears to speed formation of granulation tissue and reduce time necessary for wound healing.	Occasional pain of short duration has been reported in connection with dressing changes. Treatment of underlying condition should proceed concurrently with use of dextranomer. It is for external use only and contact with eyes should be avoided. Keep out of reach of children. Avoid spilling on the floor as it will result in a slippery surface.	When saturated, it becomes greyish yellow and should be removed. Removal is best accomplished by irrigating with sterile water or saline. Some beads may adhere to the surface, but all should be removed before a new application. Lesion should be cleansed thoroughly before application to a moist surface. At least 3 mm. of beads should be applied to the secreting area. Lightly bandage to hold beads in place. To limit cross-contamination, the container should be used with only one patient. Keep dry and store in a well-closed container.
HYALURONIDASE. *Enzyme.* Hyaluronidase, N.F. (Alidase, Diffusin, Enzodase, Hyazyme, Infiltrase, Wydase).	150 T.R.U. dissolved in 1 ml. Added to fluid or drug or injected at the site.	Used to aid absorption of fluids and drugs given interstitially.	It acts on hyaluronic acid, hydrolyzing and depolymerizing it; thus acting as a spreading factor. Action entirely local.	Tissue damage may occur. Treatment symptomatic. Should not be used when there is infection.	T.R.U. is abbreviation for turbidity reducing units.
PAPAIN. *Extract of proteolytic enzyme of Carica papaya.* Papain (Papase). (papayatin, Caroid [C]).	10,000 U. Oral or buccal.	See bromelains.	Same as other proteolytic enzymes.	Rare, but possibility of sensitivity should be kept in mind. Contraindicated in severe systemic infections or blood clotting disorders.	Safe use in pregnancy not established. Do not use with an anticoagulant.

SUBTILAINS. Derived from *Bacillus subtilis.* Subtilains (Travase).	82,000 units per gram ointment. Topical. Apply once daily.	For biochemical debridement of wounds (burns, decubitus, incisional, traumatic or pyogenic wounds) or ulcers secondary to peripheral vascular disease.	Proteolytic enzyme.	Side effects of mild transient pain, paresthesias, bleeding and transient dermatitis. Contraindications and precautions: do not let ointment come in contact with the eyes. Do not apply to wounds communicating with major body cavities or those containing exposed major nerves or nervous tissue, or fungating neoplastic ulcers. It should not be used on wounds in women of childbearing age because of lack of information concerning its effect on the fetus.	Wounds must be cleansed of antiseptics or heavy-metal antibacterials, such as silver nitrate, hexachlorophene, benzalkonium, chloride, nitrofurazone, etc., that may denature enzymes or alter the substrate characteristics. A moist environment is essential to optimal activity of the enzyme. Apply the ointment as a thin layer, assuring intimate contact with necrotic tissue and complete wound coverage, extending 5-10 mm. beyond the area to be debrided. Follow with loose wet dressing.
STREPTOKINASE-STREPTODORNASE. *Bacterial enzymes.* Streptokinase-Streptodornase (Varidase) (Bistreptase, Dornokinase [C]).	10,000 U. Streptokinase 2500 U. Streptodornase Oral or buccal tablets. 20,000 U. Streptokinase 5000 U. Streptodornase Powder for injection. I.M.	Used as physiologic agent to remove necrotic tissue, pus, blood and such material from areas of burns, infected wounds, gangrene, empyema, abscesses and similar conditions. Also used to reduce inflammation and edema.	Streptodornase liquefies viscous nucleoprotein of dead cells and pus but has no effect on living cells. Streptokinase activates a plasma factor called plasminogen, which is the precursor of plasmin; this promotes lysis of fibrin. These two promote the liquefaction and removal of clots and pus.	Pyrogenic reactions are common; allergic reactions may occur. Usual anti-allergic treatment. Contraindicated in patients with reduced plasminogen or fibrinogen or in patients with active hemorrhage. Avoid I.M. use in patients with depressed liver function or when there is evidence of a defect in blood coagulation.	

MISCELLANEOUS DRUGS (Continued)

DRUGS USED FOR BIOLOGICAL DEBRIDEMENT *(Continued)*

Name, Source, Synonyms, Preparations	Dosage and Administration	Uses	Action and Fate	Side Effects and Contraindications	Nursing Implications and Remarks
TRYPSIN. *Mammalian pancreas (crystalline trypsin).* Chymotrypsin, N.F. (Alpha-Chymar, Avazyme, Chymar, Chytryp, Enzeon, Quimotrase, Zolyse) (Alfapsin, Catarase, Chymolin, Chymar, Chymetin, Zonulyn [C]).	5000-10,000 U. Oral, I.M. 750 U. application to eye.	Used for enzymatic zonulysis for intracapsular lens extraction. See bromelains for other uses.	In vitro, trypsin digests protein material but does not affect protoplasm.	None except that allergic reactions may occur. Usual antiallergic treatment. Contraindicated in severe hepatic disorders. Use with caution if blood clotting disorders exist.	Safe use in pregnancy not established.
Trypsin and chymotrypsin (Chymolase, Chymoral, Orenzyme).	50,000-100,000 units total activity of trypsin and chymotrypsin. Oral. Ratio varies from 6:1 to 3:1 trypsin and chymotrypsin.		Proteolytic enzyme.		
Trypsin crystallized, N.F. (Tryptar, Tryptest) (Parenzymol [C]).	5 mg. I.M. Also available in topical form.		As above.	Hypersensitivity reactions may occur. Pain and induration at I.M. site. Contraindicated in severe hepatic and renal disease.	Patient should be tested for hypersensitivity before I.M. injection.

DETOXIFYING AGENTS

(See also nalorphine, levallorphan, and naloxone.)

Name, Source, Synonyms, Preparations	Dosage and Administration	Uses	Action and Fate	Side Effects and Contraindications	Nursing Implications and Remarks
Deferoxamine mesylate, U.S.P. (Desferal).	1 Gm. I.M. followed by 500 mg. q. 4 h. for 2 doses depending upon response. 500 mg. q. 4-12 h. Total not to exceed 6 Gm. in 24 hours. I.V. In iron overload 0.5-1 Gm. I.M. daily in addition to 2 Gm. I.V. administered with but separate from each unit of blood transfused.	Adjunct therapy for acute iron intoxication and in chronic iron overload due to transfusion-dependent anemias.	Deferoxamine complexes with iron to form ferrioxamine, a stable chelate that prevents the iron from entering into further chemical reactions. This chelate is readily soluble in water and passes easily through the kidneys, giving the urine a characteristic reddish color.	Contraindicated in renal disease or anuria. Side effects include erythema, urticaria and hypotension. Warning: Patients on long-term therapy should have periodic eye examinations as cataracts have been seen in patients on long-term therapy.	Only slightly absorbed orally. Should not be used in women of childbearing age or during early pregnancy unless in the doctor's judgment benefits outweigh possible hazards. Pain and induration at injection site might occur. Give I.V. injections slowly to avoid reactions of erythema, urticaria and hypotension.

Drug	Dosage	Uses	Action	Side effects	Remarks
	I.V. rate must not exceed 15 mg./kg./hr.				
DIMERCAPROL. *Synthetic.* Dimercaprol, U.S.P. (BAL, British antilewisite).	0.25-0.3 ml. (cc.) of a 10% solution/10 kg. of body weight. I.M. 2.5 mg./kg. to 5 mg./kg. I.M. Dose individually adjusted.	Used in the treatment of heavy metal poisoning, i.e., arsenic, gold and mercury. Also in the palliative treatment of multiple neuritis.	Forms a relatively stable compound with arsenic, mercury and gold, thus preventing their metabolizing with body chemicals. After intramuscular injection peak systemic concentration is reached in 30 minutes. Distributed to all tissues, with highest concentrations in liver and kidneys. Eliminated via urine and feces.	Rise in blood pressure with tachycardia, hyperpnea, tremors, nausea and vomiting. Stop drug; the barbiturates are usually ordered. In children a fever occurs in about 30% of those treated and continues throughout the treatment. Contraindicated in most instances of hepatic insufficiency and if renal insufficiency occurs during treatment.	Has a very unpleasant odor and imparts this odor to the patient's breath. Avoid spilling. The dimercaprol metal complex breaks down easily in an acid medium so an alkaline urine is desirable. Iron therapy should be deferred at least 24 h. after the last dose of dimercaprol.
EDETATES. *Synthetic.* Edetate calcium disodium, U.S.P. (Calcium disodium versenate).	1-2 Gm. In saline or dextrose solutions. I.V. 20 mg./kg. of body weight. Oral.	Used mainly in the treatment of lead poisoning.	Acts as chelating agent for the removal of metals, mainly lead. Poor oral absorption. After I.V. administration about 50% is excreted by the kidneys in the first hour, 95% in the first 24 hours.	Possible kidney damage. Anorexia, nausea, vomiting, headache, numbness, tingling, myalgia, hypercalcemia and hypotension may occur with parenteral administration. ECG changes have also occurred. With oral administration, G.I. side effects may occur.	When given to patients with lead encephalopathy, rapid I.V. infusion must be avoided to prevent increased intracranial levels and possible death. Contraindicated in patients with anuria.

Name, Source, Synonyms, Preparations	Dosage and Administration	Uses	Action and Fate	Side Effects and Contraindications	Nursing Implications and Remarks
EDETATES (Continued)					
Edetate disodium, U.S.P.	15 mg./kg./h. up to 60 mg./kg./d. Oral, I.V. 0.35%-1.85% sol. topically or by iontophoresis.	Emergency treatment of hypercalcemia or control of ventricular arrhythmias associated with digitalis toxicity. Not used for lead poisoning. Topically or by iontophoresis in treatment of corneal calcium deposits from endogenous sources or due to lime burns of the eyes.	Forms chelates with many di- and trivalent cations but has greatest affinity for calcium. Has a negative inotropic effect on the heart. Poorly absorbed from G.I. tract and not absorbed when applied topically to eyes. Too irritating to give I.M. or S.Q. Distribution data not available. Is not metabolized. After I.V. dose, rapidly excreted as calcium chelate in urine.	Rapid I.V. infusion or a high serum level may cause a sudden drop in serum calcium with subsequent hypocalcemic tetany, cardiac arrhythmias and respiratory arrest. Another serious potential hazard is nephrotoxicity. Pain and/or burning at injection site may occur. Thrombophlebitis has been reported. G.I. symptoms occur frequently. Transient circumoral paresthesias, headache and hypotension occur. Skin and mucous membrane reactions, fever, chills, anemia, glycosuria, muscle cramps or weakness, calcium embolization, hypomagnesemia, hyperuricemia and exfoliative dermatitis have been reported. Contraindicated in patients with hypocalcemia, significant renal disease, anuria, history of seizure disorders or intracranial lesions. Safe use in pregnancy not established	A source of I.V. calcium replacement should be readily available whenever edetate sodium is administered I.V. Patients should also be monitored for blood pressure, ECG, urine output, serum calcium, magnesium and potassium. In diabetics, drug has been known to lower blood sugar and reduce insulin requirements. May be the result of chelation of zinc in exogenous hormone.

EDROPHONIUM CHLORIDE. *Synthetic.* Edrophonium chloride, U.S.P. (Tensilon).	10 mg. I.V.	Used as a specific anticurare agent to terminate the action of curare. Also used in the diagnosis of myasthenia gravis.	Apparently acts by displacing curare at the myoneural junction, allowing normal reflexes to pass. Acts in 30-60 seconds and action lasts about 10 minutes.	Rare in therapeutic dosage. Side effects are chiefly those of exaggerated response to parasympathetic stimulation and may include muscarinic side effects, such as lacrimation, salivation, nausea, colic and perspiration. Stop drug and treat symptoms. Digitalization may increase the sensitivity of the heart to edrophonium. Overdosage may induce cholinergic crisis. Treatment is symptomatic in addition to administration of up to 1.2 mg. atropine sulfate I.V., repeated q. 20 min. if patient's condition warrants.	
LEUCOVORIN CALCIUM. *Biological.* Leucovorin calcium (folinic acid [C]).	3-6 mg. o.d. I.M.	Used to counteract the toxic effects of the folic acid antagonists when too much is given.	Known as citrovorum or folinic acid. It reverses the action of folic acid antagonists such as methotrexate or aminopterin.	No adverse reactions reported with recommended dosages.	
METHYLENE BLUE (Methylthionine chloride). *Synthetic coal tar derivative.* Methylene blue, U.S.P. (Hexalol, Urised).	150 mg. q.i.d. Oral. 60-130 mg. q. 4 h. Oral. 1-2 mg./kg. of body weight. I.V.	Used as a urinary antiseptic in nephritis, pyelitis and cystitis. Also used to treat methemoglobinemia. As urinary antiseptic. For methemoglobinemia.	Acts as a bacteriostatic agent. It reduces methemoglobin. Most effective in small doses I.V. Excessive doses may reverse this and turn hemoglobin to methemoglobin.	Rare in therapeutic dosage. Occasionally nausea, vomiting and bladder irritation.	Causes urine to turn greenish yellow or blue.

Name, Source, Synonyms, Preparations	Dosage and Administration	Uses	Action and Fate	Side Effects and Contraindications	Nursing Implications and Remarks
PENICILLAMINE. *Synthetic.* Penicillamine, U.S.P. (Cuprimine, Depen).	Starting dose for adults and children: 250 mg. q.i.d. 1-½ hours a.c. and h.s. Thereafter dosage individually adjusted. Infants over 6 months and small children 250 mg. daily. Given dissolved in fruit juice. Oral. Maintenance dose: 500-750 mg./day. In acute exacerbations, doses as high as 1500 mg. have been used, but dose should be increased gradually.	Used to reduce blood copper level in Wilson's disease (symptomatic and asymptomatic). Best used with a regimen designed to reduce absorption of copper through the intestinal tract. Also used to treat cystinuria. For severe, active rheumatoid arthritics who have failed to respond to conventional therapy.	A chelating agent which increases the renal excretion of copper. Also combines chemically with cystine, reducing its concentration in urine below that needed for formation of cystine stones. May dissolve existing stones. Can increase the proportions of soluble collagen in skin and other tissues; can dissociate some macroglobulins, thus reducing the viscosity of the plasma. Readily absorbed; distribution data not available. Stated to cross the placenta. Thought to be metabolized in liver; excreted in urine and feces.	Localized ecchymosis in skin, maculopapular rash, lymphadenopathy may occur. Reduce dosage or stop drug temporarily. Patients taking penicillamine may require supplemental pyridoxine. Causes allergic reactions in about 1/3 of patients. Most common reaction is dermatological, which occurs early in therapy. May be accompanied by pruritus, fever, arthralgia and lymphadenopathy. Other side effects include nephrotic syndrome, adverse hematologic reactions, ecchymosis, lupus erythematosus syndrome, glomerulonephritis. G.I. effects occur and there may be a reversible impairment of salt and sweet taste. Reported to cause accelerated sedimentation rate, increased serum alkaline phosphatase and lactic dehydrogenase; positive cephalin flocculation and thymol turbidity tests. Use has been associated with fatalities due to diseases such as Goodpasture's syndrome, myasthenic syndrome and thrombocytopenia.	Frequent blood and urine examinations advised. Review of manufacturer's pamphlet is advised. Skin and mucous membranes should be watched for allergic reactions. Temperature should be taken nightly during 1st month of therapy. Drug should be discontinued prior to elective surgery and not reinstituted until wound healing is complete. Should not be given to patients on gold therapy, taking phenylbutazone, antimalarials, or cytotoxic drugs. Should not be used during pregnancy or in women of childbearing potential. Not for R.A. patients with history of renal insufficiency.

PENICILLINASE. *Biological.* Penicillinase.	800,000-1,000,000 U. I.M. or I.V.	Used to treat hypersensitivity reactions to penicillin. More effective for pruritus than for other symptoms.	One unit of penicillinase will inactivate 1 unit of penicillin. Designed to counteract the sensitivity reactions to penicillin. It is not effective for acute emergency reactions, but does aid in delayed reactions.	Can induce sensitivity.	
PRALIDOXIME CHLORIDE. *Synthetic.* Pralidoxime chloride, U.S.P. (Protopam chloride) (2 PAM chloride [C]).	Adjusted to suit individual case. Oral and parenteral.	Used as an adjunct in treatment of poisoning by organic phosphate pesticides that inhibit cholinesterase. Treatment of cholinergic crisis in myasthenia gravis.	Antagonist to certain cholinesterase inhibitors. Metabolized chiefly by the liver and excreted in urine.	Rare in therapeutic usage.	

MISCELLANEOUS DRUGS (Continued)

THYROID INHIBITORS

Name, Source, Synonyms, Preparations	Dosage and Administration	Uses	Action and Fate	Side Effects and Contraindications	Nursing Implications and Remarks
		These are all synthetic drugs. (See also radioactive iodine, page 337.)			
Methimazole, U.S.P. (Tapazole) (thiamazole [C]). Iothiouracil sodium. Methylthiouracil, N.F. (Methiocil, Muracil). Propylthiouracil, U.S.P. (Propyl-Thyracil [C]).	5-10 mg. q. 8 h. Oral. 50-300 mg. Divided doses. Oral. 50 mg. Divided doses. Oral. 100 mg. q.i.d. Oral.	See the following. Inhibits the synthesis of thyroid hormone. Used in the treatment of hyperthyroidism. It inhibits the activity of the thyroid gland. All these drugs are used to prepare patients for thyroid surgery and to maintain those who are poor surgical risks.	These preparations interfere with the production of the thyroid hormone. This decreases the symptoms of hyperthyroidism. After discontinuance of the drug, the gland quickly regains its ability to secrete the hormone. They do not inactivate existing thyroxine and triiodothyronine stored in colloid or in the circulation. Rapid and adequate absorption from gastrointestinal tract. Duration of action only 2-3 hours. With large doses may last up to 8 hours. Exact fate is not known.	Patients on methimazole may have a decreased response to warfarin and other anticoagulants. Also see the following. Sore throat, malaise, coryza, drug fever, leukopenia, argranulocytosis and dermatitis may occur. Stop drug and treat symptoms. Breast feeding is contraindicated in mothers on thiouracil and probably should be avoided by mothers taking propylthiouracil.	Consult brochure for possible use during pregnancy and for other pertinent information. The protein bound iodine test is invalid for patients receiving iothiouracil sodium. Methylthiouracil and propylthiouracil are less apt to cause toxic symptoms than thiouracil.

VARIOUS DRUGS NOT EASILY CLASSIFIED

These are all synthetic preparations unless otherwise noted.

Name, Source, Synonyms, Preparations	Dosage and Administration	Uses	Action and Fate	Side Effects and Contraindications	Nursing Implications and Remarks
Azathioprine, U.S.P. (Imuran). Azathioprine sodium (Imuran Sodium).	3-5 mg./kg. daily. Oral. 1-5 mg./kg. daily I.V.	Adjunct therapy for the prevention of rejection in renal homograft. Other uses are investigational.	Immunosuppressant. This is an antimetabolite and interferes at the enzyme level with purine metabolism. The drug is well absorbed orally and is metabolized in the body to mercaptopurine. It is oxidized and methylated to give various	Side effects: hypersensitivity, anemia, leukopenia, thrombocytopenia and bleeding, oral lesions, skin rashes, drug fever, alopecia, pancreatitis, arthralgia and steatorrhea. Jaundice has been seen in some patients and with this extremely high alkaline phosphatase	

			degradation products. Small amounts are excreted unchanged in the urine and also small amounts of 6-mercaptopurine.	levels with slightly elevated bilirubin. A patient taking allopurinol will have a significant rise in the blood level of mercaptopurine as allopurinol inhibits the enzymatic oxidation of mercaptopurine.	
Bromocriptine mesylate (Parlodel).	Maintenance dose: 2.5 mg. b.i.d. or t.i.d. with meals. Oral. Duration of treatment not to exceed 6 mos.	Short term treatment of amenorrhea or galactorrhea associated with hyperprolactinemia due to varied etiologies, excluding demonstrable pituitary tumor.	Potent dopamine receptor agonist that inhibits prolactin secretion, with little or no effect on other pituitary hormones except in patients with acromegaly, in whom it lowers elevated blood levels of growth hormone. Suppresses milk secretion and reinitiates normal ovulatory menstrual cycles. 28% absorbed from G.I. tract. In vitro studies show 90-96% bound to serum albumin. Completely metabolized before excretion via bile and feces.	Incidence of adverse effects is high (68%), but these are generally mild to moderate. In decreasing order of frequency are: nausea, headache, dizziness, fatigue, abdominal cramps, light-headedness, vomiting, nasal congestion, constipation and diarrhea. Slight hypotension may accompany therapy. Contraindicated in patients with sensitivity to any ergot alkaloids. Because of the possibility of congenital anomalies and spontaneous abortions, drug should be discontinued immediately if pregnancy occurs.	Because treatment may result in restoration of fertility, instruct patient to use contraceptive measures other than oral drugs during therapy. As an additional precaution, a pregnancy test is recommended at least every 4 weeks during the amenorrheic period, and once menses has been reinstated, every time a menstrual period is missed.

Name, Source, Synonyms, Preparations	Dosage and Administration	Uses	Action and Fate	Side Effects and Contraindications	Nursing Implications and Remarks
Cholestyramine resin, U.S.P. (Questran).	4 Gm. t.i.d. Oral.	Relief of pruritus associated with cholestasis as occurs in biliary cirrhosis with incomplete biliary obstruction and other forms of partial obstructive jaundice. Also used as adjunctive therapy to diet in management of patients with elevated cholesterol due to primary type II hyperlipoproteinemia (patients with pure hypercholesterolemia). Not suitable for patients with type I, III, IV and V hyperlipoproteinemia.	Acts by combining with the bile salts, which are eliminated in the feces. Removal of these salts reduces the pruritus, although the underlying cause is not corrected. Aids in excretion of cholesterol.	Chronic use may be associated with increased bleeding tendency, and hyperchloremic acidosis may occur. Safe use of drug in pregnancy or lactation has not been established. Patients taking this drug may be at a greater risk of developing cholelithiasis. Most common side effects are on G.I. tract and include: constipation, especially in elderly, as well as abdominal pain, flatulence, anorexia, nausea, vomiting, diarrhea, indigestion, pancreatitis and biliary colic. With long-term therapy, absorption of fat-soluble vitamins may be impaired and patients may need supplements. Capable of binding a number of drugs and inhibiting their absorption. This includes thyroid, digitalis preparations, anticoagulants from warfarin or indandione groups, vitamin K, iron salts, phenylbutazone, thiazide diuretics, phenobarbital, and tetracycline.	Should be given at least 4 hours after other oral medications. Never take in dry form. Always mix with water or fluids before ingesting. When patients are on other drug therapies, it is advised that these drugs be taken at least 1 h. before or 4-6 h. after cholestyramine resin. Just prior to administration, the resin should be placed on the surface of 120-180 ml. of liquid and the powder allowed to hydrate for 1-2 min. without stirring. Just prior to ingestion, the mixture is stirred to a uniform suspension. After swallowing, the glass is rinsed with additional liquid and this is drunk to ensure that the entire dose has been taken. May also be mixed with highly fluid soups or pulpy fruit.
Clofibrate, U.S.P. (Atromid-S).	500 mg. q.i.d. Oral.	Used to reduce serum lipids (cholesterol and triglycerides). Also in patients with xanthoma tuberosum associated with hyperlipidemia.	Good oral absorption. Extensively bound to plasma proteins. Distribution in body limited mainly to plasma and extracellular	Side effects: most commonly nausea; also vomiting, loose stools, dyspepsia, flatulence and abdominal distress. Other side effects include	When used in conjunction with an anticoagulant drug, the dose of the anticoagulant should be reduced 1/3 to 1/2, de-

			fluid. Half-life in man approximately 12 hours. Action: it is believed to inhibit cholesterol biosynthesis in the liver in a manner similar to that of physiologic control mechanism.	headache, dizziness, fatigue, skin rash, urticaria, pruritus and stomatitis. Contraindicated in pregnancy and lactating women. Persons taking drug may have increased incidence of gall bladder disease.	pending upon *individual response,* to maintain the desired prothrombin time. Frequent prothrombin time determinations should be made until it has stabilized.
<u>Colestipol hydrochloride</u> (Colestid).	15-30 Gm. in 2-4 divided doses. Oral.	Adjunct to diet therapy in treatment of primary type IIa hyperlipoproteinemia (primary hypercholesterolemia). Investigational use in adjunct treatment of digitoxin overdosage.	Action similar to cholestyramine. An anion exchange resin that binds bile acids, forming a nonabsorbable complex excreted in feces. A compensatory increase in oxidation of cholesterol to bile acids and in hepatic cholesterol production occurs. In spite of this, plasma cholesterol and low density (beta) lipoprotein levels fall in patients with primary type II hyperlipoproteinemia.	Most common side effects are on G.I. tract, with constipation, abdominal discomfort, flatulence, anorexia, nausea, vomiting and diarrhea. Headache, dizziness, dermatitis, urticaria, muscle and joint pain, anxiety, vertigo, drowsiness, fatigue, weakness and shortness of breath have occurred, as have transient and moderate elevations of SGOT, alkaline phosphatase, serum phosphorus and chloride and decreased serum sodium and potassium. Contraindicated in patients who are hypersensitive. Safe use in pregnancy, lactation and children not established. May bind and inhibit the absorption of drugs such as tetracycline, penicillin G, digoxin. Others possibly inhibited also.	Patients on other drugs should be advised to take them at least 1 h. before or 4 h. after colestipol. Should not be taken in dry form to avoid accidental inhalation or esophogeal distress. See instructions for cholestyramine resin.

Name, Source, Synonyms, Preparations	Dosage and Administration	Uses	Action and Fate	Side Effects and Contraindications	Nursing Implications and Remarks
Cromolyn sodium (DSCG, Intal, Aarane).	20 mg. powder by inhalation. 4 times a day at regular intervals.	Used as adjunct therapy in the treatment of patients with severe perennial bronchial asthma. It is not used for acute attacks, especially status asthmaticus.	Cromolyn inhibits the degranulation of sensitized mast cells which occurs after exposure to specific antigens. It also inhibits the release of histamine and SRS-A. It has no intrinsic bronchodilator, antihistaminic or anti-inflammatory activity. It is poorly absorbed orally. After inhalation of the powder, about 8% is absorbed from the lungs and rapidly excreted unchanged in urine and bile. The remainder is deposited in the oropharynx, swallowed and excreted via the alimentary tract.	Side effects: maculopapular rash and urticaria have been reported. Cough and/or bronchospasm can occur. The latter may be serious enough to require discontinuation of the drug. Eosinophilic pneumonia has been reported. If this occurs, drug should be stopped.	One capsule contains 20 mg. Comes with special inhalater and patient must be carefully instructed as to its use.
Dinoprost tromethamine (Prostin F_2 alpha). (A prostaglandin).	40 mg. injected slowly into amniotic sac.	For termination of pregnancy during the second trimester by intra-amniotic administration.	Stimulates myometrium to contract in a manner similar to that of labor at term. Also stimulates smooth muscle tissue of G.I. tract (in man). Capable of causing vomiting and diarrhea. Elevation of blood pressure has occurred in laboratory animals, but not in clinically significant amounts in humans. Following intra-amniotic administration the drug slowly diffuses into maternal blood.	Side effects: nausea, vomiting, diarrhea. Others in order of frequency: pain (other than uterine), bradycardia, headache, flushing, backache, dizziness, dyspnea, posterior cervical perforation, chills, endometritis, diaphoresis, coughing, hot flashes, wheezing, convulsions and many others. Consult brochure for details. Contraindications: Use with caution in patients with a history of asthma,	This drug should be used only by trained personnel in a hospital. Strict adherence to dosage is essential. If abortion does not result, some other means should be used to terminate pregnancy as certain prostaglandins may have teratogenic potential. If abortion is incomplete, some other method should be used to complete the process. If saline injection is contemplated, it should

			In about 50% of the patients, contractions begin within 10-15 min. Widely distributed in maternal and fetal circulation. Rapidly metabolized in maternal lungs and liver. Metabolites completely excreted in the urine within 24 h.	glaucoma, hypertension, cardiovascular disorders or epilepsy.	not be used until uterus is no longer contracting.
Dinoprostone (Prostin E2).	20 mg. vaginally q. 3-5 h. until abortion occurs. Vaginal suppositories.	For termination of pregnancy from the 12th week of gestation through the 2nd trimester.	See above.	See above.	Must be stored in freezer not above -20°C. Bring to room temperature just prior to use.
Flavoxate (Urispas).	100-200 mg. t.i.d. or q.i.d. Oral.	Used as an antispasmodic for the urinary system.	This drug has direct spasmolytic effect on the smooth muscle of the lower urinary tract.	Nausea and vomiting, dry mouth, nervousness, vertigo, headache, drowsiness, blurred vision, increased ocular tension, disturbances in eye accommodation, urticaria, mental confusion (especially in the elderly patient), dysuria, tachycardia and palpitation. Contraindicated in patients with the following: obstructive conditions, pyloric, duodenal intestinal lesions or ileus; achalasia; gastrointestinal hemorrhage; obstructive uropathies of the lower urinary tract.	Use with caution in patients with glaucoma. Safe use during pregnancy or in children under the age of 12 years has not been established.

MISCELLANEOUS DRUGS (Continued)

VARIOUS DRUGS NOT EASILY CLASSIFIED *(Continued)*

Name, Source, Synonyms, Preparations	Dosage and Administration	Uses	Action and Fate	Side Effects and Contraindications	Nursing Implications and Remarks
Levodopa (Dopar, Larodopa).	Dosage is individually adjusted. Initial dose usually 500 mg.-1.0 Gm. daily. Slowly increased until optimal effect is obtained. The usual daily dose is from 4-6 Gm. in divided doses 3 or more times a day. Not more than 8 Gm. a day should be given. The optimal therapeutic range is usually reached in 6-8 weeks after institution of therapy.	Indicated for Parkinson's disease or syndrome. It relieves the symptoms, particularly rigidity and bradykinesia. It is sometimes helpful in tremors, dysphagia, sialorrhea and postural instability. Drug appears to be most effective during the first year of treatment.	The symptoms of parkinsonism are believed to be associated with a depletion of striatal dopamine. Since dopamine does not cross the blood-brain barrier, it is ineffective. Levodopa, which is the precursor of dopamine in the body, does cross the barrier; it is believed to have its effect by being converted to dopamine after crossing the barrier.	Because of the high incidence of adverse reactions and the necessity for individualization of therapy, the physician should be thoroughly familiar with the brochure before beginning therapy. This drug should not be given to patients with clinical or laboratory evidence of the following conditions: uncompensated endocrine, renal, hepatic, cardiovascular or pulmonary diseases; narrow angle glaucoma, unless pressure is well controlled and monitored, and blood dyscrasias.	Levodopa should not be used when a sympathomimetic amine is contraindicated. Monoamine oxidase inhibitors should be discontinued at least 2 weeks before the institution of levodopa therapy. Phenothiazines and butyrophenones may decrease the therapeutic effect of levodopa. Doses of 10-15 mg. of pyridoxine appear to reverse the effects of levodopa, so use of multivitamin compounds with this drug is not recommended unless pyridoxine can be removed.
Carbidopa (One of the ingredients of Sinemet tablets.)	Tablets contain 10 mg. carbidopa and 100 mg. L-dopa, or 25 mg. carbidopa and 250 mg. L-dopa. Maximum daily dose is 200 mg. carbidopa and 2000 mg. L-dopa.	Treatment of parkinsonism.	Carbidopa inhibits decarboxylation of levodopa in the peripheral area and, as it does not penetrate the CNS it has no central effect. This means more levodopa is available to pass into the CNS and the dose of levodopa can be decreased, which will decrease the side effects seen with the high doses of levodopa that were needed.	As above. Both therapeutic and side effects occur more rapidly with this combination.	In patients receiving L-dopa there should be at least an 8-hour interval between the last dose and the first dose of the combination. The pyridoxine reversal does not appear with the use of the combination.

Monobenzone, N.F. (Alba, Benoquin).	20% ointment. 5% lotion. Topical.	Used to reduce excessive pigmentation in patients with idiopathic vitiligo.	A melanin inhibiting agent. Depigmentation is erratic and may take 1-4 mos.	Can cause irritation and dermatitis.	In noncaucasian individuals can cause unattractive depigmentation. Exposure to sunlight reduces the depigmentation effects.
Pemoline (Cylert).	56.25-75 mg. daily. Maximum daily dose is 112.5 mg.	In treatment of MBD (minimal brain dysfunction), also called hyperkinesis in children.	Precise mechanism of action unknown. It has been shown to increase synthesis of dopamine in rat brain. It has a half-life of about 12 hours so can be given just once a day.	Anorexia and insomnia, but both recede with continued therapy. Use with caution in patients with history of seizures. Overdosage produces symptoms similar to acute amphetamine intoxication, including tachycardia, excitement, hallucinations and agitation.	
Probucol (Lorelco).	500 mg. b.i.d. with morning and evening meal.	As an adjunct to diet for reduction of elevated serum cholesterol. If triglyceride levels rise during therapy, improved diet compliance should be tried. If unsuccessful, probucol should be discontinued.	Mechanism is unknown. No increase in the cyclic precursors of cholesterol, so does not affect the later stages of cholesterol biosynthesis. During chronic administration, drug accumulates in adipose tissue, adrenals and liver. Metabolic fate unknown. In animals, is slowly excreted and appears in their milk.	Side effects include G.I. symptoms, flatulence, abdominal pain, nausea, vomiting, hyperhidrosis, fetid sweat, angioneurotic edema, idiosyncratic reaction involving dizziness, palpitations, syncope, nausea, vomiting and chest pain.	Safe use in pregnancy has not been established. The drug should be discontinued six months before the patient becomes pregnant because of persistence of the drug in the body. Safety in children has not been established. Not recommended for use in nursing mothers.
Sodium chloride 5% solution (Hypersal).	1-2 drops q. 3-4 h. in eyes.	Topical osmotherapy of corneal turgescence. Adjunctive therapy in the reduction of corneal edema. Diagnostic aid in gonioscopy, funduscopy and biomicroscopy.			

Name, Source, Synonyms, Preparations	Dosage and Administration	Uses	Action and Fate	Side Effects and Contraindications	Nursing Implications and Remarks
Trioxsalen, U.S.P. (Trisoralen).	10 mg. daily 2-4 hours before exposure to ultraviolet or fluorescent black light. Oral.	Used to facilitate repigmentation in vitiligo, increase tolerance to solar exposure and enhance pigmentation.	Exact mode of action has not been established.	Gastric discomfort has been reported. Phototoxic reactions occur when skin is overexposed to ultraviolet light or excessive amounts of drug. The drug is contraindicated in diseases associated with photosensitivity (porphyria, acute lupus erythematosus or leukoderma of infectious origin). To date safety of drug has not been established in young children (2 years or under), aphakic people, pregnant women or young women of child-bearing age.	
Tromethamine, N.F. (Tham).	Least amount of 0.3 M solution required to bring the blood to the normal pH levels.	Correction of metabolic acidosis during cardiac bypass surgery, or that associated with cardiac arrest.	A weak base, which, following I.V. administration, attracts and combines with hydrogen ions and their associated acid anions. There is a reduction of carbon dioxide tension, which is a potent respiratory stimulus. Also acts as a weak osmotic diuretic. Not metabolized appreciably. Ionized tromethamine (chiefly as bicarbonate salt) is rapidly and preferentially excreted in the urine at a rate dependent on the infusion rate.	Anuria and uremia. Used only in life-threatening cases during pregnancy. Do not use more than one day. Used cautiously in patients with renal disease and/or reduced renal output. Local irritation and tissue inflammation at site of injection, chemical phlebitis, venospasm and intravenous thrombosis. Extravasation may result in inflammation, necrosis and sloughing. Hypoglycemia and respiratory depression may occur.	Dosage must be carefully adjusted so blood pH does not increase above normal (7.4). Facilities for mechanical ventilation should be available. The following should be monitored before, during and after therapy: blood pH, carbon dioxide tension, bicarbonate, glucose and electrolytes.

Dimethyl Sulfoxide (DMSO, RIMSO-50).	50 ml. instilled into the bladder and retained for 15 min. May repeat every 2 weeks until maximum relief is obtained.	Symptomatic relief of interstitial cystitis.	Absorbed following topical application and generally distributed in tissues and body fluids. Metabolized by oxidation to dimethyl sulfone, which is excreted in urine and feces, and to dimethyl sulfide by reduction. This latter is eliminated through lungs and skin, giving a characteristic odor.	A garlic-like taste may be noted by the patient within a few minutes of instillation and may last several hours. Odor on the breath and skin may persist for up to 72 h. With use of this drug, changes in refractive index and lens opacities have been observed in monkeys. Patients should also have liver, renal, and blood studies if on long-term therapy. Occasional hypersensitivity reactions have been observed.	

RADIOACTIVE DRUGS

The dosages of all these drugs are individually adjusted. Toxicity of all drugs includes the toxic symptoms of radiation and of the specific chemical.

RADIOACTIVE ISOTOPES USED TO TREAT DISEASE					
RADIOACTIVE GOLD (^{198}Au) (Radio-Gold Colloid, Auroloid, Aureotope).	35-20 mc. Intracavitary.	Used for intracavitary injection to reduce effusions due to malignant neoplasms.	Reduce fluid accumulation.	See notation under radioactive drugs.	Fluid is first withdrawn from the cavity.
RADIOACTIVE IODINE. *Seaweed and fission products.* Sodium iodide ^{131}I, U.S.P. (radioactive iodine, Iodotope, Oriodide, Radiocaps, Theriodide, Tracervial).	1-100 microcuries. 1-100 micrograms (nonradioactive iodine). Oral. Given together as a tracer. Doses vary according to condition.	Used in the diagnosis and treatment of malignant diseases of the thyroid. Also used to treat nonmalignant thyroid conditions in older people, especially those who are poor surgical risks.	Because of the affinity of thyroid tissue for iodine, the material is concentrated in the gland or, in cases of metastatic cancer, in the metastases as well. The radioactive iodine has a half-life of 8.08 days and liberates beta particles and gamma rays.	See above.	Dosage for treatment individually adjusted.

Name, Source, Synonyms, Preparations	Dosage and Administration	Uses	Action and Fate	Side Effects and Contraindications	Nursing Implications and Remarks
Radioactive phosphorus (^{32}P) (Phosphotope, Sodium Radio-Phosphate).	2.5-5 mc. Oral, I.V., topical	Used in the palliative treatment of blood dyscrasias, especially polycythemia vera and chronic adult leukemia. Used topically for skin cancer, keloids, keratoses.	Decreases production of red blood cells. May bring about remissions which leave patient symptom-free for months. Has preferential uptake by neoplastic tissue.	See above.	
Radio-chromated serum albumin (^{51}Cr) (Chromalbin).	30-50 mc. I.V.	Used in the detection and quantitation of gastro-intestinal protein loss with hypoproteinemia associated with a variety of diseases.	See uses.	See above. Should not be administered to pregnant women or to persons under 18 years of age, unless clinical condition warrants it.	
Technetium sulfate 99m (Pertechnetate Tc 99m). Derived from molybdenum technetium 99m generators. (See column 6.)	0.5-20.0 mc (millicuries) I.V.	Used primarily for diagnosis of disorders of the brain (brain scans). Can also be used for liver, lung and spleen scans when prepared in colloidal form.	Half-life of 6 hours.	Usual precautions and side effects of radiation. However, since half-life is so short, adverse results are rare.	Molybdenum has a half-life of 80 hours. Since the half-lives of both mother and daughter isotopes are so short, this isotope must be produced where and when it is to be used. Generator kits are available from several sources. Some of these are Pertgen-99m, Technetope, and Ultratechnekow.

Radioisotope	Form Available	Uses
Chromium 51	Chromate	Spleen scan, placental localization, red blood cell labeling and survival studies.
Gallium 67	Citrate	Designate the presence and extent of Hodgkin's disease, lymphomas and bronchogenic carcinoma.
Gold 198	Colloidal	Liver scans, intracavitary treatment of pleural effusions and ascites, interstitial treatment of neoplasms.
Iodine 131	Iodide	Diagnosis of thyroid functions, thyroid scans, treatment of hyperthyroidism and thyroid carcinoma.
	Iodinated human serum albumin (Risa-131)	Blood volume determination, cisternography, brain tumor localization, placental localization, cardiac scans for determination of pericardial effusions.
	Rose bengal	Liver function studies, liver scans.
	Iodopyracet, sodium iodohippurate, sodium diatrizoate, diatrizoate methylglucamine, sodium diprotrizoate, sodium acetrizoate or sodium iothalamate.	Liver scans, kidney function studies and kidney scans.
	Fats and/or fatty acids.	Fat absorption studies.
	Cholografin	Cardiac scans for determination of pericardial effusion.
	Macroaggregated iodinated human serum albumin.	Lung scans.
	Colloidal microaggregated human serum albumin.	Liver scans.
Iodide 125	Iodide	Diagnosis of thyroid function.
	Iodinated human serum albumin.	Blood volume determination.
	Rose bengal	Liver function studies and/or kidney function studies.
	Labeled fats and/or fatty acids.	Fat absorption studies.
Iron 59	Chloride, citrate or sulfate.	Iron turnover studies.
Krypton 85	Gas	Diagnosis of cardiac abnormalities.

FORMS OF RADIOISOTOPES AVAILABLE (Continued)

Radioisotope	Form Available	Uses
Mercury 197 or Mercury 203	Chlomerodrin	Kidney scans, brain scans.
Phosphorus 32	Soluble phosphate	Treatment of polycythemia vera, leukemia and bone metastasis.
	Colloidal chromic phosphate.	Intracavitary treatment of pleural effusions and/or ascites, interstitial treatment of neoplasms.
Potassium 42	Chloride	Potassium space studies.
Strontium 85	Nitrate or chloride.	Bone scans on patients with diagnosed neoplasms.
Selenium 75	Labeled methionine.	Pancreas scans.
Technetium 99m	Pertechnetate	Brain scans, thyroid scans, placental localization, blood pool scans, salivary gland scans.
	Sulfur colloid	Liver and spleen scans.
	Diethylenetriamine pentaacetic acid (DTPA).	Kidney scans.
Thallium 201	Chloride	Test for myocardial ischemia or infarction.
Xenon 133	Gas	Diagnosis of cardiac abnormalities, cerebral blood flow, pulmonary function studies, muscle blood-flow studies.

NORMAL LABORATORY VALUES OF CLINICAL IMPORTANCE

Prepared by REX B. CONN, M.D., The Johns Hopkins School of Medicine, Baltimore

NORMAL HEMATOLOGIC VALUES

Acid hemolysis test (Ham)		No hemolysis
Alkaline phosphatase, leukocyte		Total score 14–100
Bleeding time		
Ivy		Less than 5 min.
Duke		1–5 min.
Carboxyhemoglobin		Up to 5% of total
Cell counts		
Erythrocytes: Males		4.6–6.2 million/cu. mm.
Females		4.2–5.4 million/cu. mm.
Children (varies with age)		4.5–5.1 million/cu. mm.
Leukocytes		
Total		4500–11,000/cu. mm.
Differential	*Percentage*	*Absolute*
Myelocytes	0	0/cu. mm.
Band neutrophils	3– 5	150– 400/cu. mm.
Segmented neutrophils	54–62	3000–5800/cu. mm.
Lymphocytes	25–33	1500–3000/cu. mm.
Monocytes	3– 7	300– 500/cu. mm.
Eosinophils	1– 3	50– 250/cu. mm.
Basophils	0– 0.75	15– 50/cu. mm.
(Infants and children have greater relative numbers of lymphocytes and monocytes)		
Platelets		150,000–350,000/ cu. mm.
Reticulocytes		25,000– 75,000/cu. mm. 0.5–1.5% of erythrocytes
Clot retraction, qualitative		Begins in 30–60 min. Complete in 24 hrs.
Coagulation time (Lee-White)		5–15 min. (glass tubes) 19–60 min. (siliconized tubes)

Hemoglobin		
Males		14.0–18.0 grams/100 ml.
Females		12.0–16.0 grams/100 ml.
Newborn		16.5–19.5 grams/100 ml.
Children (varies with age)		11.2–16.5 grams/100 ml.
Hemoglobin, fetal		Less than 1% of total
Hemoglobin A_2		1.5–3.0% of total
Hemoglobin, plasma		0–5.0 mg./100 ml.
Methemoglobin		0–130 mg./100 ml.
Osmotic fragility of erythrocytes		Begins in 0.45–0.39% NaCl Complete in 0.33–0.30% NaCl
Partial thromboplastin time		60–70 sec.
Kaolin activated		35–45 sec.
Prothrombin consumption		Over 80% consumed in 1 hr.
Prothrombin content		100% (calculated from prothrombin time)
Prothrombin time (one stage)		12.0–14.0 sec.
Sedimentation rate		
Wintrobe: Males		0–5 mm. in 1 hr.
Females		0–15 mm. in 1 hr.
Westergren: Males		0–15 mm. in 1 hr.
Females		0–20 mm. in 1 hr.
(May be slightly higher in children and during pregnancy)		
Thromboplastin generation test		Compared to normal control
Tourniquet test		Ten or fewer petechiae in a 2.5 cm. circle after 5 min.
Bone marrow, differential cell count	*Range*	*Average*
Myeloblasts	0.3– 5.0%	2.0%
Promyelocytes	1.0– 8.0%	5.0%

NORMAL VALUES OF CLINICAL IMPORTANCE (Continued)

NORMAL HEMATOLOGIC VALUES *(Continued)*

Cold hemolysin test (Donath-Landsteiner)	No hemolysis
Corpuscular values of erythrocytes	
(Values are for adults; in children, values vary with age)	
M.C.H. (mean corpuscular hemoglobin)	27–31 picogm.
M.C.V. (mean corpuscular volume)	82–92 cu. micra
M.C.H.C. (mean corpuscular hemoglobin concentration)	32–36%
Fibrinogen	200–400 mg./100 ml.
Fibrinolysins	0
Hematocrit	
Males	40–54 ml./100 ml.
Females	37–47 ml./100 ml.
Newborn	49–54 ml./100 ml.
Children (varies with age)	35–49 ml./100 ml.

Cell	Range	Average
Myelocytes: Neutrophilic	5.0–19.0%	12.0%
Eosinophilic	0.5– 3.0%	1.5%
Basophilic	0.0– 0.5%	0.3%
Metamyelocytes	13.0–32.0%	22.0%
Polymorphonuclear neutrophils	7.0–30.0%	20.0%
Polymorphonuclear eosinophils	0.5– 4.0%	2.0%
Polymorphonuclear basophils	0.0– 0.7%	0.2%
Lymphocytes	3.0–17.0%	10.0%
Plasma cells	0.0– 2.0%	0.4%
Monocytes	0.5– 5.0%	2.0%
Reticulum cells	0.1– 2.0%	0.2%
Megakaryocytes	0.3– 3.0%	0.4%
Pronormoblasts	1.0– 8.0%	4.0%
Normoblasts	7.0–32.0%	18.0%

NORMAL BLOOD, PLASMA AND SERUM VALUES

For some procedures the normal values may vary depending upon the methods used.

Acetoacetate plus acetone, serum	
Qualitative	Negative
Quantitative	0.3–2.0 mg./100 ml.
Aldolase, serum	0.8–3.0 ml.U./ml. (30°)
Alpha amino nitrogen, serum	3.0–5.5 mg./100 ml.
Ammonia nitrogen, blood	75–196 mcg./100 ml.
plasma	56–122 mcg./100 ml.
Amylase, serum	Less than 160 Caraway units/100 ml.
Ascorbic acid	See Vitamin C
Base, total, serum	145–160 mEq./liter
Bilirubin, serum	
Direct	0.1–0.4 mg./100 ml.
Indirect	0.2–0.7 mg./100 ml. (Total minus direct)
Total	0.3–1.1 mg./100 ml.
17-Hydroxycorticosteroids, plasma	8–18 mcg./100 ml.
Icterus index, serum	4–7
Immunoglobulins, serum	
IgG	550–1900 mg./100 ml.
IgA	60–333 mg./100 ml.
IgM	45–145 mg./100 ml.
Iodine, butanol extractable, serum	3.2–6.4 mcg./100 ml.
Iodine, protein bound, serum	3.5–8.0 mcg./100 ml. (May be slightly higher in infants)
Iron, serum	75–175 mcg./100 ml.
Iron binding capacity, total, serum	250–410 mcg./100 ml.
% saturation	20–55%
17-Ketosteroids, plasma	25–125 mcg./100 ml.
Lactic acid, blood	6–16 mg./100 ml.
Lactic dehydrogenase, serum	0–300 ml.U./ml. (30°) (Wroblewski modified) 150–450 units/ml. (Wroblewski) 80–120 units/ml. (Wacker)
Lipase, serum	0–1.5 units (Cherry-Crandall)

Calcium, serum	4.5–5.5 mEq./liter
	(9.0–11.0 mg./100 ml.)
	(Slightly higher in children)
	(Varies with protein concentration)
Calcium, ionized, serum	2.1–2.6 mEq./liter
	(4.25–5.25 mg./100 ml.)
Carbon dioxide content, serum	24–30 mEq/liter
	Infants: 20–28 mEq./liter
Carbon dioxide tension (Pco_2), blood	35–45 mm. Hg
Carotene, serum	50–300 mcg./100 ml.
Ceruloplasmin, serum	23–44 mg./100 ml.
Chloride, serum	96–106 mEq./liter
Cholesterol, serum	
Total	150–250 mg./100 ml.
Esters	68–76% of total cholesterol
Cholinesterase, serum	0.5–1.3 pH units
RBC	0.5–1.0 pH units
Copper, serum	
Male	70–140 mcg./100 ml.
Female	85–155 mcg./100 ml.
Cortisol, plasma (8 A.M.)	6–23 mcg./100 ml.
Creatine, serum	0.2–0.8 mg./100 ml.
Creatine phosphokinase, serum	
Male	0–50 ml.U./ml. (30°)
	(Oliver-Rosalki)
Female	0–30 ml.U./ml. (30°)
	(Oliver-Rosalki)
Creatinine, serum	0.7–1.5 mg./100 ml.
Cryoglobulins, serum	0
Fatty acids, total, serum	190–420 mg./100 ml.
Fibrinogen, plasma	200–400 mg./100 ml.
Folic acid, serum	7–16 nanogm./ml.
Glucose (fasting)	
blood, true	60–100 mg./100 ml.
Folin	80–120 mg./100 ml.
plasma or serum, true	70–115 mg./100 ml.
Haptoglobin, serum	100–200 mg./100 ml.
	(As hemoglobin
	binding capacity)
Hydroxybutyric dehydrogenase, serum	0–180 ml.U./ml. (30°)
	(Rosalki-Wilkinson)
	114-290 units/ml. (Wroblewski)

Lipids, total, serum		450–850 mg./100 ml.
		0.5–0.9 gram/100 ml.
Alpha$_2$		7–14% of total
Beta		0.6–1.1 grams/100 ml.
		9–15% of total
Gamma		0.7–1.7 grams/100 ml.
		11–21 % of total
Magnesium, serum		1.5–2.5 mEq./liter
		(1.8–3.0 mg./100 ml.)
Nitrogen, nonprotein, serum		15–35 mg./100 ml.
Osmolality, serum		285–295 mOsm./kg. serum water
Oxygen, blood		
Capacity		16–24 vol. % (varies with Hb)
Content	Arterial	15–23 vol. %
	Venous	10–16 vol. %
Saturation	Arterial	94–100% of capacity
	Venous	60–85% of capacity
Tension, Po_2	Arterial	75–100 mm. Hg
pH, arterial, blood		7.35–7.45
Phenylalanine, serum		Less than 3 mg./100 ml.
Phosphatase, acid, serum		1.0–5.0 units (King-Armstrong)
		0.5–2.0 units (Bodansky)
		0.5–2.0 units (Gutman)
		0.0–1.1 units (Shinowara)
		0.1–0.63 unit (Bessey-Lowry)
Phosphatase, alkaline, serum		5.0–13.0 units (King-Armstrong)
		2.0–4.5 units (Bodansky)
		3.0–10.0 units (Gutman)
		2.2-8.6 units (Shinowara)
		0.8-2.3 units (Bassey-Lowry)
		30–85 milliunits/ml. (I.U.)
		(Values are higher in children)
Phosphate, inorganic, serum		3.0–4.5 mg./100 ml.
		(Children: 4.0–7.0 mg./100 ml.)
Phospholipids, serum		6–12 mg./100 ml. as lipid phosphorus

NORMAL VALUES OF CLINICAL IMPORTANCE (Continued)

NORMAL BLOOD, PLASMA AND SERUM VALUES *(Continued)*

Potassium, serum	3.5–5.0 mEq./liter
Proteins, serum	
Total	6.0–8.0 grams/100 ml.
Albumin	3.5–5.5 grams/100 ml.
Globulin	2.5–3.5 grams/100 ml.
Electrophoresis	
Albumin	3.5–5.5 grams/100 ml.
	52–68% of total
Globulin	
$Alpha_1$	0.2–0.4 gram/100 ml.
	2–5% of total
Pyruvic acid, plasma	1.0–2.0 mg./100 ml.
Serotonin, platelet suspension	0.1–0.3 mcg./ml. blood
serum	0.10–0.32 mcg./ml.
Sodium, serum	136–145 mEq./liter
Sulfates, inorganic, serum	0.8–1.2 mg./100 ml. (as S)
Thyroxine, free, serum	1.0–2.1 nanogm./100 ml.
Thyroxine binding globulin (TBG), serum	10–26 mcg./100 ml.

Thyroxine iodine (T_1), serum	2.9–6.4 mcg./100 ml.
Transaminase, serum: SGOT	0–19 ml.U./ml. (30°)
0.17 ml.U./ml. (30°) SGPT	(Karmen modified)
(Karmen modified)	5–35 units/ml.
6–35 units/ml. (Karmen)	(Reitman-Frankel)
Triglycerides, serum	15–40 units/ml. (Karmen)
Urea, blood	18–40 units/ml.
plasma or serum	(Reitman-Frankel)
Urea nitrogen, blood (BUN)	40–150 mg./100 ml.
plasma or serum	21–43 mg./100 ml.
Uric acid, serum	24–49 mg./100 ml.
Male	10–20 mg./100 ml.
Female	11–23 mg./100 ml.
Vitamin A, serum	
Vitamin B_{12}, serum	2.5–8.0 mg./100 ml.
Vitamin C, blood	1.5–6.0 mg./100 ml.
	20–80 mcg./100 ml.
	200–800 picogm./ml.
	0.4–1.5 mg./100 ml.

NORMAL URINE VALUES

Acetone and acetoacetate	0
Addis count	
Erythrocytes	0–130,000/24 hrs.
Leukocytes	0–650,000/24 hrs.
Casts (hyaline)	0–2000/24 hrs.
Alcapton bodies	Negative
Aldosterone	3–20 mcg./24 hrs.
Alpha amino nitrogen	50–200 mg./24 hrs.
	(Not over 1.5% of total nitrogen)
Ammonia nitrogen	20–70 mEq./24 hrs.
Amylase	35-260 Caraway units/hr.
Bence Jones protein	Negative
Bilirubin (bile)	Negative
Calcium	
Low Ca diet (Bauer-Aub)	Less than 150 mg./24 hrs.
Usual diet	Less than 250 mg./24 hrs.

17-Hydroxycorticosteroids	
Male	3–9 mg./24 hrs.
Female	2–8 mg./24 hrs.
	(Varies with method used)
5-Hydroxyindole-acetic acid (5-HIAA)	
Qualitative	Negative
Quantitative	Less than 9 mg./24 hrs.
17-Ketosteroids	
Male	6–18 mg./24 hrs.
Female	4–13 mg./24 hrs.
Osmolality	38–1400 mOsm./kg. water
pH	4.6–8.0, average 6.0
	(Depends on diet)
Phenylpyruvic acid, qualitative	Negative
Phosphorus	0.9–1.3 gm./24 hrs.
	(Varies with intake)

Catecholamines	
Epinephrine	Less than 10 mcg./24 hrs.
Norepinephrine	Less than 100 mcg./24 hrs.
Chloride	110–250 mEq./24 hrs. (Varies with intake)
Chorionic gonadotrophin	0
Copper	0–50 mcg./24 hrs.
Creatine	
Male	0–40 mg./24 hrs.
Female	0–100 mg./24 hrs. (Higher in children and during pregnancy)
Creatinine	15–25 mg./kg. of body weight/24 hrs.
Cystine or cysteine, qualitative	Negative
Delta aminolevulinic acid	1.3–7.0 mg./24 hrs.
Estrogens	*Male* / *Female*
Estrone	3–8 / 4–31
Estradiol	0–6 / 0–14
Estriol	1–11 / 0–72
Total	4–25 / 5–100 (Units above are mcg./24 hours.) (Markedly increased during pregnancy)
Glucose (reducing substances)	Less than 250 mg./24 hrs.
Gonadotrophins, pituitary	5–10 rat units/24 hrs. 10–50 mouse units/24 hrs. (Increased after menopause)
Hemoglobin and myoglobin	Negative
Homogentisic acid, qualitative	Negative
Porphobilinogen	
Qualitative	Negative
Quantitative	0–0.2 mg./100 ml. Less than 2.0 mg./24 hrs.
Porphyrins	
Coproporphyrin	50–250 mcg./24 hrs.
Uroporphyrin	10–30 mcg./24 hrs.
Potassium	25–100 mEq./24 hrs. (Varies with intake)
Pregnanetriol	Less than 2.5 mg./24 hrs. in adults
Protein	
Qualitative	0
Quantitative	10–150 mg./24 hrs.
Sodium	130–260 mEq./24 hrs. (Varies with intake)
Solids, total	30–70 grams/liter, average 50 grams/liter (To estimate total solids per liter, multiply last two figures of specific gravity by 2.66, Long's coefficient)
Specific gravity	1.003–1.030
Sugar	0
Titratable acidity	20–40 mEq./24 hrs.
Urobilinogen	Up to 1.0 Ehrlich unit/2 hrs. (1–3 P.M.) 0–4.0 mg./24 hrs.
Vanillylmandelic acid (VMA)	1–8 mg./24 hrs.

NORMAL VALUES FOR GASTRIC ANALYSIS

Basal gastric secretion (one hour)	*Concentration Mean ± 1 S.D.*	*Output Mean ± 1 S.D.*
Male	25.8 ± 1.8 mEq./liter	2.57 ± 0.16 mEq./hr.
Female	20.3 ± 3.0 mEq./liter	1.61 ± 0.18 mEq./hr.
After histamine stimulation		
Normal	Mean output = 11.8 mEq./hr.	
Duodenal ulcer	Mean output = 15.2 mEq./hr.	
After maximal histamine stimulation		
Normal	Mean output	22.6 mEq./hr.
Duodenal ulcer	Mean output	44.6 mEq./hr.

Diagnex blue (Squibb):	
Anacidity	0–0.3 mg. in 2 hrs.
Doubtful	0.3–0.6 mg. in 2 hrs.
Normal	Greater than 0.6 mg. in 2 hrs.
Volume, fasting stomach content	50–100 ml.
Emptying time	3–6 hrs.
Color	Opalescent or colorless
Specific gravity	1.006–1.009
pH (adults)	0.9–1.5

NORMAL VALUES OF CLINICAL IMPORTANCE (Continued)

NORMAL VALUES FOR CEREBROSPINAL FLUID

Cells	Fewer than 5/cu. mm., all mononuclear	Protein, total	15–45 mg./100 ml.
Chloride	120–130 mEq./liter	Albumin	52%
	(20 mEq./liter higher than serum)	$Alpha_1$ globulin	5%
Colloidal gold test	Not more than 1 in any tube	$Alpha_2$ globulin	14%
Glucose	50–75 mg./100 ml.	Beta globulin	10%
	(20 mg./100 ml. less than blood)	Gamma globulin	19%
Pressure	70–180 mm. water		

NORMAL VALUES FOR SEMEN

Volume	2–5 ml., usually 3–4 ml.	Count	60–150 million/ml.
Liquefaction	Complete in 15 min.		Below 60 million/ml. is abnormal
pH	7.2–8.0; average 7.8	Motility	80% or more motile
Leukocytes	Occasional or absent	Morphology	80–90% normal forms

NORMAL VALUES FOR FECES

Bulk	100–200 grams/24 hrs.	Nitrogen, total	Less than 2.0 grams/24 hrs.
Dry matter	23–32 grams/24 hrs.	Urobilinogen	40–280 mg./24 hrs.
Fat, total	Less than 6.0 grams/24 hrs.	Water	Approximately 65%

NORMAL VALUES FOR SEROLOGIC PROCEDURES

Anti-hyaluronidase	Less than 1:200. Significant if rising titer can be demonstrated at weekly intervals.
Anti-streptolysin O titer	Normal up to 1:128. Single test usually has little significance. Rise in titer or persistently elevated titer is significant.
Bacterial agglutinins	Significant only if rise in titer is demonstrated or if antibodies are absent.
Complement fixation tests	Titers of 1:8 or less are usually not significant. Paired sera showing rise in titer of more than two tubes are usually considered significant.
C reactive protein (CRP)	Negative

Heterophile titer

	Unabsorbed	Absorbed With G.P.	Absorbed With Beef
Normal	1:160	1:10	1:160
Inf. mono.	1:160	1:320	1:10
Serum sickness	1:160	1:5	1:10

Test	Titer	Interpretation
Proteus OX-19 agglutinins	1:80	Negative
	1:160	Doubtful
	1:320	Positive
R. A. test (latex)	1:40	Negative
	1:80 –1:160	Doubtful
	1:320	Positive
Rose test	1:10	Negative
	1:20 –1:40	Doubtful
	1:80	Positive
Tularemia agglutinins	1:80	Negative
	1:160	Doubtful
	1:320	Positive

TOXICOLOGY

Arsenic, blood	3.5–7.2 mcg./100 ml.
Arsenic, urine	Less than 100 mcg./24 hrs.
Barbiturates, serum	0 Coma level: Phenobarbital approximately 11 mg./100 ml.: most other barbiturates 1.5 mg./100 ml.
Bromides, serum	0 Toxic levels above 17 mEq./liter
Carbon monoxide, blood	Up to 5% saturation Symptoms occur with 20% saturation
Dilantin, blood or serum	Therapeutic levels 1–11 mcg./ml.
Ethanol, blood	Less than 0.005%
Marked intoxication	0.3–0.4%
Alcoholic stupor	0.4–0.5%
Coma	Above 0.5%
Lead, blood	0–40 mcg./100 ml.
Lead, urine	Less than 100 mcg./24 hrs.
Lithium, serum	0 Therapeutic levels 0.5–1.5 mEq./liter Toxic levels above 2 mEq./liter
Mercury, urine	Less than 10 mcg./24 hrs.
Salicylate, plasma	0
Therapeutic range	20–25 mg./100 ml.
Toxic range	Over 30 mg./100 ml.
Death	45–75 mg./100 ml.

LIVER FUNCTION TESTS

Bromsulphalein (B.S.P.): Less than 5% remaining in serum 45 minutes after injection of 5 mg./kg. of body weight

Cephalin cholesterol flocculation: 0–1 in 24 hours.

Galactose tolerance: Excretion of not more than 3.0 grams galactose in the urine 5 hours after ingestion of 40 grams of galactose.

Glycogen storage: Increase of blood glucose 45 mg./100 ml. over fasting level 45 minutes after subcutaneous injection of 0.01 mg./kg. body weight of epinephrine.

Hippuric acid: Excretion of 3.0–3.5 grams hippuric acid in urine within 4 hours after ingestion of 6.0 grams sodium benzoate.

or

Excretion of 0.7 gram hippuric acid in urine within 1 hour after intravenous injection of 1.77 grams sodium benzoate.

Thymol turbidity: 0–5 units

Zinc turbidity: 2–12 units

PANCREATIC (ISLET) FUNCTION TESTS

Glucose tolerance tests: Patient should be on a diet containing 300 grams of carbohydrate per day for 3 days prior to test.

Oral: After ingestion of 100 grams of glucose or 1.75 grams glucose/kg. body weight, blood glucose is not more than 160 mg./100 ml. after 60 minutes, 140 mg./100 ml. after 90 minutes, and 120 mg./100 ml. after 120 minutes. Values are for blood; serum measurements are approximately 15% higher.

Intravenous: Blood glucose does not exceed 200 mg./100 ml. after infusion of 0.5 gram of glucose/kg. body weight over 30 minutes. Glucose concentration falls below initial level at 2 hours and returns to preinfusion levels in 3 hours or 1 hour. Values are for blood; serum measurements are approximately 15% higher.

Cortisone-glucose tolerance test: The patient should be on a diet containing 300 grams of carbohydrate per day for 3 days prior to test. At 8½ and again 2 hours prior to glucose load patient is given cortisone acetate by mouth (50 mg. if patient's ideal weight is less than 160 lb., 62.5 mg. if ideal weight is greater than 160 lb.). An oral dose of glucose 1.75 grams/kg. body weight, is given and blood samples are taken at 0, 30, 60, 90, and 120 minutes. Test is considered positive if true blood glucose exceeds 160 mg./100 ml. at 60 minutes, 140 mg./100 ml. at 90 minutes, and 120 mg./100 ml. at 120 minutes. Values are for blood; serum measurements are approximately 15% higher.

RENAL FUNCTION TESTS

Clearance tests (corrected to 1.73 sq. meters body surface area)		
Glomerular filtration rate (G.F.R.)		
Inulin clearance, Mannitol clearance, or Endogenous creatinine clearance	Males	110–150 ml./min.
	Females	105–132 ml./min.
Renal plasma flow (R.P.F.)		
p-Aminohippurate (P.A.H.), or Diodrast	Males	560–830 ml./min.
	Females	490–700 ml./min.
Filtration fraction (F.F.) $FF = \frac{G.F.R.}{R.P.F.}$	Males	17–21%
	Females	17–23%
Urea clearance (C_u)	Standard	40–65 ml./min.
	Maximal	60–100 ml./min.

Concentration and dilution		Specific gravity > 1.025 on dry day Specific gravity < 1.003 on water day
Maximal Diodrast excretory capacity T_{M_D}	Males	43–59 mg./min.
	Females	33–51 mg./min.
Maximal glucose reabsorptive capacity T_{M_G}.	Males	300–450 mg./min.
	Females	250–350 mg./min.
Maximal PAH excretory capacity $T_{M_{PAH}}$		80–90 mg./min.
Phenolsulfonphthalein excretion (P.S.P.)		25% or more in 15 min. 40% or more in 30 min. 55% or more in 2 hrs. After injection of 1 ml. P.S.P. intravenously.

THYROID FUNCTION TESTS

Protein bound iodine, serum (P.B.I.)	3.5–8.0 mcg./100 ml.
Butanol extractable iodine, serum (B.E.I.)	3.2–6.4 mcg./100 ml.
Thyroxine iodine, serum (T_1)	2.9–6.4 mcg./100 ml.
Free thyroxine, serum	1.4–2.5 nanogram/100 ml.
T_3 (index of unsaturated T.B.G.)	10.0–14.6%
Thyroxine-binding globulin, serum (T.B.G.)	10–26 mcg. T_1/100 ml.
Thyroid-stimulating hormone, serum (T.S.H.)	0 up to 0.2 milliunits/ml.
Radioactive iodine (^{131}I) uptake (R.A.I.)	20–50% of administered dose in 24 hrs.
Radioactive iodine (^{131}I) excretion	30–70% of administered dose in 24 hrs.
Radioactive iodine (^{131}I), protein bound	Less than 0.3% of administered dose per liter of plasma at 72 hrs.
Basal metabolic rate	Minus 10% to plus 10% of mean standard

GASTROINTESTINAL ABSORPTION TESTS

d-Xylose absorption test	After an 8 hour fast 10 ml./kg. body weight of a 5% solution of d-xylose is given by mouth. Nothing further by mouth is given until the test has been completed. All urine voided during the following 5 hours is pooled, and blood samples are taken at 0, 60, and 120 minutes. Normally 26% (range 16–33%) of ingested xylose is excreted within 5 hours, and the serum xylose reaches a level between 25 and 40 mg./100 ml. after 1 hour and is maintained at this level for another 60 minutes.
Vitamin A absorption test	A fasting blood specimen is obtained and 200,000 units of vitamin A in oil is given by mouth. Serum vitamin A level should rise to twice fasting level in 3 to 5 hours.

INDEX

An asterisk (*) appears before USP monograph title changes, which will become effective as of July 1, 1980. Following the new title is a reference to the former name and the page on which it appears in the text.

A

B

C

D

E

F

I

J

K

L

M

N

O

P

Q

R

S

T

U

V